Everyday Medical Ethics and Law

Information about major developments since the publication of this book may be obtained from the BMA's website or by contacting:

Medical Ethics Department
British Medical Association
BMA House
Tavistock Square
London WC1H 9JP
Tel: 020 7383 6286
Email: ethics@bma.org.uk
Website: bma.org.uk/ethics

Everyday Medical Ethics and Law

British Medical Association Ethics Department

Project Manager	Veronica English
Written by	Ann Sommerville
Editorial board	Sophie Brannan
	Eleanor Chrispin
	Martin Davies
	Rebecca Mussell
	Julian Sheather
Director of Professional Activities	Vivienne Nathanson

WILEY-BLACKWELL
A John Wiley & Sons, Ltd., Publication

BMA

BMJ|Books

Library of Congress Cataloging-in-Publication Data
Sommerville, Ann.
    Everyday medical ethics and law / British Medical Association Ethics Department ; [project manager], Veronica English ; [written by] Ann Sommerville ; [editors], Sophie Brannan . . . [*et al.*] ; [director of professional activities], Vivienne Nathanson.
        p. ; cm.
    Includes bibliographical references and index.
    ISBN 978-1-118-38489-3 (pbk.)
    I. English, Veronica. II. Brannan, Sophie. III. British Medical Association. Medical Ethics Department. IV. Title.
    [DNLM: 1. Ethics, Medical–Great Britain.   2. Jurisprudence–Great Britain.   3. Patient Rights–legislation & jurisprudence–Great Britain.   4. Physician-Patient Relations–ethics–Great Britain.   5. Professional Practice–ethics–Great Britain. W 50]
        174.2–dc23
            2012047947

A catalogue record for this book is available from the British Library.

Wiley also publishes its books in a variety of electronic formats. Some content that appears in print may not be available in electronic books.

Cover design by Rob Sawkins for Opta Design. Image #617669 from Istockphoto.com © 2005 Clayton Hansen

Set in 9.5/12 pt Garamond MT by Toppan Best-set Premedia Limited
Printed and bound in Malaysia by Vivar Printing Sdn Bhd

1   2013

Contents

Medical Ethics Committee

A publication from the BMA's Medical Ethics Committee (MEC). The following people were members of the MEC for the 2011/12 session.

Dr Anthony Calland, Chairman – *General practice (retired), Gwent*

Dr JS Bamrah – *Psychiatry, Manchester*
Dr John Chisholm (deputy) – *General practice, Bromley*
Dr Mary Church – *General practice, Glasgow*
Professor Bobbie Farsides – *Medical law and ethics, Brighton*
Claire Foster – *Medical ethics, London*
Professor Ilora Finlay – *Palliative medicine, Cardiff*
Professor Robin Gill – *Theology, Canterbury*
Professor Raanan Gillon – *General practice (retired) and medical ethics, London*
Dr Zoe Greaves – *Junior doctor, South Tees*
Dr Evan Harris – *Former MP and hospital doctor, Oxford*
Professor Emily Jackson – *Medical law and ethics, London*
Dr Surendra Kumar – *General practice, Widnes*
Professor Graeme Laurie – *Medical law, Edinburgh*
Dr Lewis Morrison – *General and geriatric medicine, Lothian*
Dr Ainslie Newson – *Biomedical ethics, Bristol*
Professor Julian Savulescu – *Practical ethics, Oxford*
Dr Peter Tiplady (deputy) – *Public health physician, Carlisle*
Dr Frank Wells – *Pharmaceutical physician (retired), Ipswich*
Dr Jan Wise – *Psychiatry, London*

Ex-officio
Dr Hamish Meldrum, Chairman of BMA Council
Professor David Haslam, President of BMA
Dr Steve Hajioff, Chairman of BMA Representative Body
Dr Andrew Dearden, BMA Treasurer

Thanks are due to other BMA committees and staff for providing information and comments on draft chapters.

List of case examples

Throughout this book points are illustrated with the use of case examples. Some of these are cases that have been decided by the courts (these have the case name, in italics, in the title) while other case examples are based on enquiries to the BMA or on material published by other organisations, including some disciplinary cases heard by the General Medical Council.

Chapter 2: The doctor–patient relationship

Chapter 3: Consent, choice and refusal: adults with capacity

Chapter 4: Treating adults who lack capacity

Chapter 5: Treating children and young people

Chapter 6: Confidentiality

Chapter 7: Management of health records

Chapter 8: Prescribing and administering medication

Preface

The BMA is a doctors' organisation which, among other activities, provides ethical and medico-legal advice. Other health professionals are increasingly exploring similar dilemmas to those facing doctors and BMA guidance has broadened out to reflect that. This book also summarises best practice standards, legal benchmarks and the advice published by a range of other authoritative organisations throughout the UK. This book may be useful for other health and social care professionals as well as for doctors, although naturally, they are our main audience.

Traditionally, *medical ethics* applied to the standards and principles that governed what doctors do but now often describes the obligations of all health professionals. Some people prefer a broader and, arguably, more inclusive term such as *healthcare ethics*, but we have stuck with the term *medical*. While recognising that good patient care consists of a range of skilled personnel working cooperatively, sharing the same basic values and with very similar ethical duties, our experience is primarily concerned with advising doctors. This book focuses on the daily ethical and medico-legal problems doctors face. We know what these are because, for several decades, the BMA has run an advisory service through which members can receive prompt advice on specific dilemmas. Very often, the recurring problems involve aspects of confidentiality and patient consent, such as whether an unmarried father can legally access his child's medical records or who can consent to treatment for young people. Patterns of queries alter to reflect high-profile cases reported in the media and the very significant growth of case law (judge-made law) and statute. Now many of both the mundane and the more tricky questions are covered by law, which can differ significantly across the four nations of the UK. This is reflected in the following chapters.

Case examples are also included in the text. Some of these are cases which have gone through the courts and illustrate specific points of current good practice. Others are based on dilemmas doctors have raised with us. We have summarised and anonymised real cases, but some of the examples are amalgams of many very similar scenarios, rather than one specific case. The aim is to capture the very common niggling worries that should have easy answers but often do not.

Above all, our approach is practical rather than abstract or theoretical. As each chapter is based on the problems raised with us by BMA members, many of the fascinating topics of more abstract ethical debate, beloved of philosophers and examiners – such as the moral status of the embryo and whether assisted dying should be perceived as a human right – are entirely absent from this volume. The BMA has, of course, explored all these issues in considerable depth. Readers who wish to see the full range of topics should consult the third edition of our detailed ethics handbook, *Medical Ethics Today*. A range of guidance notes are freely available to all health professionals and patients on the ethics section of the BMA's website and members can also talk through specific dilemmas either by telephone, letter or email.

1: A practical approach to ethics

Picture this . . .

A senior police officer is asking for details of all patients on a certain drug. It could be in connection with a serious crime or an unidentified corpse, but the facts are vague. What do you think? Is patient confidentiality trumped by serious crime and, if so, how serious does the crime have to be? In another part of the building, an irate father is demanding to see his daughter's record. Can he do that as a divorced dad without custody rights? Should the mother or the 12-year-old daughter herself be asked first? Another headache is that you are new to the area and keen to meet people. Surely there's no problem in going to a local barbecue? You've already had a few flirty emails from one of the organisers who wants to be your Facebook friend and happens to be a patient. It seems quite innocent or is it? On top of that, a senior colleague wants to do some research involving a change of medication for your patients with early-stage dementia. It may do them some good, but doesn't someone need to consent on their behalf or can they do that themselves? Also there's a man who always stands far too close and keeps accidentally brushing against you. He's booked in for a prostate examination and asked specifically for you to do it. Do doctors really still need chaperones? It sounds so Victorian and what if the patient objects? And you're worried about the patient with the fractured ribs who makes a habit of falling downstairs but refuses to let you tell the police that or about the cigarette burns on her arms. She has young children who don't look too good either. Shouldn't you do something? The teenager waiting for stitches in his hand also gives an odd account of the accident. Aren't you supposed to report all knife wounds even if, as he says, he was just showing off his chef's chopping technique to his mum in the kitchen?

Common enough questions but the answer may not always seem immediately obvious. That is the point of this book. In the following chapters, we pull together some of the recurring queries that doctors raise. Many dilemmas appear relatively mundane, but some touch on life-changing decisions that need to involve the courts. In fact, all health professionals are likely to face situations in which they have to pause and consider. Their initial gut reaction is not always the right one and, if challenged, they need to be able to offer a reasonable justification for the decisions taken.

Everyday Medical Ethics and Law, First Edition. Ann Sommerville.
© 2013 BMA Medical Ethics Department. Published 2013 by John Wiley & Sons, Ltd.

Does medical ethics help and how?

When professionals have to work through a problem and feel justified about the options they take or recommend, they need some consistent benchmarks. Traditionally, codes of ethics helped by setting out a framework of duties and principles. Modern medical ethics still provides the framework but also needs to take account of professional regulation, law and quasi law. Frustratingly, ready-made answers are seldom available. Careful analysis and reasoning about the particular circumstances is usually needed, so that superficially similar cases may prompt different responses. This is because an *ethical* decision is not just about providing the best clinical outcome for the patient but may also include accommodating that person's own wishes and values. It involves a search for coherent solutions in situations where different people's interests or priorities conflict. It is often as concerned with the process through which a decision is reached as with the decision itself.

Most of the issues covered in this book are not new. In many cases, the law or well-established pathways and protocols point the way forward but as health care is constantly evolving, new challenges also arise. Ethical debate and the law may then lag behind practice for a while. Often new problems can be usefully addressed by reference to parallel scenarios for which best practice has already been defined but sometimes, a solution which works well in one instance cannot be applied to another, although it appears similar. As each patient is an individual with hopes and expectations that can differ from the norm, radically different solutions may be needed. Health professionals need the skill to analyse the particular problem they face in its own context. This chapter briefly sketches out the BMA approach to medical ethics, with some practical steps on how to approach an ethical dilemma.

Key terms and concepts

Throughout history, doctors have been seen to have special obligations. Sometimes labelled *Hippocratic*, similar moral obligations were expected of doctors in diverse cultures. As other caring professions attained recognition, they reiterated the same core virtues. One of the problems, as we discuss later, is how we currently interpret traditional concepts, such as the duty to benefit patients and avoid harm (see below). Qualities doctors and other health professionals are now expected to possess include integrity, compassion and altruism as well as the pursuit of continuous improvement, excellence and effective multidisciplinary working.

Key concepts in medical ethics

Common ethical terms are generally self-evident but may require some interpretation when applied to specific cases. All of the terms listed below are explored further, with examples, in later chapters.

Self-determination or autonomy – The ability to think, decide and act for oneself is summed up in the concept of self-determination or personal autonomy. When patients have the mental capacity to make choices, their decisions should be respected as long as they do not adversely affect the rights or welfare of others. Adults with capacity who understand the options are entitled to accept or refuse them without explaining why. They can make choices that seem very harmful for them (as long as those things are lawful), but they cannot choose things that harm other people.

Mental capacity – In order to exercise their autonomy, people need to have the mental capacity to understand and weigh up the options so that they can make a choice. All adults are assumed to have this, unless there is evidence to the contrary and, in practice, most people (unless unconscious) are capable of making some decisions. Adults' decisions can still be valid when they appear unconventional, irrational or unjustified, but health professionals may need to check that patients have the mental capacity to exercise their autonomy, when such choices have major life-changing implications.

Honesty and integrity – Health professionals are required to be honest and to act with integrity. This means more than simply telling the truth. Their actions should never be intended to deceive and there should be *transparency* about how decisions are reached. One of the major challenges in this context is giving patients bad news about their prognosis, when the temptation may be to imply more hope than is justified. Good communication skills are essential. A failure to communicate effectively can undermine trust and invalidate patient consent if information the patient needs and wants to know is left unsaid.

Confidentiality – All patients are entitled to confidentiality, but their right is not absolute, especially if other people are at serious risk of harm as a result. Cases arise where an overriding *public interest* justifies disclosure, even against the patient's wishes. Although this is one of the oldest values reiterated in ethical codes, it is increasingly difficult to define its scope and limitations in practical terms, not least because notions of public interest change.

Fairness and equity – The individual patient is the main focus, but health professionals also have to consider the big picture and whether accommodating one person's wishes harms or deprives someone else unfairly. General practitioners, for example, may be confronted with situations in which the needs or interests of different patients conflict and some doctors, such as public health doctors, are necessarily concerned with groups rather than individuals. The values of fairness and equity are closely linked with the practicalities needed to prioritise and ration the use of scarce communal resources, often summarised in the term *distributive justice*. There are various ways of approaching *justice* besides the obvious one about *equality*

(Continued)

(trying to treat all similar cases the same), including the *sufficiency* view (what matters most is that everyone has essential care – although views can vary on what counts as *essential* – and beyond this, inequalities are less important). Fairness under the law is another aspect which is considered further below. Fairness to patients is also a consideration when *conflicts of interest* arise and doctors' professional judgement risks being influenced by factors such as the prospect of personal gain.

Harm and benefit – Notions of maximising benefit and minimising harm are among the trickiest aspects of modern medical ethics, although the ancient 'Hippocratic' commitment to benefit patients and to do so with minimal harm remains central to medical ethics and, indeed, to other healthcare professional codes. Keeping people alive and functioning was traditionally understood to encapsulate the obligation to avoid *harm* and promote *benefit* but, although the terminology has not changed, the interpretations have. Actions are harmful if the person experiencing them believes them to be so or has clearly rejected them. An example would be the use of invasive technology to try and prolong the life of someone who has refused it. Although they can be slippery, notions of harm and benefit continue to feature strongly in any problem-solving methodology and increasingly preoccupy the courts. There is no clear and universal definition and interpretation of the terms depends in different contexts on a number of variables, including individuals' preferences as well as legal and professional benchmarks.

Professionalism

Professionalism is closely linked to modern ethical precepts and reflects traditional core values. Defined as a set of values, behaviours and relationships that underpins the trust that the public places in health professionals, it focuses on health professionals' partnerships with patients and with each other. Some commentators express concerns about the way market models in health care might affect how we define professionalism. For example, although NHS doctors always had an ethical obligation to consider resources, their own income was generally not linked to their clinical decisions. Increasingly, the use of more commercially orientated tools, including incentives, has led to concerns about how potential conflicts of interest should be managed. (Conflicts of interest are discussed in Chapter 2.) More generally, concerns have been expressed that a broader cultural shift towards a consumer-led model of health care could undermine the core values associated with medicine. Key challenges include finding and maintaining ways in which core values, such as compassion, beneficence and a strong obligation to promote the interests of patients, can still underpin and guide practice in a commercially orientated and consumer-led health environment.

Duties and rights

Traditional ethical codes were all about doctors' duties without spelling out any explicit rights (or responsibilities) for patients. By inference, if doctors and other health professionals have certain duties, such as to avoid harm and provide benefits, logically patients have concomitant rights, but until relatively recently, health care was not primarily seen from the patient's perspective. (See Chapter 2, which discusses this change of focus, including the notion of patients' responsibilities, and Chapter 3, which describes some of the legal cases leading to the current emphasis placed on informed consent.) Now, rights – especially those linked to patient autonomy and self-determination – are often the main focus of ethics and law. A distinction can be made between moral rights and those which are legally enforceable. Many rights are moral claims which we intuitively consider appropriate ('he had a right to know his child was ill'), but because these are not always clear-cut and as the moral claims of different individuals often clash, much depends on the context of the case. In ethics (unlike law), few rights are absolute and often one person's moral rights may be overridden in exceptional cases in order to prevent a greater harm. (This is discussed in detail in Chapter 6 Confidentiality, as that is one of the areas most commonly affected by a clash of rights.) Ethical analysis can provide a useful problem-solving tool, taking into account the context of the dilemma in order to balance out such conflicts.

The public interest

The public interest is another factor which affects patients' rights and health professionals' duties as it limits individuals' freedom to act, or keep information secret, in situations where other people might be harmed. The public interest is usually defined by law and is the basis of all public health legislation, such as the duty to report infectious diseases. Other common examples of the public interest argument arise when a disclosure of information from medical records is needed to prevent accidental harm, such as when a patient with bad eyesight continues to drive, or to detect a serious crime (see Chapter 6). The General Medical Council (GMC) also advises that, in some circumstances, a disclosure without a person's consent can be justified in the public interest to enable medical research.[1] In all cases, the facts must be subject to close scrutiny as to whether there is a genuine public interest at stake. Although 'public interest' is the usual terminology and is used throughout this book, some people prefer to think of it in terms of 'the public good' to emphasise that there is a clear distinction (particularly in relation to information disclosure) between what is in the public interest and what the public is interested in.

Medical law and healthcare law

Ethical decisions in the NHS are guided by legislation, the NHS Constitution, guidance from professional and regulatory bodies, as well as local guidance and protocols at trust level. Practitioners working privately outside the NHS generally also work to the same standards. They too are bound by the law and by the rules of their regulatory body, which for doctors is the GMC. An understanding of medical law is as crucial for doctors as an awareness of ethics or of GMC rules, but the law relating to health care is fast moving, making it a challenge to keep abreast of new developments. Increasingly too, legislation differs in England, Wales, Scotland and Northern Ireland. This book draws attention to relevant legal provisions throughout the UK and to where they differ, and regular updates are provided on the BMA's website. Often, common dilemmas cannot be resolved by concentrating on the ethics because, in many cases, the law actually dictates what must be done. (See, e.g. Chapter 6 on use of patient data and Chapter 4 on who can consent for an incapacitated adult.) Law's ever-increasing role in health care can be seen in the important guidance on best practice which has evolved through court judgments. (Chapter 3 sets out, e.g. key cases on patient consent and refusal.) In practice, law and ethics are often intertwined so that judgments in legal cases draw on traditional ethical principles and moral analysis. The two are often so inseparable that it is difficult to disengage moral considerations from legal rules.

Medical law in the UK has developed significantly since the 1980s, when decisions which had previously been seen as for doctors to decide began to move into the courts. The emerging discipline of medical law borrowed from standards set out in 'family law, the law of torts, criminal law, administrative law, statutory interpretation and that unruly horse public policy'.[2] Initially, it focused on 'the relationship between doctors (and to a lesser extent hospitals and other institutions) and patients',[3] but by 2002, it was increasingly recognised that – although very important – concentrating solely on interactions between doctors and patients was too narrow. 'This is firstly because doctors are not the only health professionals, secondly because the delivery of health care in the UK is primarily the responsibility of the NHS and thirdly because it underplays the increasing importance of public health issues'.[4] Healthcare law encompassed a broader field, including the way health care is organised, preventive measures to protect against disease and the sharing of responsibility for health between patients themselves, the state, health professionals and their employers.[5]

Statute and common law

There are different types of law. *Statute* describes laws made by Parliament which govern many contentious areas such as abortion, reproductive technology and the use of human tissue as well as everyday matters such as the use of health data. Other areas of medicine are strongly influenced by *common law*. This develops as precedents set by judges in individual cases establish rules or benchmarks for other similar cases. The court's ruling in one situation can often be extrapolated to resolve disagreements in other similar scenarios. Judges are expected to abide by the precedents of earlier cases unless there are strong reasons to challenge them.

Human rights law

Human rights law is one category of statute law. It is formal, enforceable and generally non-negotiable, although some legitimate interference with people's rights is permitted, as long as it is proportionate and justifiable. Unlike moral rights, legal rights are less dependent upon context and are generally less flexible even though there can be scope for interpretation. Human rights law has some significant implications for medicine, not least in the manner in which its concepts and terminology have influenced medical ethics. The relevant Articles have also been relied upon heavily to argue medical cases before the courts. In 1998, the UK incorporated the bulk of the rights set out in the European Convention for the Protection of Human Rights and Fundamental Freedoms into British legislation. The UK's Human Rights Act came fully into force in 2000.

Convention Articles relevant to health care

- Article 2 – the right to life
- Article 3 – prohibition on torture, inhuman or degrading treatment
- Article 5 – the right to liberty and security
- Article 6 – the right to a fair hearing or fair trial
- Article 8 – respect for private and family life
- Article 9 – freedom of thought, conscience and religion
- Article 10 – freedom of expression
- Article 12 – the right to marry and found a family
- Article 14 – enjoyment of these rights to be secured without discrimination.

The significance of these rights to the way health care is provided is not always obvious. The right to life, for example, does not mean that life must be prolonged at all costs and the right to found a family does not imply a right to fertility treatment. Some interpretation is often needed. For example, legal cases about withdrawing life-prolonging treatment or arguing for euthanasia have been debated in terms of patients' rights to freedom from torture or inhuman and degrading treatment. The right to respect for private and family life is applied to cases about confidentiality and information sharing. The BMA has specific guidance on how the Human Rights Act affects health care,[6] but the fundamental message is that decisions taken by doctors on the basis of current ethical standards are likely to be compliant with the Act. Issues such as human dignity, communication, consultation and best interests, which are central to good clinical practice, are also pivotal to the Convention rights. When making decisions, however, health professionals should consider whether a person's human rights are affected and, if so, whether the interference is proportionate and justifiable. Even when there is a legitimate reason for interfering with a particular right, the anticipated outcome should justify the level of interference proposed. Where different rights come into conflict, doctors and other decision makers must be able to justify choosing one over the other.

Quasi (or soft) law

In addition to statute and common law, *quasi law* (also sometimes referred to as *soft law*) needs to be mentioned because it can also be binding on health professionals. Quasi law is not strictly legally binding and does not carry legal sanctions (although some forms of quasi law can have direct or indirect legal consequences), but it sets out the rules and guidance for good practice that health professionals are generally expected to follow. This includes the rules and professional guidance set out and policed by the regulatory bodies, such as the GMC. Such rules are backed up by serious sanctions and doctors should familiarise themselves with GMC guidance, especially with the core advice in *Good Medical Practice*.[7] Failure to comply can result in a finding of serious professional misconduct with a range of sanctions including removal of a doctor's licence to practice. Doctors often work closely with other health professionals who are bound by similar professional rules. Nurses, midwives and health visitors are personally accountable for their practice and are subject to statutory regulation by the Nursing and Midwifery Council. *The Code: Standards of Conduct, Performance and Ethics for Nurses and Midwives*[8] sets out similar principles to the GMC's guidance for doctors. Nurses, midwives and health visitors, like doctors, have a duty to acknowledge the limitations in their knowledge. All should refuse to undertake any duties or responsibilities they consider to be beyond their competence, even if asked to do so by a senior colleague. (Emergency situations when no other help is available are an exception, and these are discussed briefly in Chapter 2 in the section on recognising boundaries.)

GMC guidance on the duties of a doctor

'Patients must be able to trust doctors with their lives and health. To justify that trust, you must show respect for human life and you must:

- make the care of your patient your first concern
- protect and promote the health of patients and the public
- provide a good standard of practice and care
  - keep your professional knowledge and skills up to date
  - recognise and work within the limits of your competence
  - work with colleagues in the ways that best serve patients' interests
- treat patients as individuals and respect their dignity
  - treat every patient politely and considerately
  - respect patients' right to confidentiality
- work in partnership with patients
  - listen to patients and respond to their concerns and preferences
  - give patients the information they want or need in a way they can understand
  - respect patients' rights to reach decisions with you about their treatment and care
  - support patients in caring for themselves to improve and maintain their health
- be honest and open and act with integrity
  - act without delay if you have good reason to believe that you or a colleague may be putting patients at risk
  - never discriminate unfairly against your patients or colleagues
  - never abuse your patients' trust in you or the public trust in the profession

You are personally accountable for your professional practice and must always be prepared to justify your decisions and actions'.[7]

In many areas of modern medical practice, there is well-accepted guidance laid down in the form of NHS instructions, National Institute for Health and Clinical Excellence (NICE) guidance, circulars explaining legal requirements and current views of best practice, established care pathways and protocols. Many of these are a mixture of advice on the law, ethics and what is currently seen as clinically appropriate and may be published by professional bodies, such as the BMA and the Royal Colleges. Where relevant in the following chapters, this type of guidance is flagged up.

Ethical decision making

The law provides a framework for practice and, in some cases, gives clear direction as to what action is needed. In other cases, two or more options would be legally permissible and some analysis is required to decide what would be the best approach. Even when the principles are set out in professional guidance, the challenge for health professionals is often to apply those general principles to the individual circumstances. These are often cases where rights, duties or obligations conflict and some judgement is needed about which should take precedence. Ethical decision making involves identifying where these tensions, or conflicting rights or duties, arise and exploring them through careful assessment of all morally relevant concerns, taking account of the views and interests of all parties. This includes identification and consideration of the various options, weighing up the advantages, disadvantages, risks, benefits and implications of each. The BMA, through both its written guidance and its individual advice to doctors, aims to facilitate this process, not by telling doctors what to do but rather by helping them to identify the relevant rules or principles and to explore the issues thoroughly in order to reach a decision they can justify with soundly reasoned arguments.

Approaching an ethical problem

Many ethical queries to the BMA centre on what should be done in complex situations where the answer is far from obvious. Doctors and other health professionals need to be able to identify the main issues and weigh up the options in a reasoned manner, knowing that they may possibly have to later explain their reasoning to a court or to their regulatory body. Some situations can be resolved simply by identifying the patient's wishes, since both ethics and the law tend to emphasise personal autonomy as a default position, unless there are strong reasons for overriding it (examples of this are given in the chapters that follow). In some cases, this is impossible and, with incapacitated adults, for example, the focus switches to what would be in their best interests. In such situations it is important to stop and think. The first step must be to check the facts of the case as accurately as possible. Frequently, just this process of clarifying precisely what is at stake, and for whom, goes a long way to finding a way forward. In practice, legal boundaries and good practice protocols often determine the best option, before we begin to examine the ethical arguments. In fact, in some situations, the legally viable options are so clearly stated that it would be pointless to look beyond them when the aim is to provide practical advice. The fact that we often do persist in looking further springs from the need to ensure that ethical advice is morally consistent and justifiable in different contexts, regardless of whether or not the law has pronounced upon all the relevant scenarios. Practical ethical advice must also be consistent with society's changing expectations, especially in areas where the law is permissive or is open to interpretation.

Dilemmas arise where there are two or more possible options, neither of which is entirely ethically acceptable; this often involves circumstances in which different people's rights or wishes conflict. Various theories and methodologies exist for analysing such situations. Some focus on the consequences of taking a particular action, seeking to maximise overall benefit (consequentialist ethics); others focus on duties (deontological ethics), responsibilities (communitarian ethics) or on key principles (the four principles approach) or assess what a 'virtuous person' would do in the situation (virtue ethics). These are discussed in our ethics handbook, *Medical Ethics Today*,[9] in which there is also a section on how to apply these philosophical approaches to a practical situation. As this book concentrates very much on the practicalities, however, we do not cover them here.

The BMA's approach

Over the years the BMA has developed its own methodology for considering and analysing practical ethical dilemmas (Figure 1.1). This aims to combine an awareness of general principles, professional guidelines and previously settled legal cases but, above all, to show the thought process required to arrive at logical solutions that are workable in real life. Each case has to be considered on its own merits. How a dilemma is approached depends on the context and complexity of the question. Some can be quickly resolved by reference to GMC guidance, relevant law or established standards of best practice. In novel or complex cases, particularly where duties to different parties conflict, aspects of the dilemma need to be dissected so that irrelevant detail is removed and all perspectives are considered.

Recognise that a dilemma exists

Some avoidable problems occur because professionals fail to recognise the ethical issue or conflict of interest facing them. This may be because the way senior colleagues did things in the past has not been questioned or because staff understand the principles but do not see their relevance to a particular case. Responding to a relative's enquiry about a patient's health, without the patient's consent, is a mundane example in which a breach of confidentiality can occur unintentionally. Complex issues of clinical judgement can also have ethical dimensions, but the complexity of the clinical decision may distract attention from the underlying ethical question. Deciding whether to offer an expensive new treatment, for example, may require not only a clinical assessment of the patient but also consideration of the opportunity costs for others when resources are limited. Ethical reflection is needed when the situation

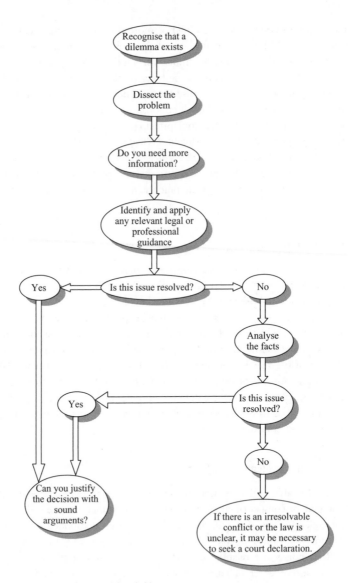

Figure 1.1 Approaching an ethical dilemma

involves a conflict of interests, values, rights or civil liberties. If the general principles that would normally be relied upon for dealing with such issues are of no help or conflict with one another, an ethical dilemma arises. These are situations where there are good moral reasons to act in two or more different ways, each of which is also in some way morally flawed.

Dissect the problem

It is always necessary to consider the context and individual circumstances of the case, but too much detail is distracting. Excess information needs to be cleared away so that the key issues are accurately identified. Once there is a clear picture of these, objective solutions become easier. Although the rights and interests of different parties clash, for example, it may still be clear which should take precedence such as when serious child protection concerns arise and parents' preferences take second place. By removing a mass of extraneous detail and isolating the crux of the problem, solutions drawn from parallel scenarios may suggest themselves.

Do you need more information?

Once the core issues have been identified, more information may be needed. You may have a lot of narrative about what has occurred but still lack key facts. In a number of dilemmas raised with the BMA, assumptions are made about how patients will react without anyone actually talking to them. The dilemma may, for example, be whether to breach confidentiality to the Driver and Vehicle Licensing Agency (DVLA) about a driver with failing eyesight or to inform the police about serious domestic violence. The difficulty of broaching the subject with the individual concerned may mean that an obvious – but not necessarily easy – solution is overlooked, which would be to support that person to take action himself or herself. Clarity is needed about the facts. If the issue is about providing contraception to a young person, for example, it is crucial to know whether the patient is mature enough to make a valid decision. If estranged parents disagree about a young child's care, it is important to know who has parental responsibility. Once you have the relevant background information, it is easier to see whether existing guidance applies.

Identify and apply relevant legal or professional guidance

Part of identifying the relevant factors includes checking whether the situation is covered by legal or professional guidance. Depending upon the complexity of the issue, information may be needed from a range of sources, including relevant

- statute or case law about the subject
- guidance from the regulatory body
- guidance from professional bodies, such as the BMA or Royal Colleges
- advice issued by health authorities in England, Scotland, Wales and Northern Ireland
- guidance from organisations legally regulating the area of enquiry
- advice from the organisations providing indemnity, such as medical defence bodies.

Analyse the facts

Having identified as much as possible the relevant facts and, where appropriate, having sounded out the patient's own views, a way forward may emerge. If information is still missing or you believe that not all angles have been considered, it may be necessary to involve a colleague or other members of the health team who may have a different perspective. The aim here is to consider all of the issues and all of the options and to make a judgement about what would be the most appropriate thing to do. In some instances, it may be helpful to discuss the case anonymously with other colleagues, a clinical ethics committee, professional associations or defence bodies before reaching a decision. In practice, however, decisions often have to be made quickly and in stressful circumstances. In such cases, health professionals are not expected to be omniscient but to act reasonably on the facts and to be able to justify their decisions. Knowing where to find professional guidance when it is needed can be good preparation for difficult dilemmas. It was with this in mind that the BMA has published on its website a range of brief 'toolkits' summarising the main points of ethics and law on a range of issues, and the BMA's more extensive text, *Medical Ethics Today*, is available to BMA members online.

Dilemmas often arise because duties owed to different parties conflict. A common enquiry, for example, concerns requests from the police for full access to patients' medical records. The duty of confidentiality has to be balanced against the duty to protect others from foreseeable harm. The questions that need to be considered in deciding how to proceed include the following:

- is it possible or desirable to obtain the patient's consent?
- is the crime or threat sufficiently serious for the public interest to prevail?
- is someone at risk of death or serious harm?
- would a refusal to disclose seriously hinder the investigation?
- is the information available elsewhere without a breach of confidentiality?
- is any information on the medical record relevant to the crime?

Based on an assessment of these types of factors, the doctor needs to decide whether to accede to the request. In some cases disclosure to the police is justified; in others it is not. Sometimes the police will seek a court order if access is refused and, unless a decision is made to challenge its relevance to the case, doctors are under an obligation to disclose the information.

Can you justify the decision with sound arguments?

Although, as mentioned above, it can be helpful to discuss the dilemma with a colleague, clinical ethics committee, professional organisation or a defence body, ultimately the clinician responsible for the patient's care has to make a decision. In the majority of cases, once a reasonable solution is reached, that is the end of the matter unless there is subsequent audit to check whether the right actions have been taken. Even where there is no audit or challenge to the decision, the clinician needs to feel able to justify it, and explain the reasoning, if called upon to do so. For example, when a decision is made to withdraw treatment that is prolonging a patient's life, the clinician should be able to explain how that decision was reached from a clinical, legal and ethical perspective. Discussions that took place with the patient should be noted in the medical record. If the patient lacked mental capacity and had no valid advance decision, the doctor needs to be able to explain why continuing treatment was not in the patient's best interests. Information should be recorded about any guidance referred to, advice sought and discussion that took place. In some cases, it is not possible for the healthcare team and the patient to resolve the dilemma either because there is an apparently irresolvable conflict or because the law is unclear. In such cases it may be necessary to seek a court declaration. When this is the case, trust lawyers, indemnifying bodies or the BMA can usually offer advice. In a limited number of cases, such as the withdrawal of artificial nutrition and hydration from a patient in a persistent vegetative state or a minimally conscious state, a court declaration is always required.

A final word on problem solving

A step-by-step approach indicates one tried and tested way of working through a dilemma, but the process is not necessarily straightforward as often some bits of the puzzle are missing. Gathering together all the information needed in order to make a proper assessment can be a challenge. Also health professionals often work in far from ideal environments, juggling many competing demands and trying to engage with patients who are often fearful and sometimes difficult. Discussion of abstract values can then seem irrelevant to the raw reality of daily practice. Large amounts of guidance, protocols and legislation have to be taken into account and the effect can appear overwhelming, especially if potentially conflicting demands are made. Health professionals are urged to put individual patients' interests first while simultaneously ensuring that limited resources are well used, patients' rights to access care and to exercise preferences are respected, and futile measures avoided. Some of these expectations are in tension with each other. An aim of the following chapters is to help practitioners to find good answers to dilemmas while recognising the pressures and limitations they often face in real life.

References

1 General Medical Council (2009) *Confidentiality*, GMC, London, para 36.
2 Kennedy I and Grubb A (1989) *Medical Law: Text with Materials*, Butterworths, London, p.77.
3 Kennedy I and Grubb A (2000) *Medical Law: Text with Materials*, 3rd edn, Butterworths, London, p.5.
4 Montgomery J (2003) *Healthcare Law*, 2nd edn, Oxford University Press, Oxford, p.1.
5 Montgomery J (2003) *Healthcare Law*, 2nd edn, Oxford University Press, Oxford, p.3.
6 British Medical Association (2008) *The Impact of the Human Rights Act 1998 on Medical Decision Making*, BMA, London.
7 General Medical Council (2006) *Good Medical Practice*, GMC, London.
8 Nursing and Midwifery Council (2008) *The Code: Standards of Conduct, Performance and Ethics for Nurses and Midwives*, NMC, London.
9 British Medical Association (2012) *Medical Ethics Today. The BMA's Handbook of Ethics and Law*, 3rd edn, Wiley-Blackwell, Chichester, pp.9–13 and 17–18.

2: The doctor–patient relationship

10 things you need to know about . . . the doctor–patient relationship

- The onus is on the doctor to make the doctor–patient relationship work.
- A doctor's duty of care for a patient can begin even before the patient is seen.
- Patients have many legal rights requiring respect, but most of these are not absolute rights.
- Health professionals should be frank and truthful, including when patients' prognosis is poor or when it is unlikely they could afford a treatment option which is only available privately.
- The onus is on doctors to recognise when a conflict of interests, or what may be perceived by others to be one, is looming for them and to deal with it openly and appropriately.
- NHS employees are prohibited from accepting gifts from patients or their relatives. Practitioners who are not NHS employees can accept gifts. If likely to benefit from a patient's will they should not be involved in assessing the patient's capacity when the will is made.
- It is unlawful to administer medication covertly to patients who have mental capacity even if they are behaving badly and they need the drugs to prevent their condition getting worse.
- Doctors have responsibility for ensuring that professional boundaries are maintained.
- If agreeing to witness patients' legal documents, doctors need to be aware that it may be assumed that they have also checked the patient's mental capacity to make the decision in question.
- Doctors have legal rights to conscientiously object to participating in some procedures, but these are very narrowly defined in law. A conscientious objection cannot justify unfair discrimination.

Setting the scene

In the previous chapter, we looked at how health professionals' moral and legal obligations to patients are set by statute, case law, regulatory bodies and various kinds of quasi law, embodied in protocols, guidelines and best practice standards. In this chapter, we look more closely at how those obligations translate into daily practice. Although focusing primarily on the role of doctors, most of these considerations also apply to other health workers.

Everyday Medical Ethics and Law, First Edition. Ann Sommerville.
© 2013 BMA Medical Ethics Department. Published 2013 by John Wiley & Sons, Ltd.

Through the advisory service it provides, the BMA keeps a log of common enquiries and areas of uncertainty. Among the queries raised are some recurring uncertainties about aspects of the doctor–patient relationship.

Common questions asked about the doctor–patient relationship

- When precisely does my duty of care for patients begin and end? What exactly does it entail?
- Who is ultimately responsible (and potentially legally liable) if something goes wrong when tasks are shared in teams or are delegated?
- What should I tell patients, without defaming colleagues, when things not my fault have gone wrong? Do I have to disclose mistakes when nobody was really hurt but telling patients means they may try to sue anyway?
- If a senior colleague tells me to do something for a patient beyond my competence, do I have to attempt it?
- What responsibility do I have for patients who are uncooperative, fail to follow advice, discharge themselves prematurely or miss appointments?
- Do I have to see people who are aggressive or threatening or can I just call the police?
- Do patients have the right to queue jump by switching between NHS and private care?
- If NHS patients say they want to see another doctor instead of me, do they have that right?
- When so many of the formal boundaries that used to exist have vanished from professional relationships, what counts as inappropriate friendliness with patients?

This chapter sets out the law, rules and principles that apply in situations concerning the doctor–patient relationship so that health professionals faced with questions or dilemmas can use this information as part of the process of ethical decision making. It will not provide answers to every question but will, hopefully, equip readers with the information they need to identify and assess the possible options and to reach a sound and reasoned decision about how to proceed.

Responsibilities for patients and the duty of care

Doctors have special responsibilities for ensuring that their relationships with patients work well.[1] Although the public has many means of accessing health information, patients are still seen as having a power disadvantage in their relationship with health professionals, who have more knowledge, experience and influence. Ethics guidance aims to balance this inherently asymmetrical relationship by giving the more knowledgeable party – the professional – a raft of duties and responsibilities. These vary according to the professional relationship.

The duty of care

The duty of care can vary, depending on the type and duration of the contact. Some health professionals only see an individual once for a specific purpose, such as writing a report or assessing eligibility for some social benefit. As is discussed later, such encounters are generally transitory and although they still involve some obligations to the person being examined, rarely involve any sense of an ongoing duty of care. When a therapeutic relationship exists, the situation is different. The duty of care can start even before a patient is seen. It is usually obvious when a relationship which entails a duty of care exists but situations can arise where there is doubt. Doctors are not under an obligation to treat a 'stranger', for example, other than in emergencies when first aid is urgently needed (emergencies are covered later in the book). Legally, doctors have a duty of care when they assume some responsibility for a patient.[2] This can be once they know of the person's need for medical services from them, or when they interact with the person in a professional capacity. In hospitals, this can be the case as soon as the patient presents for treatment.

Duty of care: *Barnett*[3]

This legal case clarified when a hospital doctor's duty of care begins. Three night watchmen drank tea which was later discovered to have contained arsenic. When they began vomiting, they went to the casualty department of the local hospital. A nurse telephoned the casualty officer, who advised that the men should go home and call their own doctors. The casualty officer himself felt tired and unwell and did not see the men. They all died from arsenic poisoning. In the subsequent court case, the judge ruled that the doctor owed the men who came to the hospital a duty of care which he had breached by failing to examine them. In brief, he owed a duty of care to people he had never seen but who had a reasonable expectation that he would look after them.

Duties of care which begin when a doctor or other health professional first engages with a patient, continue until one or other party ends the relationship. This can be when the patient moves from the area, is discharged after treatment, dies or transfers to another practitioner, for example because the relationship has broken down. Some duties to the patient – mainly those related to confidentiality – extend beyond that person's death (this is discussed in Chapter 6).

In face-to-face interactions between a patient and a health professional, it is usually clear that a duty of care exists, but it can be more nebulous when practitioners are approached by email or the internet. This can particularly be the case in relation to prescribing decisions and is discussed in Chapter 8. Once health professionals accept some aspect or episode of a patient's management, it is likely that a duty of care exists. In any consultation, they need to satisfy themselves that the patient has mental capacity, consents to examination and has sufficient information to make informed decisions. This is covered in detail in Chapter 3 and the care of patients who lack mental capacity is discussed in Chapter 4.

Case example – continuing duty of care

In a case raised with the BMA, a patient referred to hospital at the start of a programme of treatment took an immediate dislike to the female consultant responsible for his care. She did not get on with him either, not least because he made a complaint about what he termed her 'arrogant' attitude. The patient, an elderly man, was blunt to the point of rudeness with the whole health team. The consultant thought him brusque and uncooperative and did not want to see him again. It was pointed out to her that patients are entitled to make complaints and have them investigated, and the General Medical Council (GMC) puts the onus on the professional to make the relationship work. While it is generally better for patients to see a different clinician if the relationship irrevocably breaks down, a complaint does not necessarily mean that. In this case, the doctor and patient had got off on the wrong foot before getting to know each other. Although the man had a history of being demanding and outspoken when he felt patronised, he was also very worried and anxious. His behaviour was never threatening. He could not be abandoned, especially as an episode of care had begun, and so the consultant could not refuse to see him. If the relationship had broken down, the onus would have been on her to find a colleague willing to take on the patient's care but in the meantime, she had a continuing duty of care. She assumed that the patient would be reluctant to carry on seeing her, but he made clear that he was unwilling to switch to someone else. His complaint was investigated and judged to be unfounded. He more or less accepted that he had been too quick to complain and apologised. While he was far from being the ideal patient, he and the doctor managed to keep their relationship polite and respectful until his hospital care was completed.

Some patients transfer between the NHS and private treatment so that two or more health professionals share a duty of care. Consultants have a duty to patients seen by them or by their team but within the NHS, they are unlikely to have information about – or a duty towards – patients referred to them but not yet seen. In secondary NHS care, triage of such patients referred by their GP is not usually carried out by the consultant who will provide treatment but by nurses or junior doctors, or it can involve a referral management centre (RMC). The team or RMC then has a duty to ensure that appropriate action is taken. Once a consultant has accepted a patient, either by examining that person or studying the clinical details of an individual referred for treatment, a duty of care exists. Similar duties exist for specialists, such as radiologists or endoscopists, who are involved only with one aspect of a patient's investigation. When a patient has been assessed as non-urgent and placed on a list, the case still needs periodic review by those responsible for triage, if the condition is likely to deteriorate during the waiting time. If clinics are overbooked, the referring doctor should be informed so that an alternative arrangement can be made. Doctors asked by patients about waiting times obviously need to be accurate in replying.

Usually when we talk about a duty of care, it is in the context of examining or treating patients, but another aspect of the duty of care is the way in which health services are commissioned. Purchasers of healthcare services, such as clinical commissioning groups (CCGs), can be seen as having ethical obligations to continue paying for some services, even if they may not appear cost-effective but which have to be maintained as part of their duty of care to their patients[4] (see the section on managing conflicts of interest later in the chapter).

Independent assessors

When health professionals act as independent assessors, the people they examine are not their patients but are seen on isolated occasions, for example, for an insurance report. Independent assessors also carry out examinations for employment, state benefits or to report to the courts or immigration authorities. They do not have a relationship with, nor a continuing obligation to, the person examined but are paid by, and have obligations to, the agency commissioning the report. This needs to be made very clear to people being examined, who should be under no illusion that the consultation is to promote their health. They should already be well aware, but may need reminding, that their details will be reported, in the terms they have previously authorised, to the organisation which requested the examination unless they subsequently withdraw their consent.

A problem with independent examinations or assessments is sometimes a lack of openness; either the person being examined conceals information or the party commissioning the report instructs doctors not to disclose their findings to the client. In law, people have a right of access to such reports under the Data Protection Act (see Chapter 7). The GMC also advises that all doctors should usually offer to show the report to the patient before it is sent. If independent doctors discover new information significant to the management of a person's health, they should bring it to the attention of that person and, if he or she agrees, to the GP. Ideally, the organisation commissioning the report should advise the doctor in advance about how such eventualities will be handled.

Doctors who already have an ongoing duty of care to the individual, such as GPs, can also provide reports on their patients for insurance or employment purposes. Special legal provisions apply to such cases and reports cannot be sent without patients having had the opportunity, if they so choose, to see them (see Chapter 7).

Professionals with dual obligations

Some health professionals have a split responsibility to the patient and another party – usually an employer. Unlike the independent medical assessor, health professionals who work in prisons or immigration detention centres, for example, usually have an ongoing therapeutic relationship with the people they examine. They have a duty of care for them but also have to work within additional constraints. Ethical responsibilities for patients are not diminished but have to be combined with broader concerns, usually spelled out in their terms of employment.[5]

Continuity of care and patients' rights to change

Sometimes the responsibility for continuity of care rests with individual health professionals and at others it is with the healthcare establishment. Practitioners working on a sessional basis in a private clinic, for example, often believe they have an ongoing duty of care and therefore wish to take *their* patients with them when they move on or open their own clinic. They have a duty of care during the period in which they are providing treatment, as does the clinic, but it is the clinic which arranges continuity of care when practitioners leave. Clearly, employment terms of service need to make clear the rights and responsibilities of all staff but, usually in private practice, the patients' contract is with the clinic rather than the treating health professional.

When relationships work well, continuity is desirable, but patients increasingly obtain health care or advice from a range of sources and, with teamwork, continuity is often more about patients attending the same practice or service rather than seeing the same practitioner. (See also 'Breakdown of the doctor–patient relationship'.) In the past, doctors often had a strong sense of caring for 'their' patients, particularly in primary care, and it was considered inappropriate for other doctors to canvas for patients already registered with a GP. The more recent focus on patient choice means that people often combine a variety of sources of health advice and care. This can complicate notions of who has a duty of care at a particular time.

Delegation of tasks and referral of patients

Delegation involves professionals asking other staff to carry out procedures or provide care. When specific tasks are delegated, the professional arranging the delegation still retains responsibility for the patient's overall management and must ensure that tasks are delegated only to those who are competent to carry them out.

When a referral is made, responsibility for the patient is transferred, usually to someone with more specialised knowledge to carry out specific procedures, tests or treatment that fall outside the sphere of competence or of usual practice of the referring professional. In some cases, nurses, midwives and other professionals, as well as doctors, make and receive referrals, admit and discharge patients, order investigations and diagnostic tests, run clinics and prescribe drugs. Referrals are usually made to another registered health professional. If this is not the case, the person or the RMC making the referral should ensure that the professional to whom the patient is referred is accountable to a statutory regulatory body.

GMC guidance on delegation and referral

'Delegation involves asking a colleague to provide treatment or care on your behalf. Although you will not be accountable for the decisions and actions of those to whom you delegate, you will still be responsible for the overall management of the patient, and accountable for your decision to delegate. When you delegate care or treatment you must be satisfied that the person to whom you delegate has the qualifications, experience, knowledge and skills to provide the care or treatment involved. You must always pass on enough information about the patient and the treatment they need.[6]

Referral involves transferring some or all of the responsibility for the patient's care, usually temporarily and for a particular purpose, such as additional investigation, care or treatment that is outside your competence. You must be satisfied that any healthcare professional to whom you refer a patient is accountable to a statutory body or employed within a managerial environment. If they are not, the transfer of care will be regarded as delegation, not referral. This means that you remain responsible for the overall management of the patient, and accountable for your decision to delegate'.[7]

Patient autonomy and choice

Managing patients' expectations

Listening to patients and respecting their autonomy is emphasised in all ethical guidance. In the best circumstances, this is straightforward and appropriate treatment options can be matched up with the patient's preferences. When there is a mismatch, dilemmas arise. Patients who have mental capacity are entitled to decline treatment for any reason, even if their choices appear irrational, but doctors do not have to comply when patients request a particular treatment (this is discussed in detail in Chapter 3).

Do patients have choices about who provides care?

Some patients would like more say about who provides care and they may have increased expectations as a result of terminology in many official documents which emphasises their right to choose. Clearly, where it is feasible to do so, their preferences (e.g. for a male or female doctor) should be respected, but within the NHS, this is not always possible.

Case example – managing expectations

One of the queries to the BMA came from a Welsh-speaking community where some patients declined to be treated by 'foreign' doctors and thought that they should have a choice of Welsh speakers or, at least, doctors who had trained in the UK rather than in the EU. The BMA advised that trusts should have clear policies which avoid raising unreasonable patient expectations. Its advice included the following:

- trusts have obligations to provide competent, appropriately trained health professionals but cannot use unfairly discriminative judgments in their employment policies
- doctor–patient communication is important and consideration should be given to any potential impediments to it. Arrangements should be in place to deal with language or cultural differences affecting care
- attention should be given to risk management strategies where there is any foreseeable risk of harm or misunderstanding, resulting from different terms or languages being used
- patients with capacity have an absolute right to decline treatment for any reason, even if their choices appear irrational to others but they do not have comparable rights to insist on being treated by specific health personnel
- trusts should keep patients generally informed about the services provided and any relevant limitations on them
- trusts should consider their indemnity if patients suffer harm as a result of voluntarily declining treatment from a specific doctor.

It is unrealistic for patients to try to insist on seeing health professionals from a specific racial or cultural background, as the NHS provides appropriately trained professionals but cannot use racist or discriminatory policies. Private patients have more choice and can usually see the specialist they prefer but, if their care is funded by their insurer, the latter may specify where treatment is provided and designate a consultant. Patients can generally choose their GP unless local lists are full, in which case they may be allocated to a practice with capacity to accept them.

Rights of homeless people, detainees and asylum seekers

NHS GPs have an obligation to provide care on an equitable basis according to their capacity to take on new patients. They cannot exclude people whose condition requires a lot of time or resources (so-called 'uneconomic patients'), or patients who have multiple conditions. They must take into consideration the GMC's advice as well as the Equality Act's ban on discrimination.

All asylum seekers have the right to be registered with an NHS general practice, but GPs have discretion about whether they register refused asylum seekers. There is no obligation for GPs to check people's immigration status. (The BMA has specific guidance on the rights of asylum seekers to health care.[8]) In custodial settings, patients have no choice of doctor, but if they are already registered with a local doctor, remand prisoners and people held in police stations can request a visit from that GP. Whether or not the GP will agree to attend depends on the circumstances of the case. Once detainees have been convicted and are in prison, the choice of calling their own GP is no longer available.

Primary care practices sometimes ask if they have to register homeless people who have no address. If they have vacancies on their list, they must do so. Homeless patients can be registered by using the practice address. It is also unacceptable to discriminate unfairly by only registering English speakers or refusing all asylum seekers. In the private sector too, doctors should not act in an arbitrary or unfairly discriminatory manner in terms of taking on new patients. Similarly, in the hospital setting, doctors must treat all patients equitably and in a non-judgemental manner. It is not their role to verify the immigration status of patients presenting for care. This is the responsibility of overseas patient managers.

Can patients insist on having the drugs they prefer?

Requests for specific drugs, such as antibiotics, are increasingly common. Prescribing decisions have to be, as far as possible, evidence-based and should reflect established guidelines. Patients' preferences may be taken into account, but doctors do not have to comply when patients insist on options that are not clinically indicated or which cost significantly more to the NHS than other comparable regimes (this is discussed in detail in Chapter 8). Although it can be difficult to manage patients' expectations successfully, it is helpful to give clear explanations of why their preference is inappropriate or cannot be met in a specific instance.

Do patients have the right to a second opinion?

Patients' requests for second opinions are often interpreted as a sign of poor confidence in their doctor but, if reasonable, the GMC says that such requests should be implemented.[9] This is not necessarily the same as saying that NHS patients have a *right* to a second opinion and much depends on the circumstances and reasons for the request (unless the patient wants to pay for a private second opinion). In some cases, patients may be in denial about the gravity of their condition and hope to get different news from another clinician. They may need time to come to terms with the situation or more discussion about the diagnosis and options. When it would be reasonable and could be helpful to have a second view, it should be considered.

Rather than a second opinion, some patients ask the GP for a direct referral to a specialist. If there is no clinical justification for it, this needs to be explained to the patient. As mentioned below, some patients go to see a specialist privately, without a referral.

Patients' rights to combine NHS and private care

Investigations or treatment are arranged according to the clinical judgement of the doctor managing the patient's care. When more specialist assessment is needed, patients are referred appropriately and some prefer to see a specialist in the private sector. Patients with health insurance may find that the insurer specifies how, and to whom, referrals should be made. If they request referral in the absence of clinical need, the underlying reasons should be explored and an explanation given as to why it would be inappropriate. Some patients may still seek private treatment without a referral.

Patients can combine NHS and private care. Some pay initially for private investigations to get a diagnosis quickly and then switch back to the NHS for the subsequent treatment. As long as they are entitled to NHS care, such patients can opt into, or out of, NHS care at any stage and be placed onto the NHS waiting list at the same position as if their private investigations had been within the NHS. Some people think it unfair that patients who can afford to pay are able to jump the NHS queue by getting on to the treatment waiting list before those who wait for NHS investigations. Others argue that, as some people obtain a diagnosis privately, this is helpful in reducing some of the pressure on the NHS. In urgent cases, NHS patients whose clinical need is greater may join the waiting list later but still receive treatment earlier. In some circumstances, NHS patients may 'top-up' their care by paying privately for medication or treatment that is not available within the NHS. The BMA has separate guidance on this.[10]

Patients' rights to reject medical advice

Patients can be encouraged, but cannot be forced, to comply with medical advice concerning the management of their health or lifestyle. The only exception is when compulsory treatment under mental health legislation is appropriate (this is discussed in Chapter 4). For some patients, their inability, or unwillingness, to change lifestyle choices about diet, drinking, smoking or drug use may mean that they cannot be offered operations or other important interventions they need because their lifestyle endangers the chances of success. In such cases, it needs to be made clear that it is not a discriminatory decision to withhold some treatment options but rather an evidence-based assessment of the potential benefits and harms (see also Chapter 8, where concordance is discussed).

Wherever possible, the implications and consequences of ignoring medical advice should be explained to patients but ultimately, if they have mental capacity they can refuse to follow it. The BMA has discussed situations in which patients may not be deliberately rejecting or avoiding medical advice but simply do not know about it. Doctors sometimes ask if there is any duty to try to trace and pursue patients who come in for a test of some kind but then fail to pick up the results, which may have serious implications. Trying to contact the patient is not straightforward in some cases, unless an advance agreement has been made as to how they should be reached in the event of a positive test result. Examples include young patients who take a pregnancy test without asking the outcome. The BMA's general view is that reasonable efforts should be made to let patients know their test results if it is likely that they need to take some action on the basis of them.

Neither patients with or without mental capacity can be hospitalised against their will, unless they are sectioned under the Mental Health Act or deprived of their liberty using the safeguards under the Mental Capacity Act (see Chapter 4). If already in hospital, patients may discharge themselves prematurely. If they do so, or refuse important treatment, they may be asked to sign a declaration by their doctor or the trust, indicating that they understand the implications of their decision (this is discussed in Chapter 3).

What are the rights of patients who are violent or misuse services?

Whether or not health professionals are obliged to treat violent people depends on the reason for the behaviour and the urgency of the patient's need. Triggers of violence or passive aggression can be complex, arising from mental health problems, extreme distress, an unexpected reaction to medication (or not taking it) or patients' inability to cope with a challenging situation. Identifying whether there is an organic cause is obviously important when patients act out of character. Some people, however, simply use bullying tactics to get their own way or be seen quicker. Unacceptable patient behaviour includes racist or abusive remarks, words or behaviour which cause distress to other people, threats as well as physical violence. Abusive patients should not be denied urgent treatment if it can be provided safely, but this may not be an option if it puts anyone else at risk. If urgent treatment is not essential, the police can remove the patient, who may then be supervised by a forensic practitioner. Withholding treatment is seen as appropriate if patients' treatment is non-essential or their behaviour poses risks of harm to other patients or staff.

Primary care practices can request the removal from their lists of any patient who is threatening or violent (see also the section 'Breakdown of the doctor–patient relationship'). In some premises, special segregated areas or after-hours clinics deal with persistently aggressive patients in a secure environment with police or security officers on hand. Such patients should be allowed to return to normal surgeries if their behaviour improves. Some facilities use a violent patient scheme (VPS) which sets out the framework within which aggressive patients can receive treatment. For some, being included in the scheme is itself a sobering experience. A VPS review panel receives reports from doctors of all cases and the patient can be banned from the practice, or only allowed to attend with a police escort. If the patient is removed from a primary care list, other relevant practices are notified that the patient is on the VPS scheme and should not be registered by them but needs to be registered for treatment with a specific VPS provider. The VPS provider sees the patient in a secure setting which may involve police escorts and completes a report after each appointment. Patient behaviour is reviewed periodically with the intention of allowing the patient to register again in the usual manner.

Patients' rights to complain

NHS practices and hospitals must make information available about their complaints procedure. Private practitioners should also ensure that patients know how to make a complaint. Such information should make clear that patients are not disadvantaged for calling attention to problems with the service. Made in a constructive manner, complaints can help to improve the service and notification of problem areas can create opportunities to avoid future difficulties. Persistent or unfounded complaints, however, are usually indicative of a serious lack of trust. There needs to be some discussion, with patients who continually complain without good cause, to try to address the root cause and agree on how to proceed in future. They need to be aware of the potential consequences of repetitive, unjustified complaints including their possible transfer to another doctor or service (see the section 'Breakdown of the doctor–patient relationship').

Truth-telling and good communication

Good communication is about establishing positive interpersonal relationships, as well as exchanging information. In primary and secondary care, the importance of hearing and understanding patients' views is a vital part of the relationship. Clear communication is also a key element of valid patient consent (this is discussed in Chapter 3). Health professionals should try to understand patients' views without making assumptions about the importance they attach to different outcomes. Chronic diseases impact on patients' lives in various ways. People need information to manage their condition in ways compatible with their own wishes and lifestyle. Much medical information is contested knowledge even if based on statistical probability. Patients need to know what is evidence-based advice as well as the uncertainties and limitations of what is known.

Giving bad news

Even when patients suspect that bad news is coming, it is never easy to deliver or receive it. In the past, the common perception was that people could not deal with bad news and it was kinder – or even part of a doctor's duty – to keep them in ignorance. Giving difficult information or admitting to not having all the answers was thought to undermine patients' confidence in medicine and could lead them to give up the struggle when recovery might be possible. Patients and families now expect honest answers, but they may also want support in dealing with the anxiety created by greater knowledge. They have their own priorities and need as accurate information as possible about what is achievable.

One of the most difficult topics to address is the end of life. Early identification of patients approaching their last year is seen as important so that an assessment of their needs can take place and a care plan be developed with them. This is part of a wider acknowledgement that the aim of medicine is not always to postpone death but rather to make the dying process as comfortable as possible once its inevitability is recognised. For all patients, there eventually comes a stage when the aim of care shifts from trying to improve their condition to keeping the person free from distressing symptoms. The impact of early palliative care intervention in the disease trajectory has been shown to provide better quality of life and mood scores, lower depression scores and even sometimes prolong survival.[11] One of the key challenges for health professionals is to make the transition from active treatment to accepting that cure is not possible in this instance and allowing natural death to occur. Identifying when it is the right time for the team to reassess current interventions and individualise care to meet the best interests of the individual requires attention to the patient's wishes, sound clinical judgement and good communication. Discussion at an early stage gives patients the opportunity to consider issues such as organ or tissue donation as well as how they would like their end-of-life care to be managed.

Case example – failure to discuss

An 85-year-old patient fell after being discharged from hospital for cancer surgery. He was admitted to Cheltenham General Hospital, moved briefly to a different hospital for palliative care before being readmitted to Cheltenham General with pneumonia. Two Do Not Attempt Resuscitation (DNAR) orders were made while he was there, apparently without discussion with either the patient or his family. When he died, the family referred his case to the Health Service Ombudsman. The relatives complained that they had been told that the patient's condition was not immediately life-threatening, although the death certificate showed that he was known to have terminal bladder cancer. In her analysis of the case, the Ombudsman said it highlighted the importance of good communication. The patient should have been told about the severity of his condition and asked if he wanted his family to be updated, rather than being kept ignorant of his deteriorating health. Following the case, the trust drew up plans for communication training for its medical and nursing staff.[12]

In 2011, the charity Action on Elder Abuse examined the findings of the Care Quality Commission's (CQC) inspections of 100 English hospitals which focused mainly on patient nutrition and dignity.[13] It highlighted, among other failings, how older patients and their relatives were sometimes excluded from discussions about resuscitation. Criticising the sometimes 'casual disregard' of the available guidance, the charity noted that DNAR forms were sometimes routinely inserted into older patients' files on admission or decisions were left to junior doctors who did not discuss the issue with patients or their families. The CQC also criticised York Teaching Hospital NHS Trust for breaching its own DNAR guidelines.[14] Medical staff agreed on the desirability of discussion with patients or their next of kin but said that they found it a difficult topic and said that decisions to make a DNAR were often taken when relatives were unavailable to talk about them.

The clinical limitations need to be discussed, but health professionals also need to be open about any other factors that are likely to affect treatment decisions or their timing. The need to meet externally set targets for treatment, for example, may impinge on the scheduling of certain procedures. This should not be concealed from those affected by it. Health professionals provide information in order to empower patients to exercise informed choice and this is equally important when the options are limited. Obviously, difficult information has to be given with sensitivity. Traditionally, doctors were discouraged from confessing any doubts or uncertainties because this could undermine patients' morale. Now, it is recognised that patients can experience stress and anxiety precisely because information is concealed.

Telling patients about unfunded treatments

A common dilemma concerns the range of options that patients should be told about when there is no likelihood of those drugs or treatments being made available on the NHS. Patients can opt to have investigations or treatment privately in addition to their NHS care, but this does not help those who cannot afford them. Health professionals often feel embarrassed about telling patients about treatment only available privately particularly where they believe it to be out of their patients' reach financially. Many doctors want to protect their patients from this difficult situation and are concerned that this knowledge may add to their patients' stress or encourage them to get into debt in order to access the treatment. It is not appropriate, however, for doctors to withhold relevant information because they believe it is not in their patients' interests to know it. Without all relevant information, patients cannot make informed decisions and so, although it may involve difficult conversations, doctors should not withhold such information. Information should, however, be given in a balanced way and should include an accurate statement about why the NHS does not commission the treatment – whether that is because of lack of evidence of efficacy or cost or both. Ultimately, patients should be sensitively informed and morally supported so that they can make decisions for themselves.

Rationing decisions should be transparent, including telling patients when decisions have been made not to commission certain services or products, within the NHS. The situation is complicated when there is no clinical agreement about the efficacy of the treatment or where only a small improvement can be expected and the financial cost is great. Some purchasers or commissioners may pay for innovative treatments for patients who have no other options, but this perpetuates the 'postcode lottery' that most people decry. Doctors have to make clinical decisions about which treatments would be beneficial or futile in each case. Unless they specifically ask about them, there is no obligation to discuss with patients any treatments that would be clinically inappropriate or futile for their condition.

Reporting mistakes and telling patients about them

Errors should be learnt from so that changes can be implemented. Even if a mistake or near miss does not result in harm, it can provide an opportunity to tighten up procedures, if known about. This means that errors should be reported promptly and discussed through appropriate local mechanisms. The BMA publishes detailed advice about the reporting of adverse events, including mistakes occurring in poorly performing health systems. It also discusses measures to address and report errors stemming from poor performance by doctors or their colleagues.[15]

Health professionals and organisations should tell patients when mistakes have been made in treatment or diagnosis. Once aware that they themselves have made an error, doctors usually seek advice from their defence body about how best to handle the situation but, as a general principle, action should include coming up with a strategy to let the patient know. Sometimes, no physical harm has been caused, but the patient's life has still been affected by a great deal of anxiety or uncertainty. The GMC says that, when patients suffer harm or distress, doctors should act immediately to put matters right if that is possible.[16] They should explain fully and promptly to the patient what has happened and the likely long-term and short-term implications. If the injured person is an incapacitated adult or a young child, an explanation needs to be given to the carer or parent.

Sometimes very difficult and sensitive cases arise in which clinicians discover that previous doctors have either missed important signs of a serious condition or laboratory tests have been misinterpreted. In any situation where substandard practice has occurred, there is an obligation to do something about it. This did not generally happen in the past, as doctors were wary about appearing to defame a colleague or undermine patient trust in the health service. Attitudes have changed considerably and the GMC emphasises the duty to act as a whistle-blower and give patients information they need to act on past errors or to complain. In many cases, patients who have suffered the consequences of mistakes are keener to have an apology and assurances that steps are taken against a recurrence, rather than trying to get compensation, but the option of court action is available in some cases. The GMC also reminds doctors that when patients complain, they have the right to a prompt, honest and constructive response, and an apology, where appropriate.[17] A complaint must not be allowed to affect the care or treatment provided.

An important consideration must also be whether the error was likely to have been a one-off occurrence or part of a pattern of mistakes that may mean an ongoing risk of harm. Whistle-blowing involves drawing mistakes to the attention of the person or agency who can remedy them, as well as ensuring that those who have suffered from them are informed. Where there is a pattern of error in secondary care, it is usual for the hospital to set up a system for contacting patients and informing them. Audit and notification of significant events may expose incidents of substandard care, but doctors should also monitor their own performance so that they can spot errors and address the implications.

Reporting errors: *Froggatt*

A patient's breast biopsy was confused with someone else's sample by the histopathologist, with the result that a healthy patient had a mastectomy and suffered distress, believing herself at risk of premature death. The mistake was suspected by a consultant oncologist who contacted the histopathologist and asked him to review the slides. This revealed normal tissue without evidence of malignancy. The patient's GP was informed and it was agreed that the situation should be explained to the patient at the hospital by the surgeon who had operated on her, with two nurses to provide support. Telling patients that they have undergone unwarranted distress and surgery is clearly difficult. The patient said it was easier to accept the mastectomy when she thought she had cancer, but she felt worse knowing that it had been unnecessary. She became depressed and thought constantly about the operation. The patient developed a serious psychiatric disorder which seemed unlikely to improve. In court, the patient was awarded £350,000 damages and lesser sums were awarded to her family for the trauma they had undergone.[18]

Mistakes are hard to acknowledge and traumatic for patients to learn about. Even when sensitively handled, the situation can seem worse rather than better as a result of disclosure, but this does not justify secrecy. Patients need support to cope with such information and to understand the difference between errors and legitimate differences of clinical opinion. Clearly, it is important to recognise when a past diagnosis was appropriate, given the knowledge available at the time, even when hindsight shows it was wrong. Clarifying the past involves contacting previous clinicians and reviewing old samples and records.

If it is obvious that an error was made, there should be discussion about how the patient can sensitively be prepared for that information and who should take responsibility for doing so. When a mistake has been instrumental in causing a death, people close to the deceased need to be informed sensitively and the events investigated. If a child has died, the circumstances should be explained to the parents or people with parental responsibility. If the cause of death is misadventure or is not fully known, the coroner or procurator fiscal must be involved. Even when there is no evidence of error, an elective (or hospital) post-mortem examination may be requested by the deceased's clinician, with the family's consent, to verify the diagnosis or assess the effect of treatment.

Keeping patients' trust

The ideal professional relationship is one in which there is mutual trust and truthfulness. At times, patients can be less than frank, especially if worried about how their information might later be used, but health professionals should always be open and should act with integrity. Patients can lose trust in them if they feel they have not been given accurate information or if decisions affecting them have been motivated by other considerations – such as a financial incentive for the health professional – rather than benefit for the patient.

Managing conflicts of interest

The usual definition of a conflict of interest is 'a set of conditions in which professional judgement concerning a primary interest (such as patients' welfare or the validity of research) tends to be unduly influenced by a secondary interest (such as financial gain)'.[19] Not all conflicts of interest are avoidable but, if they cannot be avoided, they need to be carefully managed. The onus is on doctors and other health professionals to identify for themselves where a real or perceived conflict of interest exists, or is likely to arise in their planned activities, and to take steps to manage it. The effect of perceived conflicts can be as bad as that of real ones: the belief that doctors' advice is biased to further their own interests is damaging, even if unfounded. When health professionals have an investment in a product, clinic, care home or other health facility which they would like to recommend to patients, they need to be open about their financial interest. Patients should be aware when professionals treating them stand to benefit personally from a particular option. A common example is when doctors (or their close relatives) invest in a residential nursing home and want to refer patients to it. They should declare their financial interest and, ideally, provide information about alternatives. In some circumstances being open about a conflict of interests is not enough and the doctor should exclude him or herself from any situation where a conflict is likely to occur. Doctors who hold pharmaceutical shares are advised to exercise caution when switching their patients' medication to a product of that drug company because even if done in good faith, this can *appear* as self-interest and patients are rarely in a good position to evaluate the choices. This is an example of where just being open with patients about a conflict of interest is not necessarily enough, if they cannot reasonably assess the options for themselves. For this reason, doctors are generally advised not to invest in companies whose products they are likely to want to prescribe for their patients in the future.

In some cases, doctors can have a blind spot about the potential for conflict, particularly if a long-accepted practice has never been questioned. They may also genuinely believe that their clinical judgement is unaffected by some financial incentive, but the evidence can show the contrary.[20] Although conflicts of interest are often portrayed in terms of financial benefits, they can also occur when there are conflicts of loyalties (e.g. when the duty owed to a patient in prison clashes with the duty owed to the prison authorities) or when personal kudos is at stake (such as by a researcher duplicating existing findings to gain a publication). If in doubt, the so-called 'Paxman' test can be useful; 'if you might be embarrassed if asked to explain a situation to an investigative journalist or reporter, a conflict of interest probably exists'.[21] Openly acknowledging that conflicts of interest exist is often the first step to managing them. This allows attention to be given to ensuring that they are addressed fairly and appropriately and in a way that is proportionate.

Conflicts when commissioning services

Any agency commissioning services needs robust mechanisms for managing real and perceived conflicts of interest. Choices that are in the interests of the majority of local people, the commissioning body and taxpayers may not be good for patients needing expensive care. Solutions are required that not only save public money but also ensure fairness and equity. A balance needs to be achieved and the impact of decisions should be proportionate. Unlike commercial enterprises whose responsibility is to maximise profits for shareholders, healthcare commissioners have a responsibility both to patients and the wider public. Commissioning groups may want to discontinue services which seem insufficiently cost-effective, but they may have a moral responsibility to ensure that the service is still provided by someone, if some patients need it.[22] Core services, even when apparently not cost-effective, may have to be continued as part of the duty of care owed to patients.

The Royal College of General Practitioners has guidance for CCGs on managing conflicts of interest in commissioning[23] and making difficult decisions.[24] Having interests in the local healthcare economy both as purchasers and providers, CCGs are likely to have conflicting priorities and obligations. Doctors may also have a personal vested interest in preferring some solutions over others. 'The fact that in their provider and gatekeeper roles, GPs and their colleagues could potentially profit personally (financially or otherwise) from the decisions of a commissioning group of which they are also members, means that questions about their role in the governance of NHS commissioning bodies are legitimate'.[21] Here as elsewhere, if conflicts of interest are unavoidable, the important thing is to identify, record and try to manage them appropriately in order to avoid the kind of bad decision making that could result in legal challenge or damage to doctors' reputations.

Payment for referrals or recommendations

Doctors should not accept or offer payment for a referral.[25] Accepting inducements, gifts or hospitality as a reward from another practitioner, agency or company for referring patients or arranging their care has long been judged unacceptable. Similarly, payment for endorsing other practitioners to patients is ruled out. Payment for referral to solicitors or other non-health professionals is also seen as unacceptable. Basically, any measure that seems to be a variation on the concept of payment in exchange for recommendation or endorsement should generally be avoided. It may be that some attitudes are changing as some aspects of health care become more commercially orientated and doctors test the limits of what is permissible. When testing boundaries, health professionals need to be careful and take advice.

Accepting gifts and bequests

Doctors are warned by the GMC not to encourage patients to offer loans, gifts or donations,[26] but patients often spontaneously ask if they can make a donation or if they can name their doctor as a beneficiary in their will. NHS employees are prohibited from accepting substantial gifts, but small tokens of gratitude are permissible. GPs and any other health professionals who are not NHS employees can accept unsolicited donations, but it should always be made clear to patients that the quality of care is not influenced by a donation. Transparency is important. In England and Wales, the Health and Social Care Act 2001 made provision for a reporting and recording system for gifts by GPs, and equivalent rules operate in the other UK countries. Regulations concerning GPs' acceptance of gifts from patients came into force in March 2004.[27] These require individual GPs and contractors to keep a register of gifts from patients (or patients' relatives) which have a value of £100 or more unless the gift is unconnected with the provision of services. The register must include certain information such as the names of the donor and recipient, the nature of the gift and its estimated value.[28]

Case example – accepting a bequest

Typical of many enquiries to the BMA was one from a group of GPs who had been left a house and a substantial legacy, on the death of a patient who had been with the practice for many years. The senior partner was advised by colleagues that he should set up a separate bank account and use the legacy to improve patient care. In this situation, doctors often think they are obliged to use patients' donations to improve their equipment or premises, but much depends on the stated wishes of the donor. If, as in this case, the deceased did not specify a purpose for which the money should be used, all options are open. This practice decided to use part of their legacy to buy equipment and improve the patients' waiting area, but some of it paid for a party to which patients were invited. Setting up a separate account for gifts which will be used to enhance services in the practice seems to be common, especially when the donor patient has been cared for by several members of the primary care team. Sometimes all the staff have a say in how a donation is used, if the donor did not specify a purpose. In all cases, transparency is important and the donation must be declared for tax purposes.

GPs are often aware that a patient whom they have looked after intends to leave them a substantial amount of money or a property in their will, even though the doctor has made clear that the patient's care was not influenced by it. Problems can arise if the beneficiary of the patient's gift has also been involved in assessing that patient's mental capacity. If a patient who wants to make a gift needs an assessment of capacity, this should be undertaken by a health professional who has no financial interest in the outcome.

Covert medication

Health professionals should never mislead people about the purpose of their medication or withhold information about it from people who have mental capacity. The temptation to skip giving a proper explanation of what the patient's tablets are for seems to occur most when staff are hard pressed for time and looking after patients who are either elderly and forgetful or people whose behaviour is challenging. Various reports have described how some patients are routinely given medication without discussion of the purpose of them or, in some cases, are over-medicated to make their care easier to manage.[29]

In some areas, covert medication appears to be more common among older people in care homes than in hospitals.[30] Covert medication for adults with capacity is unethical, unlawful and falls into the definition of abuse.

There are instances where it can be in the best interests of people who lack mental capacity to give them their essential drugs covertly, if their refusal to have them would damage their health (this is discussed in Chapter 4 and Chapter 8). The practice should not be routine, even if deemed to be in the best interests of an incapacitated patient in some particular circumstances. Prescribing and the administration of medication are discussed in more detail in Chapter 8.

Recording consultations

Patients sometimes tape-record consultations for a variety of reasons. Usually, it is to help them remember and cooperate with important advice or share it accurately with other family members, but it can also indicate a lack of trust. Some patients may want a record so as to make a complaint later if anything goes wrong. In the enquiries raised by doctors with the BMA, most anxiety is expressed about patients attempting to record the interview clandestinely. Ideally, recording should not be banned but should be done openly rather than secretly. Recording by either side can significantly alter the consultation and contribute to inhibitions felt by both parties.

Doctors too sometimes record consultations or make visual recordings of operations. Such audio or visual recordings may be used for staff training or audit, but prior patient consent is needed. If young children are recorded, the permission of parents or people with parental responsibility is a prerequisite. The GMC has published detailed guidance,[31] which is discussed in Chapter 6.

Covert recording and surveillance

Surveillance cameras are often used as part of security arrangements, but the public need to be made aware of their use. Doctors must obtain subject consent to use any recording made for reasons other than the patient's treatment or assessment, unless the secondary purpose only requires anonymised material and uses recordings made as part of the individual's treatment.[32] (Secondary uses of patient material are covered in detail in Chapter 6.) An exception is the use of covert video surveillance (CVS) to detect induced illness in children. In health settings, CVS is sometimes used, as part of a formal child protection multi-agency strategy, to monitor children receiving in-patient care when there are grounds to suspect relatives or carers of causing the child's condition. It takes place without the knowledge and consent of families in cases where children would otherwise be at significant risk of harm but can only be undertaken by the police acting under the Regulation of Investigatory Powers Act 2000.[33] The law requires the police first to obtain authorisation from the chief constable. Detailed guidance on the use of CVS has been issued by the Royal College of Paediatrics and Child Health (RCPCH),[34] which says that if the child is likely to remain in the care of a suspected perpetrator, because there is insufficient evidence of abuse to ensure the child's protection, and a high risk of future harm, CVS might be acceptable as part of evidence gathering. Each case must be considered on its merits. The RCPCH guidance also sets out the steps that have to be taken first, including working with the police, involving the trust chief executive and detailed discussion with the staff caring for the child. Health professionals need to seek expert advice about any situation in which the use of CVS is proposed.

In connection with compensation claims for injury, covert monitoring may be proposed to verify whether patients are as disabled as they claim and identify those who may be acting fraudulently. The GMC says that, even when doctors are acting as expert witnesses or producing a medico-legal report and therefore have a primary duty to the court, this does not negate the duties they owe to the individual being examined.[35] It advises that doctors should not collude with covert recordings other than very exceptional cases where it is in the patient's interest and should not arrange secret surveillance on the premises where they work. They should take legal advice if they believe that the filmed material that they have been asked to view or comment on is likely to have been improperly obtained.

Chaperones and accompanying persons

Even when there is a mutually trusting relationship, patients often want to have someone accompany them if they expect to be given complicated information or need moral support. A chaperone should also be available for situations in which patients undress. Complaints of indecent assault are made by patients of both sexes and are not restricted to allegations against a doctor of the opposite sex. Chaperones should be offered for intimate examinations of patients of either gender and in other situations where patients are likely to feel uncomfortable. Such occasions can arise when it is necessary to darken the room for retinoscopy, for example. Young patients who are unaccompanied by a parent or other adult may need a chaperone[36] and so may people with learning difficulties. A chaperone is also recommended for patients whose religion or culture imposes strict limitations on how they may be physically examined. These matters are addressed in detail in the NHS guidance.[37] Ideally, the option of having a chaperone or accompanying person should be discussed with patients in advance, particularly if they need to bring a relative or friend.

GMC guidance on chaperones

'Wherever possible, you should offer the patient the security of having an impartial observer (a "chaperone") present during an intimate examination. This applies whether or not you are the same gender as the patient.

A chaperone does not have to be medically qualified but will ideally:

- be sensitive, and respectful of the patient's dignity and confidentiality
- be prepared to reassure the patient if they show signs of distress or discomfort
- be familiar with the procedures involved in a routine intimate examination
- be prepared to raise concerns about a doctor if misconduct occurs.

In some circumstances, a member of practice staff, or a relative or friend of the patient may be an acceptable chaperone.

If either you or the patient does not wish the examination to proceed without a chaperone present, or if either of you is uncomfortable with the choice of chaperone, you may offer to delay the examination to a later date when a chaperone (or an alternative chaperone) will be available, if this is compatible with the patient's best interests.

You should record any discussion about chaperones and its outcome. If a chaperone is present, you should record that fact and make a note of their identity. If the patient does not want a chaperone, you should record that the offer was made and declined'.[38]

Intimate examinations

The GMC and medical defence bodies recommend that a chaperone always be offered for intimate examinations. The Royal College of Obstetricians and Gynaecologists (RCOG) has also emphasised the importance of having a chaperone, regardless of the gender of the doctor.[39]

GMC guidance on intimate examinations

'It is particularly important to maintain a professional boundary when examining patients: intimate examinations can be embarrassing or distressing for patients. Whenever you examine a patient you should be sensitive to what they may perceive as intimate. This is likely to include examinations of breasts, genitalia and rectum, but could also include any examination where it is necessary to touch or even be close to the patient.

Before conducting an intimate examination you should:

- explain to the patient why an examination is necessary and give the patient an opportunity to ask questions
- explain what the examination will involve, in a way the patient can understand, so that the patient has a clear idea of what to expect, including any potential pain or discomfort

(Continued)

- obtain the patient's permission before the examination and record that permission has been obtained
- give the patient privacy to undress and dress and keep the patient covered as much as possible to maintain their dignity. Do not assist the patient in removing clothing unless you have clarified with them that your assistance is required.

During the examination you should: explain what you are going to do before you do it and, if this differs from what you have already outlined to the patient, explain why and seek the patient's permission; be prepared to discontinue the examination if the patient asks you to; keep discussion relevant and do not make unnecessary personal comments'.[40]

During and in advance of carrying out an intimate examination, it is essential for the health professional to explain fully what is involved. Complaints are sometimes made by patients who feel that health professionals behaved inappropriately during an intimate examination when the root of the issue is poor communication and the patient being unaware of what precisely would happen.

Recognising boundaries

Managing personal relationships with patients

In many of the cases raised with the BMA, boundaries in the doctor–patient relationship have been crossed, unintentionally. As many old taboos and social distinctions within society have disappeared, doctors and patients can find themselves naturally socialising together or working closely with each other in campaigns.

Case examples – maintaining professional boundaries

A GP who was standing for election to the local Council asked some of her patients to display posters or distribute leaflets to support her campaign. She invited others who she thought would be interested in volunteering, to help out with routine tasks in the party's campaign offices. She only approached people who she thought would be supportive or who were likely to need a friend on the Council to lobby in their own areas of interest, such as maintaining special clubs for children and the elderly. The BMA was asked to advise and said that doctors should avoid asking patients to take any action unrelated to their medical care. By asking them to help her in her private life, the doctor may be seen as using her influence inappropriately and exceeding the boundaries of the doctor–patient relationship, especially

(Continued)

when the activity that patients may feel pressured to undertake is completely divorced from health care. The doctor may argue that she is not exerting pressure but, in many complaint cases, the patients have tended to see the request in a rather different light and may be concerned about the possibility of annoying the doctor and affecting their future care by not agreeing. In brief, the doctor's medical role should be kept completely separate from her political role or any other aspect of her personal or social life.

In another case, a GP involved with a homeless charity provided temporary help to a series of ex-prisoners who were homeless. One of these had long been a patient of the GP's practice and, like others before him, lived with the doctor's family after release. The main difference between this man and other ex-prisoners was his reluctance to leave the GP's house or register with another practice for medical services. His physical and emotional dependency on the family increased as time went on, but the doctor was reluctant to appear to 'reject' him as he thought this was likely to undermine all the progress the patient had made in overcoming addiction to drugs and alcohol. The doctor realised, however, that the situation muddled the doctor–patient relationship and a more intimate connection of a close family friend. He persuaded the patient to register with another practice and widen his support network while the doctor continued to provide support but as a friend rather than a medical advisor.

Doctors sometimes enquire whether it is permissible to give apparently innocuous gifts, such as flowers or concert tickets, to patients who they know are having a difficult time, but they need to be wary about how that might be interpreted. Personal gifts between health professionals and patients can mean that professional boundaries cease to be seen as significant. Any emotional dependence between doctors and their patients, or the close relatives of patients, should be discouraged. Doctors have access to health information about their patients and see them when they are feeling vulnerable, all of which puts patients at a disadvantage. Some patients also come to see their doctor as someone who will help them with a range non-medical tasks and paperwork that they find difficult. While this is not prohibited, it can become very onerous and can lead to situations where the doctor is expected to help out with all manner of problems. Families may perceive the doctor as a friend rather than a professional and a significant degree of dependency can develop, if unchecked.

When a friendship becomes inappropriate

Classic examples of inappropriate situations are those where the doctor and patient meet socially and decide they want to form an intimate relationship. The GMC says that doctors must not use their professional position 'to establish or pursue a sexual or an improper emotional relationship with a patient or someone close to them'.[41] While it is widely recognised that an emotional or sexual relationship between patients and their doctors is inappropriate, it is sometimes difficult to identify where precisely the boundaries lie with other forms of social interaction. Doctors sometimes ask whether it is acceptable to attend social events, such as fund-raising parties or art exhibitions, when specifically invited to accompany a patient involved with the event. The GMC's advice certainly does not prohibit this, but it may be advisable to think about the *intention* behind such an invitation: is it a date or just a chance for people with similar interests to attend a public event? Much depends on the circumstances and whether a casual social contact is likely to develop into something more serious. Some doctors only think that the patient should transfer to another practitioner if the relationship has either broken down or become sexual, but in some cases, a friendship with a very vulnerable patient can also give cause for concern.

Case example – personal relationships

In several cases raised with the BMA, GPs had struck up personal relationships with people undergoing a crisis. Acting as volunteers in charitable church groups or community support organisations, they had played a mentoring role for troubled teenagers or helped asylum seekers draft their appeals. This personal relationship subsequently became problematic when the person being helped needed them to write an 'independent' doctor's report for some state benefit. Another doctor who had rebuilt his career after alcoholism joined a network offering support to others struggling with similar problems. This was unproblematic when the relationship was entirely separate from the doctor's working life but not when the individuals needing befriending were his patients. Keeping a clear boundary between their professional and private life became impossible.

Intimate relationships

Some circumstances need to be particularly carefully handled, such as when patients consult a doctor for emotional difficulties after a loss or bereavement. Any intimate or close personal relationship which develops in such circumstances is problematic and is likely to be seen as cause for disciplinary proceedings. Patients' relatives are also particularly vulnerable during the progress of a patient's acute or terminal illness. Doctors must ensure that inappropriate attachments are not allowed to develop. The BMA is occasionally contacted by doctors who, having acted completely properly, are concerned that during the progress of a long illness the spouse or close relative of a patient has become inappropriately dependent upon them. This can occur gradually over time if the doctor becomes the main focus for an otherwise isolated carer. Such situations are delicate and relatives may be particularly emotional, anticipating bereavement. Nevertheless, it is essential that an emotional distance is maintained. Wherever possible, other health and social care professionals should be involved and it may assist relatives to be put in touch with patient support groups. In the case of terminal illness, other members of the primary healthcare team and hospice outreach services may be able to share in providing support.

Although personal relationships can arise in good faith when doctors and patients meet in a purely social setting, it is essential that doctors take steps to establish and maintain clear boundaries. If they discover that a person with whom they are developing a relationship is also their patient, they should immediately cease the relationship or ensure that medical care is transferred to another doctor. In a secondary care setting, doctors must not embark on a personal relationship with a patient or a person close to a patient while they are responsible for an episode of care. Doctors sometimes ask for advice on how to handle a situation in which they feel attracted to a patient or the close relative of a patient and therefore need to ask that person to transfer to another doctor before it is clear whether or not a personal relationship is likely to grow. It can seem very presumptuous to ask patients to transfer, but this is advisable at an early stage if a personal relationship is intended.

Use of social media

Social media can blur the boundary between doctors' private and professional lives. Personal material uploaded onto social networking sites such as Facebook and Twitter intended for friends can be accessible to a wider audience, including patients. Employers too show increasing interest in the content of blogs, internet fora and other forms of social networking, when recruiting staff. Health professionals and medical students can find that provocative comments they posted for a contained audience at one stage of their career come back to haunt them later when applying for jobs.

In 2011, the BMA became concerned about the use of social media by doctors and medical students.[42] Some exposed themselves to risk by uploading personal material about their own lives, or repeated stories patients had told them about their own relationships. Although such media provide opportunities to discuss aspects of clinical practice, great caution is required if mention is made of specific cases. Disclosing information about patients which could be identifiable, without consent, breaches GMC standards and can give rise to legal complaints. Informal discussion which mentions patients should always be avoided. In some cases, there can be a temptation to include on a blog accessible only to friends a funny story about a patient or a clinical case which has been particularly stressful. Even when all the information is anonymised, it is difficult to control the spread of such messages and any flippant or derogatory remarks could undermine public trust. In 2012, the GMC was worried enough to announce it would be issuing specific advice about social media.[43]

Doctors sometimes divulge personal information about themselves when talking to patients face-to-face, but the potential disclosure via social media can go far beyond what they would normally allow. Examples have arisen of patients attempting to strike up a personal relationship after discovering information about their doctor through a social networking site.[42] Entering into informal relationships with patients on social media can increase the likelihood of inappropriate boundary transgressions and difficult ethical issues can arise if, for example, doctors acquire information about patients that has not been disclosed in a clinical consultation. Doctors and medical students who receive 'friend requests' from patients are advised to decline. Some sites have privacy settings that put restrictions on access, but not all users activate these and not all content on the web can be protected in this way. Medical students need to be conscious about the image they present on social media. Guidance published jointly by the GMC and the Medical Schools Council (MSC) reminds them that because they 'have certain privileges and responsibilities different from those of other students . . . different standards of professional behaviour are expected of them'.[44] American research into the material posted online by medical students found patient confidentiality violations; instances of discriminatory language and profanity; and depictions of intoxication and illicit substance use, which in some cases resulted in official warnings from medical schools and even dismissal.[45]

Doctors and medical students should also be aware of their ethical obligations if they recommend or mention online any healthcare organisation or pharmaceutical product in which they have a financial interest. Even if they blog anonymously, such material may be viewed by the public as an objective recommendation. Failing to declare conflicts of interest could undermine public trust, compromise the professionalism of authors and risk referral to the GMC. People can often feel less inhibited when posting comments online and as a result may say things they would not express in other circumstances. Posting comments under a username does not guarantee anonymity as comments can be traced back to the original author. Doctors and medical students need to exercise sound judgement when posting online and to avoid making gratuitous, unsubstantiated or unsustainable comments about individuals or organisations. Defamation law can apply to any comments posted on the Web, irrespective of whether they are made in a personal or professional capacity. Defamation is the act of making an unjustified statement about a person or organisation that is considered to harm their reputation. If an individual makes a statement that is alleged to be defamatory, it could result in legal action against either the individual or the organisation they are representing.

Health professionals acting as witnesses to legal documents

Patients often ask health professionals to countersign or witness a passport application or other similar document. A distinction needs to be made here between paperwork which has no connection with health care (such as a passport application) and therefore could be equally well signed by any person of good standing and cases where the document's validity may partly depend on medical judgement. In cases where the signatory could be any person of good standing unrelated to the applicant, doctors may agree to countersign as long as they know the individual well enough. They are not obliged to do so and should avoid countersigning if they have any doubts about the identity of the applicant or about the information the applicant has given.

Advance decisions about medical treatment

Some documents benefit from medical input, such as patients' advance decisions about treatment. Doctors are often also asked to witness them and may later be called upon to say why they believed the patient was informed enough and had the mental capacity at the time to make the decision (see the case of *XB* in Chapter 3).

It is often seen as desirable that doctors or other health professionals should witness a range of other legal documents, such as a will, in situations where the drafter's mental capacity may later be questioned. Practitioners need to be aware that, by acting as signatory to any legal document of this kind, it is likely to be assumed that they also checked the patient's mental capacity. They should not presume that they are just witnessing the authenticity of a signature. As discussed in Chapter 3, everyone is assumed to have capacity unless evidence suggests otherwise. If there is no reason to doubt a patient's capacity, it is not necessary to carry out a formal assessment, but where doubt exists, an assessment is needed. Health professionals should be wary of witnessing documents for patients whom they suspect may be suffering from some impairment, without considering whether an assessment of mental capacity is needed.

Acting as a legal advocate for a patient

In England and Wales, the Mental Capacity Act introduced a new lasting power of attorney (LPA) allowing an individual (the donor) to authorise someone else (the attorney) to make decisions on the donor's behalf once mental capacity is lost. As the name suggests, a health and personal welfare LPA covers welfare decisions, including those about medical treatment. Patients may request that doctors or other health professionals act as their attorney, which may be problematic if the attorney also manages some aspect of the patient's care; doctors should bear this in mind when deciding whether to take on this role.

Firearms certificates

The job of deciding whether or not an individual is safe to have legal possession of a shotgun or other firearm rests with the police. For this they need to make certain enquiries. Patients applying for a licence to hold such weapons agree to this and to their GP disclosing any relevant matter in their medical record. Current practice is for GPs to be automatically informed when one of their patients applies for a licence or a renewal of a licence so that any anxieties the GP has can be noted by the police, who can also request additional information in cases when genuine doubts arise.

As a separate issue, any person of good standing, including a doctor, can be asked to countersign patients' firearms or shotgun applications or be their referee in relation to such an application. The referee or countersignatory is not expected to give a medical opinion but simply confirms knowledge of the applicant. Despite this, supporting an application from their own patients might be interpreted as an expression of confidence in the patient's stability and so should be avoided unless the doctor knows the person well enough in a personal capacity to have that confidence.

Health professionals' personal beliefs

When patients face serious life-changing events, they often have emotional, psychological and social needs. If they wish to do so, opportunities should be available for them to discuss their anxieties with appropriate counsellors or other professionals. The main thing is to listen to patients rather than make assumptions. Although not limited to terminal care, one of the areas of treatment where psychological or spiritual support is often welcomed is at the end of patients' lives. Not all patients want such support, however, and such discussion should be initiated by patients, not by health professionals. The GMC has detailed guidance[46] which makes clear that doctors should not normally discuss their own personal beliefs and values at work nor impose them on patients. If they think that their personal moral views could affect their advice or treatment, doctors should give patients the option of seeing someone else. Doctors who oppose contraception or the termination of pregnancy, for example, should inform patients who want those services how they can access them from another doctor.

In some cases, habits such as smoking, drug or alcohol addiction have clinical implications for the effectiveness of any proposed treatment. These need to be discussed candidly, in a non-judgemental manner, as part of informing patients. Health professionals should avoid saying anything that implies discrimination.[47] Some health professionals see prayer or religious comment as part of the routine provision of support to patients, but such matters should not be raised unless the patient requests them.

Case example – personal beliefs

In 2008, Caroline Petrie, a nurse and an evangelical Christian, was suspended after offering to pray for a patient. Although the patient was not offended, the nurse's remarks were reported to her employers. She was summoned to a disciplinary hearing on a charge of failing to demonstrate a professional commitment to equality and diversity. North Somerset Primary Care Trust subsequently reinstated Mrs Petrie.[48] Subsequent guidance from the Department of Health and the GMC made clear that offering prayers is only acceptable when patients ask for them.

The Department of Health emphasises the importance of respecting religious diversity.[47] It bans discrimination, highlighting the rights of NHS employees and patients to observe their own religion or lack of it. The guidance criticises attempts at proselytising when NHS staff attempt to convert others, intimidate them or comment disparagingly about their lifestyle. It says that such behaviour in the workplace 'could be construed as harassment under the disciplinary and grievance procedures'.[49] The guidance is clear that all other religious observation should be respected and facilitated. Praying is not prohibited if the patient initiates it, but health professionals should not assume it is acceptable as it may be offensive to some people. Consensual discussion is not prohibited if patients initiate it and it does not constitute proselytising or harassment.

Case example – religious beliefs

A GP was given a formal warning by the GMC for discussing his religious beliefs during a consultation in a way that distressed the patient and for seeking to impose his own beliefs on his patient in breach of GMC guidance. Under cross-examination the doctor admitted using words to the effect that if the patient did not turn towards Jesus and hand Jesus his suffering, the patient would suffer for the rest of his life. He also admitted making refer-

(Continued)

ence to the devil, and the GMC found that he had used words to the effect that the devil haunts people who do not turn to Jesus. The GMC also found that the doctor had told the patient that he was not offering him any medical help or tests because there was no other answer and he would keep suffering until he was ready to hand his suffering to Jesus. The doctor admitted telling the patient that his own religion could offer him no protection and that no other religion could offer him what Jesus could offer. The GMC held that the doctor's actions were both inappropriate and not in the patient's best interests.[50]

Conscientious objection

Patients have rights to high-quality care, provided in a non-judgemental manner. Doctors and other health professionals have rights to opt out of some lawful procedures, as long as doing so would not endanger a patient's welfare. In an emergency situation, they must provide appropriate care despite any conscientious objection. Statutory opt-out clauses cover the right not to participate in abortion and fertility treatment, but this right must be applied in a non-discriminatory manner. Some doctors who provide services, such as fertility treatment, may want to restrict it to certain patients who match their own criteria for family life, by excluding gay patients, for example. The Equality and Human Rights Commission has warned that such action would constitute direct discrimination on grounds of sexual orientation.[51] In other areas of their routine practice too, health professionals should not discriminate against patients for reasons such as their social situation. This means that doctors who are willing to prescribe contraception for married people, for example, should not refuse to do so for unmarried patients who need it.

BMA policy is that doctors should only claim a conscientious exemption to those procedures where statute recognises their right (abortion and fertility treatment) and to withdrawing life-prolonging treatment (in cases where there is another health professional willing to take over the patient's care). The BMA's policy is to support doctors' rights to conscientiously object to carrying out non-emergency procedures in these limited instances. The GMC's guidance is more permissive, allowing doctors to claim a conscientious objection to a wider range of procedures provided, in doing so, they are not discriminating against particular groups of patients. The GMC also emphasises that in urgent cases, doctors must follow good practice guidance and provide appropriate care, regardless of their personal beliefs. Both the BMA and the GMC advise that, in the event of patients seeking advice on something to which the doctor has a conscientious objection, the doctor should immediately make this clear to the patients and inform them of their right to see another doctor. They should ensure that patients have sufficient information to exercise their right to receive advice elsewhere. If patients want to transfer but cannot readily make their own arrangements to see another doctor, the practitioner they have consulted must ensure that arrangements are made, without delay, for another doctor to take over their care. This should be done in as seamless a way as possible so that the patient is not disadvantaged.

Breakdown of the doctor–patient relationship

Relationships can break down for many reasons and when this happens, patients generally transfer to another doctor (either to another GP or another consultant). In cases of violence or misuse of services, there may be no other option than for the doctor to transfer the patient elsewhere but whenever possible, there should first be some discussion and a prior warning should be given. GPs have always had the right to remove patients from their lists, which reciprocates the right of patients to change GPs. While it is not in anyone's interests for an unsatisfactory relationship to continue, removal should not be a knee-jerk response. Practices should not remove patients for reasons such as their treatment is costly or on grounds of age or the fact that a complaint has been made. Nor should an automatic decision be made to remove a whole family if one member is difficult. Wherever possible, attempts should be made to resolve any problems through discussion.

Case example – deregistration on grounds of cost and disability

A GP practice in South West London was criticised for deregistering 48 patients with complex health needs who were all residents of a local nursing home. The reason given for this decision was the 'significant funding constraints' on the practice and the 'high demand for GP services from the care home'. The patients were not given any warning of their deregistration. An Internal Review concluded that the patients had been removed from the practice list because of their age and disability in breach of the practice's Personal Medical Services (PMS) contract. NHS South West London issued a breach of contract notice to the practice.[52]

In 2011, the NHS Ombudsman expressed concern that a rising number of patients in England were struck off GPs' lists without any advance warning.[53] She emphasised that NHS contracts require GPs to give a warning unless this would be unreasonable, impractical or too risky in terms of maintaining safety. The Ombudsman's report said that zero tolerance policies were sometimes being applied without consideration being given to the circumstances of the case.

Case example – removal without warning

Miss F was a registered nurse who, with her sister, cared for their terminally ill mother at home. When the battery failed on the device administering the mother's medication, Miss F changed it and restarted the device instead of waiting for the district nurse, who then reported the incident to the family's GP. As a result the practice concluded that the relationship with the family had broken down and the three family members should be removed from the practice list. This was said to have left the terminally ill patient distraught and she died soon after. The NHS Ombudsman was critical of the practice, concluding that it had failed to warn the family about the risk of removal, had not communicated properly with the women and failed to consider any alternative to removal. The terminally ill patient had been removed even though she had been uninvolved and was close to death. The practice apologised for the distress caused to the family and reviewed its procedures to avoid a recurrence of the failings.[54]

GMC guidance on ending a professional relationship with a patient[55]

'In rare circumstances, the trust between you and a patient may break down, and you may find it necessary to end the professional relationship. For example, this may occur if a patient has been violent to you or a colleague, has stolen from the premises, or has persistently acted inconsiderately or unreasonably. You should not end a relationship with a patient solely because of a complaint the patient has made about you or your team, or because of the resource implications* of the patient's care or treatment.

Before you end a professional relationship with a patient, you must be satisfied that your decision is fair . . . You must be prepared to justify your decision. You should inform the patient of your decision and your reasons for ending the professional relationship, wherever practical in writing.

You must take steps to ensure that arrangements are made promptly for the continuing care of the patient, and you must pass on the patient's records without delay.

*If you charge fees, you may refuse further treatment for patients unable or unwilling to pay for services you have already provided'.

Limits or boundaries on advertising services

This is an issue about which the BMA still receives enquiries, although most of the limitations on how health services can be advertised to the public have long since disappeared. Historically, the GMC placed many restrictions on advertising. A distinction was made between advertising by GPs, which was limited but permitted, and by specialists, which was not allowed. The restrictions were intended to prevent patients being overly influenced by marketing techniques. In the 1980s, this came to be seen as paternalistic. Patients were taking a bigger role in managing their health and wanted ready access to factual information about medical services. The GMC relaxed the advertising prohibition so that all doctors were able to advertise. Now, factual advertising is allowed, irrespective of the medium, including the internet, newspapers and practice leaflets. Doctors can make prospective patients aware of the services available as long as the information is factual, verifiable and does not make unjustifiable claims about the quality or outcomes of the service. It must not exploit patients' lack of knowledge nor put pressure on them by, for example, arousing ill-founded fears.[56]

Some practices explore new or unconventional ways of marketing their services. While the GMC has not so far prohibited any innovative ways of drawing attention to a doctor's services, the main purpose of advertising should be to give patients information about their options. The Advertising Standards Authority (ASA) is the UK's advertising regulator. It requires substantiation of claims in the health sector and has specific guidance on marketing health-related products and services. Its remit includes marketing through UK websites. Practitioners offering homeopathy or services such as cosmetic treatments, including slimming products, particularly need to ensure that they comply with ASA codes of practice as complaints about these services appear to be relatively common. In spring 2011, for example, the ASA received 150 complaints about advertisements for homeopathy in which unsubstantiated claims were made.[57]

Treating oneself, friends and family

Self-diagnosis and treatment

Among health professionals, there has often been the assumption that they should carry on working even when unwell. In the past, few doctors registered with a GP. Efforts have long been made to change this culture, but time pressure, unease about adopting the role of a patient and worries about confidentiality still often lead to self-treatment. Although doctors must monitor their own health, especially in terms of whether they may pose any health risk to others, self-treatment for any potentially serious condition should be avoided. If exposed to a communicable disease, they must seek and follow professional advice without delay, rather than relying solely on their own assessment. The hazards of such self-diagnosis are many, but particular concerns include the temptation to extend oneself beyond one's competence and the possibility of denial in the face of serious illness. All health professionals should be registered with a GP, rather than treating themselves or informally asking a colleague to do so.

GMC guidance on self-treatment

'You should be registered with a GP outside your family to ensure that you have access to independent and objective medical care. You should not treat yourself.

You should protect your patients, your colleagues and yourself by being immunised against common serious communicable diseases where vaccines are available.

If you know that you have, or think that you might have, a serious condition that you could pass on to patients, or if your judgement or performance could be affected by a condition or its treatment, you must consult a suitably qualified colleague. You must ask for and follow their advice about investigations, treatment and changes to your practice that they consider necessary. You must not rely on your own assessment of the risk you pose to patients'.[58]

Treating family or close friends

Guidance from the GMC emphasises that, where feasible, doctors should avoid providing medical care to anyone with whom they have a close personal relationship.[59] They should not get involved in treating their friends or families, other than for very minor ailments. To do so obviously deprives the sick person of confidential treatment but also repeats some of the same hazards as can arise in trying to self-treat. Ominous symptoms can be unintentionally misinterpreted and decisions can be influenced by emotion rather than being strictly objective.

Staff who are also patients

When selecting new staff, primary care practices should avoid discriminating against people who apply for the job but are already on their practice list as patients. In small communities, it is often unavoidable for staff to be patients but, where there are other options, it is not an ideal arrangement for either party. Conflicts and difficulties most often arise in relation to patient confidentiality. Some problems can be avoided by discussing them frankly in advance, or both sides may conclude that this is unlikely to be problematic, once thought has been given to potential difficulties, such as the management of situations where the patient/employee needs a lot of sick leave. Situations in which disciplinary procedures need to be invoked can be challenging as the patient/employee's health record may hold relevant information, known to the employer only by virtue of being the employee's doctor. As a general principle, patient records should not be used without consent for purposes other than the provision of care. Employees' permission is needed for them to be disclosed in the event of an employment dispute.

In some rare cases, patients have tried to use the opportunity of working in a surgery to look at friends' or relatives' records or to alter their own to remove information about sensitive topics such as depression, violence or termination of pregnancy. The computerisation of primary care records has made it harder to attempt to alter records without being detected. All staff must be trained about confidentiality issues and be made aware that it is a dismissible offence to look at the medical records of relatives, neighbours, or friends. All information is confidential and available only to those working in the practice on a strict 'need to know' basis. If an employee's relatives are worried about the possibility of the employee having access to their records, they should be reassured about the strict confidentiality measures in place or, if feasible, they may choose to move to another practice. Confidentiality is discussed in detail in Chapter 6.

Providing a safe service

Part of the duty owed to patients is to ensure that they are not exposed to harm. All health staff have roles in ensuring a safe service and have obligations to blow the whistle when care is substandard or a colleague puts patients at risk.

Whistle-blowing

Prompt discussion is needed about any concerns that health professionals have about colleagues' performance or about systemic problems which threaten patient safety. Steps must be taken without delay so that problems can be properly investigated. The GMC tells doctors to make attempts to rectify any situation where patient safety seems to be compromised and to keep a record of the action taken.[60] A series of steps have also been set out by the GMC as to how issues should be raised, by first alerting a manager or an appropriate officer of the employing or contracting body.[61] The BMA makes clear that it is part of doctors' duty to protect patients, colleagues and themselves from unprofessional conduct or acts of clinical negligence.[15] To take appropriate action is a professional obligation and not just a matter of personal conscience. (The BMA has guidance for doctors working in secondary care[62] and also publishes specific guidance for medical students.[63])

A first step in drawing attention to problems should generally be to discuss concerns locally but, if the situation cannot be resolved, the issue may need to be aired more widely. In England, Wales, and Scotland, the Public Interest Disclosure Act aims to support whistle-blowers. In Northern Ireland, similar provisions are covered in the Public Interest Disclosure (Northern Ireland) Order. The regulations apply to people who report concerns about criminal activity, negligence, any danger to health and safety, or attempts to cover up such things. The legislation applies to trainees, including medical students, and protects whistle-blowers who disclose information in good faith. Within the NHS, disclosure to the Department of Health is protected in the same way as internal disclosure. The provision of information to the police, media or Members of Parliament is protected, when this is 'reasonable', not made for personal gain and meets one of three conditions. These are that whistle-blowers

- think they would be victimised if they raise concerns internally or with a prescribed regulator
- believe a cover-up is likely and there is no prescribed regulator
- have already raised the matter internally or with a prescribed regulator.

If whistle-blowers are victimised, they can bring a claim to an employment tribunal for compensation. If sacked, they can apply for an interim order to keep their job. So-called 'gagging clauses' in employment contracts are void insofar as they conflict with the legislation. In 2011, the BMA urged that policies relating to whistle-blowing be strengthened so that NHS trusts could not pressure staff who report concerns. Responding to a Department of Health consultation,[64] the Association called on the government to ban gagging clauses by law and urged the clearer regulation of whistle-blowing policies, which are left for NHS trusts to manage. It said that a change in attitudes and behaviour is needed to protect the reputations of whistle-blowers. The BMA can provide advice to its members in individual cases. All NHS organisations should have a policy setting out how concerns should be addressed within the organisation.

Emergency situations

While some countries have legislation requiring doctors and other health professionals to offer 'Good Samaritan' assistance in an emergency, there is no comparable legal obligation in the UK, but there is a general expectation that they should help when they can. The GMC tells doctors that 'in an emergency, wherever it may arise, you must offer anyone at risk the assistance you could reasonably be expected to provide'.[65] What is *reasonably expected* can vary with the context of the emergency and the likelihood of other help becoming available. The BMA has detailed advice about different kinds of emergencies[66] but also says that generally, doctors should be willing to identify themselves and offer what help they can at the scene of a road accident, for example, or in an aircraft emergency.

All health professionals have a duty to act within their normal sphere of expertise and not be tempted or pressured to exceed it. While refusing to step beyond what they are confident they can do to a good standard is the correct response in daily practice, other considerations are likely to come into play in emergencies. It can be a very difficult call to try and decide whether to intervene when ill-prepared and poorly equipped. Some health professionals may be willing to stretch themselves to the limit if no more specialised assistance is available and there are many anecdotes of lives being saved against the odds as a result. Others are more reluctant and unwilling to take any risk, especially when lacking the equipment usually needed. They may also worry about their liability if they exceed their competence and things go wrong, but there is no evidence that litigation has ever been mounted in the UK against any doctor attempting to provide first aid in such circumstances, even when errors are made. Advice from a medical defence body is that 'if you are trying to do the right thing by using your professional expertise to help a fellow human continue to live . . . the chances of facing legal action are so low they are almost non-existent'.[67]

Ensuring competence in daily practice

Junior doctors can be particularly vulnerable in terms of being expected to perform, without appropriate supervision, tasks for which they lack expertise. If asked to take on tasks with which they are unfamiliar, doctors need to acknowledge if they are out of their depth and talk to senior colleagues. Except in emergency situations, doctors should resist any pressure or temptation to act outside their normal sphere of expertise.

Case example – doctors working outside their sphere of expertise

While examining a patient who wanted advice on hormone replacement therapy, a gynaecologist noticed several unsightly skin lesions. He asked the patient whether she wanted them removed under a general anaesthetic. She agreed but was not warned about possible scarring. The gynaecologist carried out the procedure but when the sutures were removed, some of the wounds gaped and Steri-Strips were applied. No follow-up treatment was given. The patient developed keloid scarring and successfully sued the gynaecologist. Following the case, the Medical Protection Society emphasised the importance of doctors not acting outside their area of professional practice but of referring patients to a colleague in the relevant specialty.[68]

Locums, out-of-hours services and arranging medical cover

The GMC tells doctors that when off duty, they must be satisfied that suitable arrangements have been made for patient care. The arrangements should include effective hand-over procedures and good communication beforehand with colleagues. If the cover arrangements appear inadequate to ensure patient safety, the doctor has a duty to either put the matter right or draw it to the attention of the employing or contracting body.[69] Employers must ensure that the staff they employ are competent and properly supported by a thorough induction if the setting is unfamiliar to them. Inexperienced doctors and those new to the UK should not be left facing decisions beyond their clinical competence. Following the implementation of the European Working Time Directive in 2009, there was increased demand for locums at a time when some employers had difficulty finding doctors who were familiar with NHS practice. In 2010, there was considerable media debate about the potential risks posed by some overseas doctors working as locums in the NHS where the work was different from their usual practice.

> ### Case example – out-of-hours cover
>
> In February 2008, Daniel Ubani, a German doctor providing out-of-hours cover, administered 10 times the clinically indicated dose of diamorphine to David Gray, who died as a result. Dr Ubani said he was tired, stressed and unfamiliar with the drug. Errors were also made in the treatment of two other patients in the same shift. The GMC later said there had been wide-ranging, serious and persistent failings in his basic competence. Dr Ubani had only undergone a brief induction and the assessor had warned that there was insufficient time for a full appraisal. Dr Ubani said that the fatal mistake derived from a confusion between two drugs, one of which was not used by on-call services in Germany. Other German doctors had also been in difficulties with the same drug. Dr Ubani was given a 9-month suspended prison sentence in Germany for negligence. In Britain, he was struck off in June 2010 by the GMC, which said that he had showed a persistent lack of insight into the seriousness of his actions and had not attempted to improve his skills. The GMC also called for EU doctors to be tested on their clinical skills and language abilities.[70]

Locums must ensure their own competence. Agencies and employers must also ensure that relevant pre-employment checks have been carried out and employers should only use agencies that have reliable quality control systems.

Vetting and barring

Health professionals have a responsibility to speak out if they consider that colleagues present a risk. Delays have sometimes occurred in preventing harm to patients because health professionals think that they need knowledge of more than one incident involving a colleague before action can be taken.[71] This is not the case. When doctors employ colleagues or other staff, or accept volunteers, they must take steps to ensure that these people are safe and reliable, especially those working with children or vulnerable adults. Traditionally, in the primary care setting, it was left to each practice to decide what checks to make. In 2002 in England and Wales, guidance was published regarding pre-and post-appointment checks for anyone working in the NHS, whether as an employee, volunteer or contracted service provider. This included the need to check with the Criminal Records Bureau (CRB).[72] In 2006, the Safeguarding Vulnerable Groups Act (England and Wales) was passed as a result of the Bichard Inquiry into the Soham murders of two schoolgirls by a school caretaker in 2002 (similar provisions were introduced in Northern Ireland in 2007[73]). It introduced a formal system of vetting and barring for all those working with vulnerable people, including health and social care workers. It placed a statutory duty on employers and regulators to provide certain information to the Independent Safeguarding Authority (ISA). It is a criminal offence to employ someone who has been barred from working with vulnerable groups in that capacity. In Scotland, general guidance was published in 2005 by the Northern Constabulary on best practice in protecting vulnerable adults.[74] The Adult Support and Protection (Scotland) Act 2007 made provision for safeguarding adults deemed to be at risk of harm including those with impaired capacity. It set out principles on when intervening in the adult's affairs would be justifiable, set out a system of banning certain individuals from attending the adult and rules about notification to the sheriff of an adult thought to be at risk. This was backed up by the Protection of Vulnerable Groups (Scotland) Act 2007, which barred certain people from working with children or vulnerable adults and required Ministers to keep lists of such barred individuals.

In 2011, the Government announced new recommendations for the future of the Vetting and Barring Scheme and criminal record checks in England, Wales and Northern Ireland. The Protection of Freedoms Act 2012 introduces a revised barring scheme; the key changes are

- a large reduction of the number of positions requiring checks to just those working most closely and regularly with children and vulnerable adults (from September 2012)
- merging of the CRB and the ISA to form a Disclosure and Barring Service (DBS) from December 2012
- portability of criminal record checks between jobs with the introduction of an online system to allow employers to check if updated information is held

on an applicant (from early 2013 in England and Wales but slightly later in Northern Ireland).

Information on the new scheme can be found on the BMA's website.

When offering employment, GP practices routinely check the colleague's indemnity and registration details. For other information, they generally rely heavily on references provided. The importance of providing accurate testimonials is paramount. Trusts carry out health screening and pre-employment checks on all staff and similar checks are made in relation to volunteer workers. In addition, all staff, volunteers and people such as students doing work observation must be aware of the obligation to maintain patient confidentiality and should be asked to sign a declaration to that effect.

Students, shadowing and work experience

Young people reaching the end of secondary education and thinking of applying to medical school sometimes ask to observe a doctor's practice (shadowing). Sitting in on consultations will give them access to some confidential medical information. As with all employees and volunteers, it is the doctor's responsibility to emphasise to those on work experience the importance of patient confidentiality, and the doctor retains ultimate responsibility for any breaches. Doctors must be satisfied that the observer is sufficiently mature and responsible to understand the principles of confidentiality. It is good practice for the doctor to obtain a signed commitment that the young person will maintain strict confidentiality. Medical students and young people who are shadowing a doctor should only be present during consultations when patients have consented. Patients should be given time to consider such requests without the potential observer present and it must be made clear to patients that a refusal will not influence their treatment.

Writing references for colleagues

When doctors write references for colleagues, they must give an honest and factual appraisal of performance. Bland or uncritical references should not be given in order to encourage the mobility of underperforming colleagues.

Case example – writing references

A consultant anaesthetist was found guilty of serious professional misconduct by the GMC for an opinion he had provided. He had been asked by
(Continued)

a colleague for advice about the professional performance of a locum doctor in order to write a reference but failed to disclose that the locum had been involved in a serious incident that was the subject of a pending enquiry. The GMC said that doctors who have reason to believe that a colleague's conduct or professional performance poses a danger to patients must act to ensure patient safety. Before taking action, they should do their best to establish the facts. Where there is doubt, it is unethical for a doctor to give a reference about a colleague, particularly if it may result in the employment of that doctor elsewhere. References about colleagues must be carefully considered; comments made in them must be justifiable, offered in good faith and intended to promote the best interests of patients.[75]

A last word on the doctor–patient relationship

In public opinion polls, doctors, nurses and other health professionals usually figure among the most trusted and respected groups in society. Patients and the general public greatly appreciate what they do and protest if they see the healthcare system threatened. But they often also look for someone to blame when things go wrong in individual cases. In this chapter, we have pointed out how the onus is on the health professional to make all contacts with patients work well, whatever the circumstances of the case, and to speak out when there are risks of things going awry. The ideal professional relationship is one in which there is mutual trust and truthfulness. It is clear that this is not always easy to achieve, not least as changes in the way health care is delivered can mean that patients see many different professionals for different aspects of care. Continuing relationships between one doctor and one patient, common in the past, still exist but are rarer. Whatever changes come and even in less than ideal circumstances, health professionals have to keep up their side of the bargain and act with integrity and compassion.

References

1 General Medical Council (2006) *Good Medical Practice*, GMC, London.
2 Jackson E (2010) *Medical Law: Text, Cases and Materials*, 2nd edn, Oxford University Press, Oxford, p.104.
3 *Barnett v Chelsea and Kensington Hospital Management Committee* [1969] 1 QB 428.
4 Centre for Innovation in Health Management (2012) *National Inquiry into Organisational Ethical Decision Making in the NHS*, University of Leeds, Leeds, p.35.

5   The BMA publishes detailed advice on dual responsibilities in: British Medical Association (2012) *Medical Ethics Today. The BMA's Handbook of Ethics and Law*, 3rd edn, Wiley-Blackwell, Chichester, chapters 16 and 17.

6   General Medical Council (2006) *Good Medical Practice*, GMC, London, para 54.

7   General Medical Council (2006) *Good Medical Practice*, GMC, London, para 55.

8   British Medical Association (2008) *Access to Healthcare for Asylum Seekers and Refused Asylum Seekers*, BMA, London.

9   General Medical Council (2006) *Good Medical Practice*, GMC, London, para 3(e).

10 British Medical Association (2009) *The Interface between NHS and Private Treatment: a Practical Guide for Doctors in England, Wales and Northern Ireland*, BMA, London; British Medical Association (2009) *The Interface between NHS and Private Treatment: a Practical Guide for Doctors in Scotland*, BMA, London.

11 Temel JS, Greer JA, Muzikansky A, *et al.* (2010) Early palliative care for patients with metastatic non-small-cell lung cancer. *N Engl J Med* **363**, 733–742.

12 Parliamentary and Health Service Ombudsman (2011) *Listening and Learning: the Ombudsman's Review of Complaint Handling by the NHS in England 2010–11*, The Stationery Office, London, p.10.

13 Action on Elder Abuse (2011) Regulatory activity in hospital settings: a critical analysis of the Care Quality Commission's Dignity and Nutrition Inspection of 100 English hospitals, *Clinical Effectiveness Bulletin for NHS Primary Care in North Staffordshire* 57.

14 Anon. (2011) York Hospital criticised over patient resuscitation. *BBC News Online* (Oct 27). Available at: http://www.bbc.co.uk/news (accessed 8 June 2012).

15 British Medical Association (2012) *Medical Ethics Today. The BMA's Handbook of Ethics and Law*, 3rd edn, Wiley-Blackwell, Chichester, chapter 21.

16 General Medical Council (2006) *Good Medical Practice*, GMC, London, para 30.

17 General Medical Council (2006) *Good Medical Practice*, GMC, London, para 31.

18 *Froggatt v Chesterfield and North Derbyshire NHS Trust* [2002] All ER(D) 218; [2002] WL 31676323.

19 Thompson DF (1993) Understanding financial conflict of interest. *N Engl J Med* **329**, 573–576.

20 Royal College of General Practitioners (2012) *Managing Conflicts of Interest in Clinical Commissioning Groups*, RCGP, London, p.5.

21 Royal College of General Practitioners (2012) *Managing Conflicts of Interest in Clinical Commissioning Groups*, RCGP, London, p.4.

22 Centre for Innovation in Health Management (2012) *National Inquiry into Organisational Ethical Decision Making in the NHS*, University of Leeds, Leeds, p.20.

23 Royal College of General Practitioners (2012) *Managing Conflicts of Interest in Clinical Commissioning Groups*, RCGP, London.

24 Royal College of General Practitioners (2012) *Making Difficult Choices – Ethical Commissioning Guidance for GPs*, RCGP, London.

25 General Medical Council (2006) *Good Medical Practice*, GMC, London, para 74.

26 General Medical Council (2006) *Good Medical Practice*, GMC, London, para 72.

27 The National Health Service (General Medical Services Contracts) Regulations 2004, SI 2004/291.

28 The BMA has detailed guidance about the contractual and ethical aspects of accepting a gift. British Medical Association (2007) *Accepting Donations from Patients*, BMA, London.

29 See, for example: House of Commons Health Committee (2004) *Elder Abuse Second Report of Session 2003–4*, The Stationery Office, London, vol 1, para 65; Joint Committee on Human Rights (2007) *The Human Rights of Older people in Healthcare. Eighteenth Report of Session 2006–7*, The Stationery Office, London, vol 2, evidence sessions 173 and 222.

30 Mental Welfare Commission for Scotland (2006) *Covert Medication: Legal and Practical Guidance*, Mental Welfare Commission for Scotland, Edinburgh.

31 General Medical Council (2011) *Making and Using Visual and Audio Recordings of Patients*, GMC, London.

32 General Medical Council (2011) *Making and Using Visual and Audio Recordings of Patients*, GMC, London, paras 11–12.

33 The Regulation of Investigatory Powers Act 2000 covers England, Wales and Northern Ireland. Scotland is covered by the Regulation of Investigatory Powers (Scotland) Act 2000.

34 Royal College of Paediatrics and Child Health (2009) *Fabricated or Induced Illness by Carers (FII): a Practical Guide for Paediatricians*, RCPCH, London, pp.27–28 and 50.

35 General Medical Council (2003) Covert video recording is unacceptable. *GMC News* 17, 8.

36 General Medical Council (2007) *0–18 Years: Guidance for All Doctors*, GMC, London.

37 Department of Health Clinical Governance Support Team (2005) *Guidance on the Role and Effective Use of Chaperones in Primary and Community Care Settings*. Available at: http://www.lmc.org.uk (accessed 1 October 2012).

38 General Medical Council (2006) *Maintaining Boundaries*, GMC, London, paras 10–13.

39 Royal College of Obstetricians and Gynaecologists (1997) *Intimate Examinations*, RCOG, London.

40 General Medical Council (2006) *Maintaining Boundaries*, GMC, London, paras 9, 14 and 15.

41 General Medical Council (2006) *Good Medical Practice*, GMC, London, para 32.

42 British Medical Association (2011) *Using Social Media: Practical and Ethical Guidance for Doctors and Medical Students*, BMA, London.

43 At the time of writing this guidance was in draft form. Up-to-date information can be found on the GMC's website available at: http://www.gmc-uk.org (accessed 1 August 2012).

44 General Medical Council, Medical Schools Council (2009) *Medical Students: Professional Values and Fitness to Practise*, GMC, London, para 3.

45 Chretien KC, Greysen SR, Chretien JP, *et al.* (2009) Online posting of unprofessional content by medical students. *JAMA* **302**(12), 1309–1315.

46 By late 2012, the General Medical Council was scheduled to update its 2008 guidance, entitled *Personal Beliefs and Medical Practice*. Available at: http://www.gmc-uk.org (accessed 21 September 2012).

47 Department of Health (2009) *Religion or Belief: a Practical Guide for the NHS*, DH, London.

48 Gledhill R (2009) Victory for suspended Christian nurse. *The Times* (Feb 7). Available at: http://www.timesonline.co.uk (accessed 8 June 2012).

49 Department of Health (2009) *Religion or Belief: a Practical Guide for the NHS*, DH, London, p.22.

50 General Medical Council Investigation Committee Hearing, 11–14 June 2012.

51 Equality and Human Rights Commission. *Your Rights: Sexual Orientation*. Available at: http://www.equalityhumanrights.com (accessed 1 August 2012).

52 Ramesh R (2012) GP practice 'offloaded vulnerable patients to save money'. *The Guardian* (May 31). A copy of the Internal Review can be seen at: http://www.guardian.co.uk (accessed 7 June 2012).

53 The Parliamentary and Health Service Ombudsman (2011) *Listening and Learning: the Ombudsman's Review of Complaint Handling by the NHS in England 2010–11*, The Stationery Office, p.16.

54 The Parliamentary and Health Service Ombudsman (2011) *Listening and Learning: the Ombudsman's Review of Complaint Handling by the NHS in England 2010–11*, The Stationery Office, p.18.

55 General Medical Council (2006) *Good Medical Practice*, GMC, London, paras 38–40.

56 General Medical Council (2006) *Good Medical Practice*, GMC, London, paras 60–62.

57 Advertising Standards Authority (2011) *First Letter to Homeopathy Advertisers*. Available at: http://www.asa.org.uk (accessed 21 September 2012).

58 General Medical Council (2006) *Good Medical Practice*, GMC, London, paras 77–79.

59 General Medical Council (2006) *Good Medical Practice*, GMC, London, para 5.

60 General Medical Council (2006) *Good Medical Practice*, GMC, London, para 6.

61 General Medical Council (2012) *Raising and Acting on Concerns about Patient Safety*, GMC, London.

62 British Medical Association (2009) *Whistle-Blowing: Advice for BMA Members Working in NHS Secondary Care about Raising Concerns in the Workplace*, BMA, London.

63 British Medical Association (2008) *Whistle-Blowing: Guidance from the Medical Students Committee (MSC)*, BMA, London.

64 Department of Health (2011) *The NHS Constitution: The Introduction of New Expectations and Commitments around Whistleblowing*, DH, London.

65 General Medical Council (2006) *Good Medical Practice*, GMC, London, para 11.

66 British Medical Association (2012) *Medical Ethics Today. The BMA's Handbook of Ethics and Law*, 3rd edn, Wiley-Blackwell, Chichester, chapter 15.

67 Kirkpatrick A (2002) Come join the good Samaritans. *Stud BMJ* **10**, 89–130.

68 Medical Protection Society (1999) Act within the limits of your expertise. *UK Casebook*, 13, 12.

69 General Medical Council (2006) *Good Medical Practice*, GMC, London, paras 6 and 48.

70 General Medical Council Fitness to Practise hearing, 18 June 2010.

71 Anon. (2009) Sexual abuse allowed to carry on, report shows, *Health Care Risk Report*, vol 15, issue 5.

72 NHS Employment Policy Branch (2003) *Pre-employment checks for NHS staff [extract taken from HSG 98/064.]* NHS Employment Policy Branch, Leeds. National Assembly

for Wales (2003) *Pre and post-employment checks for all persons working in the NHS in Wales*, National Assembly for Wales, Cardiff.

73   Safeguarding Vulnerable Groups (Northern Ireland) Order 2007.

74   Northern Constabulary (2005) *Protecting Vulnerable Adults: Good Practice Guidance and Procedures*, Highland Council, Inverness.

75   General Medical Council Professional Conduct Committee hearing, 14–18 March 1994.

3: Consent, choice and refusal: adults with capacity

10 things you need to know about . . . patient consent and refusal

- Patient consent is not an optional extra but a core part of examination and treatment.
- All adults are assumed to have mental capacity to consent to or refuse treatment, unless there is evidence to the contrary.
- Consent by a person with capacity is valid when it is adequately informed and voluntary.
- Information cannot be imposed on adults with capacity who do not wish to receive it, but failure to accept basic information may invalidate the consent.
- Health professionals should check that patients consent before examining or treating them, unless it is an emergency or compulsory treatment is given under mental health legislation.
- Patients can give explicit consent or refusal orally, in writing or by gesture. They can imply consent or refusal non-verbally, by complying with, or resisting, what is proposed.
- Adults with capacity can refuse treatment, even when serious harm or death will result. Such decisions are likely to be binding on health professionals.
- An adult patient with capacity can refuse treatment even if that would result in the death of a viable fetus.
- People can make decisions about their current and future treatment, but advance decisions must meet certain criteria in order to be valid.
- Valid advance refusals of treatment are legally binding on health professionals.

Setting the scene

This chapter focuses on consent and refusal by adults who have the mental capacity to make whatever decision is needed at the time. It involves a process through which the doctor's clinical knowledge and expertise and the patient's individual needs and preferences are shared, in order to agree upon the best treatment option. Patient consent is then the trigger that allows treatment or examination to take place. Seeking consent from patients therefore forms a crucial part of the practice of almost every doctor.

Everyday Medical Ethics and Law, First Edition. Ann Sommerville.
© 2013 BMA Medical Ethics Department. Published 2013 by John Wiley & Sons, Ltd.

In order for consent to be valid the patient must
- have capacity
- be offered sufficient information to make an informed decision
- be acting voluntarily and free from undue pressure
- be aware that he or she can refuse.

Consent need not be in writing. As long as patients understand what is proposed, a verbal indication of acceptance is sufficient, but written authorisation is advisable for higher risk or innovative treatments and is legally required for some procedures.[1] It is also good practice to document treatment refusals, and the discussions that have taken place, particularly where the consequences are likely to be serious. Although checking whether patients are willing to proceed with what is proposed is an important preliminary step, consent is not a one-off event but rather a part of an ongoing process. This is particularly the case when patients have a long-term condition or one that is subject to change. People often change their minds as their perspectives evolve during the course of a long illness. What seems unacceptable to them at one stage may be requested at another or vice versa. It is important not to make assumptions about what patients want based on their past choice but to encourage them to assess and re-evaluate their options over time.

There is a considerable amount of detailed advice available on consent throughout the UK.[2] Among the common queries raised with the BMA, many focus on patient consent or lack of it. This chapter sets out the rules and principles relating to the most common enquiries around consent and refusal of treatment. In some cases, the answer to the question is legally straightforward even though it might seem to raise difficult ethical questions. Refusal of treatment can be particularly challenging for health professionals. Many doctors struggle to accept a refusal of life-prolonging treatment by an adult with capacity where they believe that, with treatment, the individual would be able to achieve a good quality of life. With a strong focus on personal autonomy, the law is clear, however, that an adult with capacity has the right to refuse any treatment even if that treatment results in his or her death (see the case of *Re B* later in the chapter). Doctors can and should try to understand the reasons for the refusal and to ensure that the patient has fully understood the situation but they cannot seek to impose their own views and wishes on their patients. Such cases are relatively rare but raise difficult issues for health professionals who often feel frustrated by their inability to do what they perceive to be the best for their patient. Ultimately, however, it is for each individual to decide where his or her best interests lie.

Much of this chapter focuses on the practical aspects of consent – the rules governing the amount of information needed, who should obtain consent, whether consent needs to be in writing, and so on. Where dilemmas arise that require more detailed analysis it will be helpful to return to these guiding principles as part of the decision-making process.

Common questions asked about consent and refusal

- How much information has to be given in order for the patient's consent or refusal to be valid?
- Should I mention risks that are very unlikely to occur?
- Is verbal agreement or refusal enough or should patients sign something?
- How long is consent valid for?
- If a patient refuses to receive information about a procedure, is the consent still valid?
- If a patient has signed a consent form, does that mean that treatment must proceed?

The importance of information

People over the age of 16 are legally assumed to be able to make medical decisions for themselves unless there is evidence to the contrary (but see the section on refusals of treatment by those under the age of 18). They can be confused, forgetful, depressed or have some other form of mental difficulty and still have decision-making capacity, if they understand the options and can weigh them up. Making an unusual choice, such as a decision to postpone or refuse crucial treatment, does not necessarily mean that their capacity is impaired, but if there is any significant doubt about it, a formal assessment is likely to be needed. (Mental capacity is discussed in detail in Chapter 4.) By the same token, some highly functioning people can be incapable of valid decisions if, for example, they are misinformed or being coerced by someone else. When they have mental capacity and relevant information, patients can also make choices about how they want to be treated in the future at a time when their decision-making capacity becomes impaired.

Offering information for contemporaneous and advance decisions

In order to make valid choices individuals need information to understand what is proposed and why, so that they can decide whether to give consent. Giving people information about their options, discussing their wishes and checking their agreement to proceed are therefore the usual first steps in the consent process. This is both a legal and a moral requirement as society places considerable emphasis on personal autonomy and on individuals making the decisions that are right for them.

Most people are keen to have information about the proposed treatment and its likely outcome. If they are not, or are simply not ready to have it yet, they still need to know that the information is on offer and should be encouraged to keep their decision to refuse, or limit, information under review. All patients need to be aware of the core facts or their consent may be considered invalid. They also need the facts to be given in a way they understand. A bland menu of options is generally unhelpful and can be difficult for patients to assess in a meaningful way. Advice about what is likely to be most effective or appropriate for their particular situation is often more helpful. Sometimes, it is unclear how much the patient is taking in, particularly when the news is bad, unexpected or very complicated. In such cases, the health team should give people time to reflect and encourage them to ask questions (see also the sections in Chapter 2 on giving bad news and recording consultations). Support groups, helplines and information leaflets can be useful but cannot replace discussion with the clinician.

Except for short-term and self-contained episodes of treatment, patients' consent is part of an ongoing process. Information may need to be repeated, reviewed or periodically updated. If a time gap occurs between the consent and the procedure, the details may need to be reviewed with the patient and the consent reaffirmed. This would obviously be the case if the individual's condition or the options available have altered. A patient's consent or refusal applies to the particular treatments discussed but not to alternatives that might seem obvious to a clinician but were not discussed with the patient. Health professionals should flag up in advance any reasonably foreseeable problems that could arise when the patient is anaesthetised or otherwise unable to discuss preferences. It is only usually justifiable to proceed without prior authority to avoid death or serious harm to the patient.[3] In the past, medical students were sometimes permitted to learn some procedures, such as intimate examinations, on unconscious patients whose consent had not been sought. This has long been considered completely unacceptable.

Case example – exceeding consent during surgery

A consultant obstetrician was found guilty of serious professional misconduct for his management of a patient's total abdominal hysterectomy and bilateral salpingo-oophorectomy. The General Medical Council (GMC) found that, during the operation, the doctor realised that the patient might be pregnant but continued anyway. This possibility had not been mentioned in advance so that the pregnancy was ended, without the woman having any say in the matter. The GMC ruled that the consultant knew, or should have known, that the patient had not agreed to a termination of pregnancy and needed to be consulted. He was severely reprimanded.[4]

Translation and signing services

Information is only useful when the recipient understands it. This can be particularly difficult to ensure when the options are complex and a decision is urgently needed. Even more complicated are those cases where the patient is not an English speaker or is deaf and needs signing services. Translation and signing services should be provided whenever possible. Even when such services are provided, however, it can be difficult for health professionals to be sure that the choices have been accurately described and understood. Where hospitals have a significant number of non-English speakers, written information on common procedures in a range of languages can help to ensure that these patients understand what is proposed and are empowered to make informed choices.

Case example – problems conveying information accurately

A patient from overseas arrived at hospital in labour. Among the complicating factors were the baby's breech position and the fact that the mother was unaccompanied and had no knowledge of English. A caesarean section was strongly advised, but no translator who knew the patient's dialect was available to explain this and to tell her she was likely to need a blood transfusion. Repeated attempts were made to outline the options to her, including the use of visual aids. On arrival, the patient showed the staff a multilingual card, implying that she was a Jehovah's Witness who refused blood products, but it did not state whether she would be willing to have blood, or alternatives to blood products, in a life or death situation. The healthcare team were very doubtful about whether any consent or refusal would be valid, given the ambiguity about her understanding of the choices. Without consent to any other course of action, the hospital staff felt they had no option but to try to manage a vaginal delivery. In the event, this was successful but at the cost of a very difficult labour for the mother and added risk for the child.

In this case, the health team were concerned that they had not done their best for their patient, but given that the mother was an adult with mental capacity, they felt unable to carry out a caesarean section without her consent. Although she carried a card refusing a blood transfusion, it did not make clear that this should apply even if her life was at risk and so would not be a legally binding refusal of treatment in those circumstances. Her wishes about the caesarean section were unknown. The individual factors of the case are very relevant, such as what efforts had been made to find ways to communicate with the woman and whether she was showing any signs of either acquiescence or resistance. It is likely to be very rare where it is genuinely impossible to gain any indication of the patient's wishes but in such circumstances, a doctor who does what is clinically best for the patient is unlikely to be criticised. In such circumstances, however, where time permits it would be advisable to seek specific legal advice.

What type of information?

Patients not only need to be told about their medical condition and the options for managing it but also the implications of accepting or refusing any of the choices on offer. The GMC sets out a useful list of the kind of information that patients should have prior to any intervention (other than in an emergency situation where discussion with the patient is impossible). Patients are also likely to have specific questions related to their own particular circumstances.

Information to be provided

The GMC advises that the information given to patients should cover the following points:

- the patient's diagnosis, prognosis, uncertainties about the condition, the potential (if any) for further investigations and, where appropriate, the option of getting a second opinion
- options for treating or managing the condition, including the option of non-treatment
- the purpose of the proposed investigation or treatment and what it involves
- the potential benefits, risks, burdens and likelihood of success of each option, including, if available, information about whether the benefits or risks are affected by the choice of doctor or organisation to provide care
- whether a proposed investigation or treatment is part of a research pro-gramme or is an innovative treatment designed specifically for the patient's benefit; information should include how the proposed treatment differs from standard care, why it is offered and its risks or uncertainties
- the identity and roles of those involved in, or responsible for, the patient's care
- whether students may be involved and the patient's right to decline par-ticipation in teaching or research
- any bills patients have to pay and any conflicts of interest that the doctor, or healthcare organisation, may have
- any treatments that the doctor believes have greater potential benefit for the patient than those that the doctor, or his or her healthcare organisa-tion, can offer.[5]

As well as general information when treatment is planned, more specific details usually need to be repeated closer to the procedure. Although patients are often given most of the information for surgery, for example, at a preoperative assessment clinic, they often have specific questions later for the anaesthetist. (Detailed guidance for anaesthetists and information for patients are available from the Association of Anaesthetists.[6])

Although some patients may not want all the information available, most do want to understand as much as possible. Even those who hesitate to have the whole picture need to know the basic points. Patients should also be asked before medical students or other observers attend any examination or treatment. Their consent should not be taken for granted, even in teaching hospitals.

In addition to information about a particular intervention, the provision of information is also important for patients with long-term or progressive illnesses to enable them to decide about future care options. Such wishes are discussed with the healthcare team and are recorded in the patient's medical records. This is a standard part of good medical practice.

Information to make an advance decision

People who are clear that they would not wish to have particular interventions or treatment may decide to make a formal advance decision. An advance decision refusing treatment, which meets the necessary legal criteria, will be legally binding on health professionals. Their options, and the likelihood of their choices being implemented, are greater when patients have a diagnosis with a predictable disease path, involving loss of mental abilities. Patients making advance decisions should take advice so that they understand the course their condition will take and the treatments available for it. Input from health professionals generally results in a better informed advance decision. Making an advance decision in anticipation of future illness or accident is far more complex since it is very difficult for patients to anticipate the conditions they are likely to experience or the treatments that will be offered. Some patients may gain peace of mind in making provision for their future, but their advance decisions are never implemented, as they retain their mental agility until the end of their lives and can thus consent to, or refuse, treatment at the time a decision is needed. The biggest risks are that patients fail to update their recorded wishes when their views or treatment options change or that they fail to foresee some situation in which they would want a treatment which they have refused in advance.

In giving advice, the aim is not to influence patients but to help them to think through their wishes and concerns and to state their intentions clearly in a way that meets the legal criteria (where that is the patient's intention). Patients need to have realistic expectations about the extent to which the end of anyone's life can be controlled. Uncertainties need to be explained and discussed, as the colleagues who may ultimately have to try to interpret and implement patients' wishes rely on them being properly informed and clearly formulated.

Case example – advance decision made on the basis of incomplete information

A patient in her 70s stated that she would not wish resuscitation to be attempted in the event of a heart attack or stroke. A do-not-attempt cardiopulmonary resuscitation (DNACPR) notice was placed on her record with her consent. When she went into hospital for a minor procedure requiring anaesthesia, this triggered an unexpected cardiorespiratory instability, which had never been discussed with her. Her medical notes said her choice was for resuscitation not to be attempted, but she had not anticipated an easily reversible cause of potential cardiorespiratory arrest. In the belief that her advance decision had never been intended for this eventuality, resuscitation was successfully given. The BMA agreed that this was the right thing to do as the circumstances which arose were far different from what the patient anticipated when she made her advance refusal.

Information about participating in a research project

When people give consent to be part of a research programme, they need to know its purpose and what is involved. It may simply be that their records are used and their health monitored or the research may involve changes to an existing treatment regime. Where consent has been given to participate in a research programme, whether as a patient or a healthy volunteer trying out new drugs, research participants need to be told of any known risks, side effects, potential complications and areas of uncertainty. In relation to risk, they should be given information about the nature of the risk, its magnitude, its probability and its imminence. As with consent for examination or treatment, people participating in research programmes vary in how much detail they want. Patients with an existing condition should be told whether or not their treatment will be randomised as part of a trial and what the implications might be for them if a successful new drug or other treatment emerges from it. They also need to be clear that the quality of their care will be unaffected, regardless of whether or not they decide to participate.

How much information?

Different patients require varying amounts of information about their condition and the treatment options available. Some want as much as possible and many arrive with information drawn from the media or Web-based resources, which may or may not be accurate or applicable to their case. The default position should be to offer patients relevant facts and clinical opinions about their condition and options while responding to additional issues they have. Their questions should be answered as truthfully as possible without glossing over uncertainties. The GMC says that when deciding how much information to give, attention should focus on the patient's wishes: 'the amount of detail offered should be in proportion to the patient's condition, the complexity of the proposed investigation or treatment, and the gravity of any side effects, complications or other risks'.[7]

The duty to warn about risks

The legal duty to inform patients appropriately, as part of a doctor's duty to exercise reasonable care and skill, was established by the House of Lords in 1985.[8] The case arose at a time when there was anxiety that attempting to reveal every possible risk could make patients reluctant to have any beneficial procedure, even if the risks they were warned about very rarely materialised. What many doctors wanted to know at the time was where the benchmark should be set in terms of what to disclose routinely. Should it be permissible to withhold information if the likelihood of the damage occurring was extremely low – a risk of less than 2%, say? The classic judgment expressed in the *Sidaway* case is still often quoted and subsequent important legal cases have built on it.

Duty to warn about risks: *Sidaway*

Mrs Sidaway had recurrent pain in her neck, right shoulder and arms. To rectify this, she underwent surgery, but even when carried out with care and skill, the operation bore inherent risks. These were estimated to be about a 2% risk of damage to the nerve roots and a less than 1% risk of damage to the spinal cord. The surgeon reportedly warned Mrs Sidaway of the risk of nerve damage but did not mention the risk of spinal injury, which was what actually occurred. She was left disabled and claimed damages for negligence against the hospital and the estate of the surgeon (by then deceased) on the grounds that she had not been properly informed of the risks. The case was taken to the House of Lords, but Mrs Sidaway's claim was rejected.[8] Despite giving different reasons for rejecting her assertion that she should have been warned about the risk of damage to her spinal cord, there was a general agreement among the judges on the approach that had been taken in the earlier case of *Bolam*.[9] This had set out the rule that doctors would not be considered negligent if their practice conformed to that of a responsible body of medical opinion held by practitioners skilled in the field in question. Although not shared by other judges at the time, the
(Continued)

opinion of one judge – Lord Scarman – was that the standard for the amount of information to be given was not necessarily what the medical profession thought appropriate but what the individual patient required or what the average 'prudent patient' would want to know. He argued that

'Ideally, the court should ask itself whether in the particular circumstances the risk was such that this particular patient would think it significant if he was told it existed. I would think that, as a matter of ethics, this is the test of the doctor's duty. The law, however, operates not in Utopia but in the world as it is: and such an inquiry would prove in practice to be frustrated by the subjectivity of its aim and purpose. The law can, however, do the next best thing, and require the court to answer the question, what would a reasonably prudent patient think significant if in the situation of this patient. The 'prudent patient' cannot, however, always provide the answer for the obvious reason that he is a norm (like the man on the Clapham omnibus), not a real person: and certainly not the patient himself'.[10]

Lord Scarman's basic argument was that it should be patients rather than doctors who decide on what information is given or withheld. His view represented a patient-centred approach, which later gained prominence in ethics guidance. Much debate focused on how much information should be routinely given about very exceptional risks. It was also recognised that the main issue was not solely how likely it was that damage might occur but how grave or important it would be for that particular patient if the rare occurrence happened.

Duty to warn about risks: *Pearce*

In the 1998 case of *Pearce v United Bristol Healthcare NHS Trust*, an action was brought by a couple whose child died in utero when almost 3 weeks overdue. The mother had asked the consultant either to induce the birth or carry out a caesarean section. He advised against both, citing the high risks associated with induction and the long recovery time from caesarean section, but at the same time failed to discuss with her the risks of fetal death in the womb as a result of delayed delivery. In the Court of Appeal, Lord Woolf held that

'if there is a significant risk which would affect the judgment of a reasonable patient, then in the normal course it is the responsibility of a doctor to inform the patient of that significant risk, if the information is needed so that the patient can determine for him or herself as to what course he or she should adopt'.[11]

This judgment marked a further shift in emphasis, from what the 'reasonably prudent medical man' saw as a significant risk, towards how a 'reasonable patient' interpreted the same information. The degree of information needed for informed consent was again considered by the House of Lords in 2004, in a further seminal case concerning a surgeon's omission to forewarn a patient of a risk that a back operation could cause paralysis even though the patient had specifically asked about the risk.

Duty to warn about risks: *Chester*

The patient, Miss Chester, experienced lower back pain, for which she was referred to Mr Afshar, a consultant neurosurgeon, who recommended spinal surgery. The operation took place with the patient's consent but resulted in nerve damage, which left her partially paralysed. Although the procedure carried a small (1–2%) risk of such damage, the surgeon had not mentioned it despite the patient having asked about such risks. The courts found that there had been no question of negligence in the way the operation was carried out, but there was negligence in terms of not having obtained properly informed consent. It was noted that Miss Chester might have investigated other alternatives, had she known of the risk, although it was also argued that she would probably have gone ahead anyway, if she had known. Mr Afshar was judged to have failed in his duty to mention a relevant risk and get properly informed consent and this was upheld by the House of Lords.[12]

This case discussed the *purpose* of warning patients about risks, which was seen as being to enable them to make informed choices. Although the fact that Miss Chester was unaware of the risk made no difference to the likelihood of it occurring, she was seen as having been denied a choice in the matter. One of the judges, Lord Steyn, talked about the need for doctors to ensure that 'due respect is given to the autonomy and dignity of each patient'.[13] He said that 'a patient has a *prima facie* right to be informed by a surgeon of a small, but well established, risk of serious injury as a result of surgery'.[14] The GMC subsequently emphasised that patients should be told of any possible significant adverse outcomes of a proposed treatment and pointed to how, in this case, a small but well-established risk of a serious adverse outcome was considered by the House of Lords to be 'significant'.[15] This was echoed by Department of Health guidance that 'the health practitioner should try to ensure that the person is able to make an informed judgment on whether to give or withhold consent . . . It is therefore advisable to inform the person of any "material" or "significant" risks or unavoidable risks, even if small, in the proposed treatment; any alternatives to it; and the risks incurred by doing nothing. . .'.[16]

The overall legal message is that failure to warn patients about risks associated with their treatment can give rise to negligence claims if the risks materialise, even when the actual procedure is skilfully carried out. To meet the legal and ethical requirements, health professionals need to inform patients both about significant risks inherent in the treatment but also about risks particularly important to those patients. If they can do this, they are likely to satisfy two standards set out by the courts when considering information provision and patient consent: firstly, the 'professional standard', which looks to a responsible body of medical opinion to determine what patients should be told in order to give valid consent, and secondly, the 'patient standard', where the amount of information required by the individual patient determines how much information he or she needs in order for consent to be obtained.[17] In all cases, the risks and benefits of alternatives and of non-treatment need also to be explained. More recent case law suggests that unless patients are informed of the comparative risk of different procedures, they are unable to give fully valid consent to one procedure rather than another.[18] As patient consent can only be valid if it is based on adequate information, including about the range of choices and the consequences of making one choice over another, health professionals should ensure that patients are informed of the comparative risks associated with any alternative treatments or procedures.

While failure to give enough relevant information could result in health professionals facing legal challenge, time and resource constraints mean there is inevitably a degree of selectivity about the information provided in many cases. It would be impractical for every detail to be explained, but it is important that patients can be confident of being offered information relevant to them and know that they can ask for more details if they wish.

Can information be withheld?

A generation or so ago, oncologists rarely told patients that they had cancer and similar attitudes prevailed for other life-threatening conditions. Giving patients bad news was seen as imposing distress and lowering morale. Often, only relatives were told when the patient's disease would be fatal. Now, the high value placed on self-determination in most western societies requires that patients are not left in ignorance, even when the choices facing them are difficult. In practical terms, people generally cope better with very challenging situations if they have a sense of being in control. For this, they need to know what options are available and the likely impact of the choices they make. Some seriously ill people say that they would have preferred to live in hope rather than know that they only have very limited time left, but it should be assumed that people want to know unless they indicate to the contrary. Obviously, this can be difficult, but all health professionals, and especially those working with patients with life-limiting conditions, should have ongoing training in communication skills. They need to develop techniques for sensitively conveying the core information and then exploring options, together with the individual.

Special attention is needed in very rare situations where providing information could be damaging to the person receiving it. Situations where this would be the case are likely to be rare and the prospect of harm needs to be genuine. Such decisions cannot be made lightly and need to be kept under review in case information could be given later without causing serious harm.[19] The reasons justifying withholding information should be noted in the patient record. Any professional making such a decision needs to be able to explain it, if challenged. Regulators and courts may accept the justification where it is clear that the circumstances warrant it, but 'the mere fact that the patient might become upset by hearing the information, or might refuse treatment, is not sufficient'.[20]

Medical research is an area where some information is routinely withheld with the explicit agreement of the patient. Randomised controlled trials are a common method of comparing treatments when it is unclear which is best or most effective. New drugs are often tested against existing ones, a placebo or no treatment at all. Participants in the research need to know in advance that they cannot choose which option they receive. The placebo effect can be quite successful but only if patients are unaware that they are receiving an inert substance rather than an active drug. In a placebo-controlled trial, patients need to be told explicitly what their chance is of not getting the active drug/intervention. The information provided to research participants should be scrutinised by a research ethics committee (REC) which also examines other aspects of the consent process.[21]

Can patients refuse information?

In some cases, patients initially refuse information or say that they want a decision made on their behalf by their relatives or their doctor. People cannot be forced to listen and some need time before they are ready to handle information about their illness. They may already suspect that the news is bad or they may be in denial about the seriousness of their condition. Health professionals need to try to find out why they are fearful and explain that treatment choices will need to be made, about which they may have preferences, and so they need to understand the options. When patients have mental capacity, the law requires that they have basic information before treatment is given. What counts as 'basic' differs according to the circumstances, including the severity of the patient's condition and any risks associated with treatment. (See also the previous sections on the amount and type of information to be given.) For their consent to be valid, people also need to know what the treatment is intended to achieve, and what it involves.[22] When people refuse to have even basic information, or are unable to be given it (as in the case example of the overseas patient mentioned earlier), serious questions arise about the validity of their consent. People unwilling to listen to core information need to know that this will affect what treatment can be provided. They should be encouraged to accept the information available and be aware that they can change their minds. In this situation, it is important that the offer, and refusal, of information is documented. Given time and support, most people deal with even very difficult choices, particularly if they can control how or when details are provided. Written material or advice about how to contact voluntary organisations, advocacy services, expert patient programmes or support groups for people with specific conditions can help, although these are not a substitute for discussion between patient and health professional.

Refusal of treatment

Adults with capacity have the right to refuse examination or treatment, except where compulsory treatment is authorised under mental health legislation. Where the patient's capacity fulfils the legal requirements, treatment for the mental disorder may be provided without consent even if the patient seems capable of refusing.[23] In all other cases, adults with capacity can make a valid decision, contemporaneously or in advance, to refuse treatment even when that will result in their own death or disability, or that of a fetus in the uterus. Patients are not obliged to justify their decisions to refuse treatment, but health professionals should attempt to discover why the patient is refusing treatment in order to determine, as far as possible, that they have based their decisions on accurate information and to correct any misunderstandings. Patients sometimes refuse treatment, for example, because they have unfounded fears that can be allayed by providing more information or reassurance. Ideally patients should have the same amount of information when refusing treatment as when giving consent, although neither information nor treatment can be imposed on an adult with capacity.

A refusal of one treatment does not imply a refusal of all treatments and measures to keep patients comfortable should still be offered. Patients can change their minds at any time, as long as they have the capacity to do so. If not providing treatment soon would significantly limit their future options, patients need to know that. They should be told, for example, if a cancer operable now will be inoperable later, if surgery is postponed.

It can be very difficult for health professionals providing life-prolonging treatment to accept a situation where a patient with mental capacity makes an informed and explicit choice to discontinue it. When a patient with capacity refuses treatment in full knowledge of the likely consequences, this decision must be respected by health professionals. If there is any doubt, legal advice should be sought, but it is not acceptable for treatment to continue in the face of a valid refusal.

Refusal of life-sustaining treatment: *Re B*

Ms B suffered a haemorrhage of the spinal cord in her neck. Admitted to hospital, she was diagnosed with a condition caused by a malformation of blood vessels in the spinal cord (cavernoma). At that point, she made an advance decision refusing treatment if she later lost capacity when she was suffering from a life-threatening condition, but when her condition improved, she returned to work. Ms B later sustained further damage to her spinal cord, as a result of which she became tetraplegic and required ventilator support. Although aware that she would die once artificial ventilation was removed, Ms B repeatedly asked for her ventilator to be switched off and formal instructions were given to the hospital to this effect by her solicitor. The clinicians were unwilling to do as she asked and suggested gradually reducing her ventilation with the hope that she might eventually breathe on her own. Ms B rejected this and also rejected efforts at rehabilitation because it offered her no chance of recovery. She was assessed by consultant psychiatrists and found not to be depressed and capable of making a valid decision to discontinue treatment. Despite her refusal, ventilation was continued and Ms B applied to the High Court for a declaration that it represented unlawful trespass. The trust argued that Ms B did not have the capacity to make the decision to stop treatment. The court held that Ms B had the capacity to make all relevant decisions about her medical treatment, including the decision to seek withdrawal of artificial ventilation. The judge also found that Ms B had been treated unlawfully by the trust.[24] Ms B died in her sleep a month later when her ventilation was withdrawn.

Doubts about capacity can arise if the person has a history of mental disturbance or if the choice seems to be part of a pattern of contradictory behaviour. In such cases, it can be very difficult for health professionals to assess whether the refusal is valid.

Case example – valid refusal of treatment following a suicide attempt

In 2007, 26-year-old Kerrie Wooltorton was admitted to hospital after consuming a fatal quantity of antifreeze. Previously diagnosed with an untreatable personality disorder and said to be depressed at her inability to have a child, she had done the same thing nine times before. In each case, she had been successfully treated in hospital, with her consent. On this last occasion, she refused treatment and gave the health staff a written declaration repeating her refusal. Her purpose in calling an ambulance was not to be saved but to avoid dying alone or in pain. After much discussion and a
(Continued)

second opinion from another consultant, the doctor in charge of her care judged that she had capacity to refuse treatment. He later said he could have treated her against her will, but that would have been wrong.[25] Her choice was respected and she died. This was seen as highly controversial, given the patient's history of mental illness. McLean pointed out, however, that although on previous occasions the patient accepted treatment after swallowing antifreeze, she had the right to make a different decision this time. Also, 'as she was able to make a contemporaneous refusal of treatment on admission to the hospital, her doctors were legally unable to provide it. The fact that she apparently had some form of personality disorder is not in itself persuasive evidence that she lacked capacity. It is well established in law that even the presence of mental illness is not a bar to the presumption of capacity'.[26] An inquest in 2009 upheld the doctor's decision not to treat her without consent. In his summary, the coroner said that Kerrie Wooltorton 'refused . . . treatment in full knowledge of the consequences and died as a result'.[25] Treatment by doctors in the face of a competent verbal refusal, unless mental health legislation was engaged, would have been unlawful.

Although a refusal of life-sustaining treatment from a patient with a history of serious mental disorder presents doctors with a significant ethical challenge, this case reaffirmed that the presence of a mental disorder is not synonymous with a lack of decision-making capacity.[27] Had the doctors felt it appropriate, however, detention and treatment under mental health legislation may have been an option. Such cases are immensely difficult, and in reaching decisions about how to proceed, health professionals need to apply the relevant laws, rules and guidelines, consider all of the facts, interests and options, and make a judgment about the best course of action in the particular circumstances of the case.

Seeking consent

Patients have choices about what is or is not done to them, but they cannot insist on having drugs or procedures considered clinically inappropriate. Rather, they should be able to choose between the options judged by health professionals to be potentially beneficial for them.

Who should seek the patient's consent?

Ideally, the professional recommending a procedure should seek consent, after explaining to the patient what is involved, including the prognosis, risks and any alternative options. The GMC, for example, says that a doctor under-taking an investigation or treatment has the responsibility of discussing it with the patient.[28] In some cases, this is impractical and the task can be delegated but only to someone who is suitably trained and qualified, familiar with what is being proposed and able to answer patients' questions. Junior hospital staff are sometimes expected to obtain patients' consent when they themselves do not have full knowledge and understanding of the condition, treatment and risks, and so cannot answer patients' queries. This is inappropriate. Health professionals who carry out this role 'must be competent to do so: either because they themselves carry out the procedure, or because they have received specialist training in advising patients about this procedure, have been assessed, are aware of their own knowledge limitations and are subject to audit'.[29] GMC advice also reminds doctors who delegate that they remain responsible for 'making sure that the patient has been given enough time and information to make an informed decision, and has given their consent' before the investiga-tion or treatment starts.[28]

In addition to the health professional who originally seeks consent, other colleagues can have a duty to check that it has been obtained. For example, one clinician may discuss an option and obtain the patient's consent, but if another carries it out, that practitioner needs to check that the patient's agreement was properly informed. Clinicians specialising in one procedure, such as anaesthesia, should check that consent is obtained for that aspect of treatment. The profes-sional with overall charge of a patient's care also has responsibilities for ensur-ing that correct procedures are followed and that valid consent has been obtained.

What type of consent or refusal is valid?

Implied decisions and explicit or express decisions

People often indicate consent or refusal through actions and body language rather than words. For example, they may ready themselves for an injection or may actively resist it. Consent or refusal indicated in this way is 'implied' and applies only to the immediate procedure, and not necessarily to any later tests or treatment. Passive acquiescence is not the same as implied 'consent'. It is not any form of consent at all unless patients are aware of what the interven-tion entails and that there is an option of refusing it.

Consent or refusal given verbally, in writing or in any other unambiguous way is commonly referred to as 'explicit' or 'express'. Explicit consent or refusal by an informed adult, following discussion of the various options, is the most reliable indication of what that person wants.

Written and verbal decisions

Most contact between patients and health professionals works on the basis of a verbal agreement rather than a formally signed document. In most cases, following discussion, the health professional will make a note of the conversation and a record of any tests or treatments agreed to in the patient's medical notes. In serious, controversial or risky cases, it is preferable to have a specific written record of the patient's consent or refusal. In particular, an advance refusal of future treatment needs to conform to specific legal criteria, including, where it applies to life-prolonging treatment, being in writing, signed and witnessed. Merely getting patients to sign a consent form does not necessarily mean that their consent is valid. It is unlikely to be so if they lacked a crucial bit of information. For most people, being asked to put their signature to a decision generally reinforces the point that an important choice is being made so that a signature is seen as evidence that some discussion took place. Ultimately, what counts is the quality and clarity of the information provided and the lack of any undue pressure on the patient.

Voluntary and pressured decisions: Do patients mean what they say?

In addition to having information and the mental capacity to make a valid decision, the patient's choice must also be voluntary. Various pressures, such as family influence, can affect a patient's choice and raise questions about the validity of the decision. The key question for health professionals is, at what point does an influence become so strong that it undermines a person's ability to make a free choice?

Undue influence

In some cases, trying to assess whether the patient can decide freely or is subject to some coercion or undue pressure can be very difficult and there is little guidance on how to do it. In many situations, health professionals simply do not have reliable evidence to make a judgement, but they should bear in mind the possibility of undue influence if patients make unexpected decisions which conflict with their known wishes or appear out of character. When people are out of their normal environment and tired, depressed or in pain, they can be more vulnerable to pressure, especially if the person persuading them is someone they perceive as authoritative. Most patients rely on family and friends for advice when faced with particularly hard choices, without that being seen as any kind of pressure. The usual example given of undue pressure is a legal case from 1992 which highlighted unacceptably intrusive family influence in a patient's decision to refuse treatment.

Refusal and undue influence: *Re T*

A 20-year-old woman, identified in court as 'T', was injured in a traffic accident when 34 weeks pregnant. Her mother was a Jehovah's Witness, although T was not known to be of that faith. In hospital, T refused a blood transfusion on various occasions, after spending time with her mother. A stillborn child was delivered, but T was unconscious by the time that her need for a blood transfusion became urgent. T's father and boyfriend did not believe she had made a genuine choice to refuse blood and went to court to challenge the validity of her advance refusal. Their challenge was successful and the blood transfusion was given. The Court of Appeal noted that while it was to be expected for patients to take advice before making a decision about treatment, in some situations their own wishes could be overborne by pressure from other people.[30] In such a situation, the patient's choice would be invalid. Lord Donaldson, Master of the Rolls, said that

'A special problem arises if at the time the decision is made the patient has been subjected to the influence of some third party. This is by no means to say that the patient is not entitled to receive and indeed invite assistance from others in reaching a decision, particularly from members of the family. But the doctors have to consider whether the decision is really that of the patient. The real question in each case, is does the patient really mean what he says or is he merely saying it for a quiet life, to satisfy someone else or because the advice and persuasion to which he has been subjected is such that he can no longer think and decide for himself? In other words, is it a decision expressed in form only, not in reality?'[31]

Where possible, health professionals should talk to patients privately to assess if pressure or coercion is a factor. The benefit of talking privately to the patient is demonstrated by a case that was brought to the BMA's attention. In this case the patient appeared to accept his family's view that he would not wish to have a blood transfusion, if needed, but privately expressed a wish to have it.

Case example – a pretence of refusal

An elderly patient had been admitted to hospital after a bad fall. A widower, he was at the centre of a close and caring family who were keen to be involved in all decisions affecting his care. On admission with his sons present, it was noted that he was a Jehovah's Witness and therefore refused all blood products. Once his family had left, however, the patient made clear that he was not committed to the religion in the way his children were and as his late wife had been. He asked that his medical record should be amended to show his willingness to have blood if that should prove necessary, but he stressed this decision should not be mentioned to his family. When they were present, he felt obliged to avoid upsetting them and did this by maintaining a pretence. He felt under pressure to refuse all blood
(Continued)

products. When having private discussions with health professionals, he was able to discuss the issue in a less constrained way and his confidential medical notes made clear his own views. His doctor pointed out that, if the family were kept in ignorance, they might give the wrong information in future if called upon to express what they believed to be his own wishes but, even so, the patient considered it would be too divisive within the family to attempt to talk frankly to his children.[32]

Another way in which undue pressure can be exerted is if health professionals themselves have strong feelings about what should happen and are not strictly objective, or if they inadvertently introduce an element of pressure by the very positive or negative manner in which they explain some options.

Alleged influence from a health professional: *Mrs U*

Mr and Mrs U hoped to have a child together. After an earlier vasectomy, Mr U agreed to the surgical retrieval of his sperm to be used in an IVF procedure, but the two consent forms he initially signed authorised different things. One was the form used by the centre providing the IVF treatment and this indicated that it would not perform posthumous insemination, if Mr U died before treatment had been completed. The second form he completed was that required by the Human Fertilisation and Embryology Act 1990 and authorised the continued storage and use of sperm after the donor's death. When Mr and Mrs U had a planning meeting with the centre's specialist nursing sister, she asked Mr U to alter this second form and withdraw his permission for the continued storage and use of his sperm in the event of his death. He did so. Mr U then unexpectedly died after the first unsuccessful IVF procedure and Mrs U argued that the retraction of his consent to his sperm being stored after death was invalid due to the nursing sister's undue influence. The fact that the nurse personally supported the centre's opposition to posthumous insemination was not in dispute, but Mrs U argued that this health professional had given them the impression that the IVF treatment could not proceed unless Mr U withdrew his consent to posthumous storage and use. Even if Mr U had been given that impression, the court of first instance decided that it did not amount to undue influence. It rejected the assumption that he no longer thought for himself when he signed it, given that Mr U had been an able, intelligent and educated man, in good health at the time.

On appeal, Mrs U argued that the test for undue influence had been set too high and the real issue was whether or not Mr U thought he had a choice to stick by his first decision. The appeal court rejected this too and did not believe that the nursing sister exerted undue pressure. It drew a distinction between this kind of case and others in which someone uses their influence because they have something to gain; the IVF centre did not benefit from Mr U's withdrawal of consent. It said that the letter of the form refusing sperm storage should be relied upon, unless it could be demonstrated that it was invalid as a result of something like forgery, the use of duress or a mistake about the nature of the form being signed.[33]

Although the court concluded that, in this case, the nursing sister had not pressured the patient, health professionals should be alert to the susceptibility of some vulnerable patients to decide in a way that pleases others, including their relatives or the medical staff. Patients who feel greatly indebted to the clinician treating them can be motivated to comply with whatever that person suggests. There can also be a temptation for health professionals to try to persuade patients to agree to things which pose no harm to them but significantly help someone else. An example is seeking consent to test a patient's blood samples after a doctor has sustained a needlestick injury. If the patient refuses, that must be respected. People detained by the police or immigration services are often unaware of whether or not they have the right to refuse some tests or procedures, like intimate body searches.[34] Information should always be given in a balanced way, and if a particular treatment or course of action is being recommended, it should be explained to the patient why this is the case.[35]

Patients agreeing to a procedure to benefit someone else may be doing so voluntarily or they may be subject to emotional pressure. Volunteering for genetic tests to help a family member, donating tissue or gametes, or acting as a surrogate mother are the kinds of scenario when emotional pressure can be an issue. Health professionals should therefore be sensitive to this.

Cultural influences

Health professionals also need to be sensitive to cultural issues that may impact on the consent process. In some cultures, for example, it is common practice for a woman's husband or father to make all important decisions including those concerning health care. If adults with capacity wish to involve others in the decision-making process, then this wish should be facilitated. Legally, however, it is still important that the patient himself or herself gives consent to the procedure and that the consent is voluntarily given and free from pressure.

The influence of incentives

Healthy volunteers are usually paid to participate in clinical trials run by commercial organisations. In these cases, consent can be influenced by the offer of financial or other incentives. The RECs, which scrutinise research protocols, need to ensure that the financial or other benefits given to participants are proportionate to the time and effort involved so that healthy volunteers, in particular, are not unduly tempted or 'induced' to take part. 'Inducement' implies offering a temptation for people in need of money to act contrary to their better judgement by accepting risks that they would not otherwise take or to volunteer more frequently than is advisable. Patients with a serious condition may also effectively be coerced if they are led to believe that participation in research might give them early access to new treatment or better care and attention. People in a situation of dependency can be vulnerable to pressure, possibly without being aware of it. Residents in a care home or other institution might feel obliged to agree to be included in research, for example, or worry that they will be seen as uncooperative if they do not agree. It is a clear responsibility of RECs to minimise the likelihood of these instances arising.

Documenting the decision

It is unnecessary to document patient consent for every treatment or test provided, but it is advisable to record the patient's agreement to anything controversial, risky or very complex. Patient refusals are rarer but can have very significant ramifications and so should be documented, especially when they concern withdrawing or withholding life-prolonging treatment.

Documenting consent

In many cases, there is no need for a consent form, but written consent should be obtained when

- 'the investigation or treatment or procedure is complex or involves significant risks
- there may be significant consequences for the patient's employment, or social or personal life
- providing clinical care is not the primary purpose of the investigation or treatment
- the treatment is part of a research programme or is an innovative treatment designed specifically for the patient's benefit'.[36]

Some other situations legally require a signed consent form, including some procedures covered by the Human Fertilisation and Embryology Act.[37] Doctors and other health professionals whose role involves seeking patient consent should familiarise themselves with guidance relevant to their area of practice.

Documenting refusal

As discussed in Chapter 2, patients can reject medical advice or decide to discharge themselves from care prematurely. Sometimes they are asked to sign a declaration that they refuse treatment and accept responsibility for declining what was recommended. Courts have said that, for their own protection, hospital authorities should keep a copy of patients' written assurances that they understand the nature of the treatment and the reasons why it was proposed, as well as the risks and likely prognosis resulting from the decision to refuse it. When patients are unwilling to sign such a declaration, their refusal of treatment should be noted in the health record, showing that a discussion took place about the implications of refusing.[38]

Many Jehovah's Witnesses refuse any treatment involving the use of blood or blood products and carry a card making their position clear. Ideally, their medical notes should indicate whether or not they would be willing to accept their own blood donated in advance (predeposit) or the use of blood salvage equipment that recycles their blood in a continuous circuit. Patients refusing blood products should be given the opportunity to discuss other possible options, such as 'bloodless' medical procedures. While health professionals should not make assumptions about what patients might want, they should ensure that refusals are clearly documented in the records, including whether the refusal is to apply even where life is at risk. Documentation is only useful if it is properly reviewed by those managing the patient's care.

Treatment without consent: *Patrick McGovern*

The Royal Devon and Exeter Hospital paid out of court compensation to a patient who was a Jehovah's Witness after a failure to take proper note of the fact that he opposed all use of blood products. The patient had been attending the hospital for 20 years and, as was clearly documented in his record, he had repeatedly refused blood transfusions in various life-threatening situations during that time. In 2001, when needing treatment for a renal condition, he was given a transfusion in error without his consent. Although dialysis and a blood transfusion would have been the usual procedures for his condition, an assumption about its acceptability should not have been made without asking him or consulting his medical record, which showed that he was unlikely to agree.[39]

Documenting views about future medical treatment

In some situations, verbal statements can ensure that patients are not given treatment they do not want. When nearing the end of life, for example, treatment plans and their preferences are generally discussed with patients so that the palliative care team is aware of them and the verbal wishes are recorded in patients' notes. In other circumstances, verbal refusals, if witnessed or supported by other strong evidence, can be hugely important (see the case of *XB* later in this chapter).

In many cases, people express – but fail to document – their wish not to be kept alive if they had no hope of recovery from an incapacitating injury. Most people never imagine it will happen to them and so do not make formal provision for it. If it does occur, the courts may have to rule on whether the individual's remarks were a genuine decision or a passing reaction to some news item. In the absence of clear documentation, a judgement has to be made about how much weight should be placed on what may only have been intended as a casual remark. When patients have a confirmed intention to refuse treatment, and they want to ensure it will be respected when they lose capacity, they need to make a formal advance decision refusing treatment which complies with the legal requirements.

Failure to make a formal advance decision: *Re M*

In 2003, a woman known as 'M' contracted viral encephalitis, which left her with extensive brain damage. She was first diagnosed as being in a vegetative, and then a minimally conscious, state which left her totally dependent. She received clinically assisted nutrition and hydration which her family eventually asked for a court order to withdraw. The case was heard in the Court of Protection where M's family reported her as having said on various occasions that she would not want to be kept alive in such a condition but she had made no formal advance decision refusing treatment. Nor had she appointed a health and welfare attorney with the power to make the decision on her behalf. (This option is discussed in Chapter 4.) The Court ruled that it would be unlawful to withdraw M's nutrition and hydration.[40] In the absence of a clear and valid advance refusal of treatment, the judgment made clear that health professionals have a strong obligation to preserve life.[41] The judgment also reiterated the requirement for court review of all decisions relating to withdrawing or withholding clinically assisted nutrition and hydration from patients in a vegetative or minimally conscious state.

To avoid doubt, some people document their preferences about medical treatment for a future time when they have lost mental capacity. If they retain capacity, the advance decision has no effect. Advance choices are always superseded by patients' current views, as long as they have the mental capacity to make the decision in question.

Advance requests

Some people draft general statements, while others make a specific request for some kind of care. Either can be helpful when health professionals later assess what would be in the person's best interests, but only valid advance decisions refusing treatment are legally binding. Patients can specify in advance the kinds of care they would like to receive. Sometimes, this can be the basis of a care plan agreed in advance between clinicians and patients with a known diagnosis. While health professionals bear all treatment requests in mind, they are not obliged to implement them if there are clinical reasons, or other strong arguments, for not doing so. Advance statements cannot authorise anything that individuals could not expect to receive if their request was contemporaneous, so they cannot demand treatment that is not clinically appropriate.

Request for treatment: *Burke*

Mr Burke had cerebellar ataxia with peripheral neuropathy, a progressively degenerative condition that follows a similar course to multiple sclerosis. As his illness progressed, he knew he would lose the ability to swallow and would need clinically assisted nutrition and hydration. The evidence was that he was likely to retain his mental capacity until close to death, but he was worried that if he became incapable, his wish to receive artificial feeding might be ignored. GMC guidance at that time implied that the decision would rest with his doctors and they would have the discretion to withhold or withdraw clinically assisted nutrition and hydration if they felt that was appropriate. Mr Burke argued that the GMC's advice was incompatible with the European Human Rights Convention and the judge at first instance agreed, but this was overturned by the Court of Appeal. It was argued that there was no question of Mr Burke being denied clinically assisted nutrition and hydration because he had made clear in advance that he wanted them. The court said that autonomy and the right to self-determination do not entitle the patient to insist on receiving a particular medical treatment, regardless of the nature of the treatment. The doctor's duty of care, however, included the obligation to take reasonable steps to prolong a patient's life when that was known to be the patient's wish.[42]

The duty to provide life-prolonging treatment in compliance with a patient's known wishes does not extend to treatment which doctors believe is not clinically appropriate. What is reasonable in each situation needs to be judged in the context of each case.

Advance decisions refusing treatment: The law in England and Wales

The law on advance decisions refusing treatment varies across the UK and, where legal criteria are spelled out in statute, patients' wishes may not necessarily be carried out if the documentation does not meet the legal requirements. In England and Wales, the legal criteria are set out in the Mental Capacity Act 2005. The Act's powers apply to advance *refusals* of treatment which are as legally effective as a contemporaneous refusal if

- those who made advance refusals have lost their mental capacity but were mentally capable adults (aged 18 or older) when they made the decision;
- they clearly specified (in lay terms if necessary) the treatment they wanted to refuse and the circumstances in which their refusal would apply;
- they did not change their minds while they had the capacity to do so;
- after the decision was made, they did not appoint an attorney to make the specified decision;
- they have not subsequently done anything inconsistent with that refusal or which would imply the decision should be disregarded;
- if the advance refusal applies to life-sustaining treatment, it must be in writing, signed, witnessed and must contain a statement that it is to apply even where life is at risk.[43]

The Mental Capacity Act code of practice suggests that advance refusals should include

- the name, address and date of birth of the person making the advance decision
- the name and address of the person's GP
- a statement that the document should be used when the person lacks capacity
- a clear statement of the decision, the treatment to be refused and the circumstances in which the decision will apply
- the date the document was written and the date of any subsequent reviews
- the signatures of the person making the decision and of a witness.[44]

In the case of women of childbearing age, unless the documentation clearly spells out that it is intended to apply during pregnancy, it is unlikely to be valid if the patient is pregnant when she loses capacity.

Documentation of advance refusal: XB

An unusual case concerning refusal of life-prolonging treatment was decided by the courts in spring 2012. A man, known as XB, suffering from motor neurone disease, had made clear his advance refusal of life-prolonging treatment in November 2011, despite only being able to communicate by eye movements. His wife had found a template for it on the internet and the issue of treatment refusal had been discussed with the patient on various occasions. XB used eye movements to express his wishes that life-prolonging treatment not be given, and this decision was witnessed by his wife, a doctor, a social worker and a carer. Another of XB's carers, however, had reservations as to whether he had really agreed to the treatment not being provided and the case went to court. Mrs Justice Theis ruled that XB had the mental capacity to make the decision when the document was drawn up in 2011 and emphasised the vital importance of clarity in such documents.[45]

Advance refusals in Scotland

In Scotland, there is no specific legislation covering advance decisions refusing treatment, but the code of practice accompanying the Adults with Incapacity (Scotland) Act says that where an explicit advance refusal of treatment exists and applies to the patient's circumstances, it may be binding.[46] It is likely to carry weight if made orally or in writing to a solicitor, health professional or other independent professional person. To avoid any confusion, it is advisable to include similar information to the points listed earlier for England and Wales, but the statement should at least make clear

- that the person was an adult with mental capacity when the statement was made
- that the person had access to sufficient, accurate information to make an informed choice
- the decision, in terms of the treatment to be refused and the circumstances in which the decision is to apply
- that no undue influence was brought to bear on the person making the decision.

Advance refusals in Northern Ireland

As yet, Northern Ireland has no legislation on this topic and English precedents (such as the *T* case mentioned previously) are not binding there, but it is likely that Northern Ireland courts would still take a similar approach. Patients wanting to make an advance refusal are generally advised to document them in a similar way as they would do if in England or Wales, that is, to make clear that the decision was made by an informed adult with mental capacity who was not under pressure to choose that option. The statement should also specify the circumstances in which the refusal will apply.

Implementing the decision

Does having consent mean the procedure must proceed?

Once obtained and (where appropriate) documented, patients' consent or refusal needs to be put into effect. The fact that patients have authorised or requested something does not necessarily mean it has to be provided, but their consent opens up the opportunity to deliver that treatment, if it is clinically appropriate, affordable and available. A relatively common example is that of patients requesting that resuscitation be attempted if they suffer a cardiac arrest, even when they know that there is little chance of it succeeding in their particular circumstances. Health professionals need to consider whether it is possible to comply with patients' wishes, without causing harm either to the patient or, by wasting limited resources, to others awaiting treatment. In some cases the clinical situation may change so that a procedure for which the patient has given consent is no longer deemed to be clinically appropriate. There is no obligation to provide treatment simply because consent has been obtained.

When the treatment requested is life-saving, health professionals have a legal and ethical duty to assess whether it should go ahead. Article 2 of the European Human Rights Convention imposes an obligation to protect life, but its scope is limited; life does not have to be prolonged in all cases and at all costs, but factors such as the individual's known wishes and the likelihood of the treatment succeeding are key considerations. In some circumstances, advance requests for specific life-prolonging treatment, such as clinically assisted nutrition and hydration, should be followed (see the case of *Burke* mentioned previously). The law in this area is complex and so it is advisable to take legal advice in such situations.

A last word about patient consent and refusal

Patient consent has long been seen as a cornerstone of medical ethics. Refusal of treatment is relatively rare and often takes health professionals by surprise, despite some very high-profile legal cases. We are accustomed to the idea that respect for autonomy means a focus on valid consent and are sometimes less able to envisage how it equally means respecting a patient's refusal. Accepting patients' rights to refuse can be challenging and immensely difficult in cases like that of Kerrie Wooltorton, whose life could have been saved, if only she had agreed. In this chapter, we have tried to give equal attention to consent and refusal. We acknowledge the fact that, as medical technology develops ever more sophisticated techniques for prolonging life and society emphasises self-determination, people are more aware of their rights to limit what is done to, and for, them especially at the end of life.

References

1 For example, consent forms are a legal requirement under certain parts of the Human Fertilisation and Embryology Act 1990 (as amended).

2 See, for example: General Medical Council (2008) *Consent: Patients and Doctors Making Decisions Together*, GMC, London; Department of Health (2009) *Reference Guide to Consent for Examination or Treatment*, 2nd edn, DH, London; Scottish Executive Health Department (2006) *A Good Practice Guide on Consent for Health Professionals in*

NHS Scotland, SEHD, Edinburgh; Welsh Assembly Government (2009) *Reference Guide for Consent to Examination or Treatment*, WAG, Cardiff; Department of Health, Social Services and Public Safety (2003) *Reference Guide to Consent for Examination, Treatment or Care*, DHSSPS, Belfast; The Medical and Dental Defence Union of Scotland (2007) *Essential Guide to Consent*, MDDUS, Glasgow.

3   General Medical Council (2008) *Consent: Patients and Doctors Making Decisions Together*, GMC, London, para 79.

4   GMC Professional Conduct Committee hearing, 27–30 May 2002.

5   General Medical Council (2008) *Consent: Patients and Doctors Making Decisions Together*, GMC, London, para 9.

6   Association of Anaesthetists of Great Britain and Ireland (2010) *Pre-operative Assessment and Patient Preparation: the Role of the Anaesthetist*, AAGBI, London.

7   General Medical Council (2008) *Consent: Patients and Doctors Making Decisions Together*, GMC, London, p.5.

8   *Sidaway v Board of Governors of the Bethlem Royal Hospital* [1985] AC 871.

9   *Bolam v Friern Hospital Management Committee* [1957] 2 All ER 118.

10 *Sidaway v Board of Governors of the Bethlem Royal Hospital* [1985] AC 871:888-9.

11 *Pearce v United Bristol Healthcare NHS Trust* [1998] EWCA Civ 865.

12 *Chester v Afshar* [2005] 1 AC 134.

13 *Chester v Afshar* [2005] 1 AC 134:144.

14 *Chester v Afshar* [2005] 1 AC 134:143.

15 General Medical Council (2008) *Consent: Patients and Doctors Making Decisions Together*, GMC, London, p.34.

16 Department of Health (2009) *Reference Guide to Consent for Examination or Treatment*, 2nd edn, DH, London, para 18.

17 Mason JK and Laurie GT (2011) *Mason and McCall Smith's Law and Medical Ethics*, 8th edn, Oxford University Press, Oxford, p.108, para 4.108.

18 *Birch v University College London Hospital NHS Foundation Trust* [2008] 104 BMLR 168.

19 General Medical Council (2008) *Consent: Patients and Doctors Making Decisions Together*, GMC, London, para 17.

20 Department of Health (2009) *Reference Guide to Consent for Examination or Treatment*, 2nd edn, DH, London, p.13, para 20; Department of Health, Social Services and Public Safety (2003) *Reference Guide to Consent for Examination, Treatment or Care*, DHSSPS, Belfast, p.7, para 4.8.

21 The BMA produces detailed guidance in: British Medical Association (2012) *Medical Ethics Today. The BMA's Handbook of Ethics and Law*, 3rd edn, Wiley-Blackwell, Chichester, chapter 14; The GMC also publishes guidance on research ethics: General Medical Council (2010) *Supplementary Guidance: Good Practice in Research and Consent to Research*, GMC, London.

22 General Medical Council (2008) *Consent: Patients and Doctors Making Decisions Together*, GMC, London, para 14; British Medical Association (2009) *Consent Tool Kit*, 5th edn, BMA, London, card 3.

23 Treatment must be under the direction of the approved clinician in charge of the treatment, which must be for the patient's mental disorder or the symptoms of it

(Mental Health Act 1983, s 63), or in respect of certain treatments under the Mental Health Act 1983, s 62.

24 *Re B (Adult: Refusal of Medical Treatment)* [2002] 2 All ER 449.

25 Anon. (2009) Doctors 'forced' to allow suicide. *BBC News Online* (Oct 1). Available at: http://www.bbc.co.uk/news (accessed 30 August 2012).

26 McLean S (2009) Sheila McLean on advance directives and the case of Kerrie Wooltorton. *BMJ Group blogs* (Oct 1). Available at: http://blogs.bmj.com (accessed 30 August 2012).

27 *Re C (Adult: Refusal of Medical Treatment)* [1994] 1 All ER 819; Mental Capacity Act 2005, s 2; Department for Constitutional Affairs (2007) *Mental Capacity Act 2005 Code of Practice*, The Stationery Office, London.

28 General Medical Council (2008) *Consent: Patients and Doctors Making Decisions Together*, GMC, London, paras 26–27.

29 Department of Health (2001) *Good Practice in Consent Implementation Guide: Consent to Examination or Treatment*, DH, London, p.20, para 3; Welsh Assembly Government (2002) *Good Practice in Consent Implementation Guide: Consent to Examination or Treatment*, WAG, Cardiff, p.17, para 3.

30 *Re T (Adult: Refusal of Treatment)* [1992] 4 All ER 649.

31 *Re T (Adult: Refusal of Treatment)* [1992] 4 All ER 649:662.

32 The implications of this case are discussed further in: British Medical Association (2009) *The Ethics of Caring for Older People*, 2nd edn, Wiley-Blackwell, Chichester, p.16.

33 *Centre for Reproductive Medicine v Mrs U* [2002], unreported. Discussed by: Stewart C, Lynch A. (2003) Undue influence, consent and medical treatment. *J R Soc Med* **96**, 598–601.

34 The medical care of people in various forms of detention is discussed in detail in: British Medical Association (2012) *Medical Ethics Today. The BMA's Handbook of Ethics and Law*, 3rd edn, Wiley-Blackwell, Chichester, chapter 17.

35 General Medical Council (2008) *Consent: Patients and Doctors Making Decisions Together*, GMC, London, para 19.

36 General Medical Council (2008) *Consent: Patients and Doctors Making Decisions Together*, GMC, London, para 49.

37 See, for example: Human Fertilisation and Embryology Act 1990, (as amended), Sch 3.

38 *St George's Healthcare NHS Trust v S, R v Collins and others, ex parte S* [1998] 3 All ER 673.

39 *Patrick McGovern v Royal Devon & Exeter Healthcare NHS Trust* [2004], unreported.

40 *W (by her litigation friend, B) v M (by her litigation friend, the Official Solicitor) and others* [2011] EWHC 2443 (Fam).

41 *W (by her litigation friend, B) v M (by her litigation friend, the Official Solicitor) and others* [2011] EWHC 2443 (Fam) at 249.

42 *R (on the application of Burke) v General Medical Council* [2005] 2 FLR 1223.

43 Department for Constitutional Affairs (2007) *Mental Capacity Act 2005 Code of Practice*, The Stationery Office, London, p.167.

44   Department for Constitutional Affairs (2007) *Mental Capacity Act 2005 Code of Practice*, The Stationery Office, London, p.164.

45   *The X Primary Care Trust v XB & Anor* [2012] EWHC 1390 (Fam).

46   Scottish Executive (2010) *Adults with Incapacity (Scotland) Act 2000 Code of Practice (Third Edition) for Practitioners Authorised to Carry Out Medical Treatment or Research under Part 5 of the Act*. SG/2010/57, SEHD, Edinburgh, para 2.30.

4: Treating adults who lack capacity

10 things you need to know about . . . treating adults who lack capacity

- All adults are assumed to have capacity unless there is evidence to the contrary.
- Unwise decisions are not in themselves evidence that an adult lacks capacity.
- Patients should be encouraged to make all the decisions they can for themselves and all reasonable efforts should be made to enhance their decision-making capacity.
- Mentally disordered patients may still have decision-making capacity.
- Patients' capacity has to be commensurate with the gravity or complexity of the decision.
- If a patient's incapacity is temporary or fluctuating and the decision can reasonably wait until there is some improvement, it should be deferred.
- Decisions made on behalf of adults lacking capacity should be based on their best interests (in England, Wales and Northern Ireland) or what would benefit them (in Scotland).
- Actions on behalf of adults who lack capacity should be the less restrictive option.
- In some instances, incapacitated adults can be treated using either mental capacity or mental health legislation.
- Care or treatment of an incapacitated adult that amounts to a deprivation of liberty requires special safeguards.

Setting the scene

When patients lack the mental capacity to make a specific choice, someone else has to make the decision for them, based on a judgement of their best interests (in England, Wales and Northern Ireland) or what would benefit them (in Scotland). Caring for such patients presents challenges. They should be supported to decide as much as they can for themselves but because of their vulnerability, they also need to be protected. The nature of the doctor–patient partnership changes from focusing mainly on patient autonomy to a more welfare-oriented approach. Health professionals have to balance encouragement for patient self-determination with a willingness to intervene, if necessary, to safeguard the welfare of those whose capacity is impaired.

Everyday Medical Ethics and Law, First Edition. Ann Sommerville.
© 2013 BMA Medical Ethics Department. Published 2013 by John Wiley & Sons, Ltd.

Factors that contribute to a conclusion that patients have capacity include the following:

- they have the ability to make a choice between the available options
- they understand what is being asked and why a choice is needed
- they are able to remember information essential to the decision
- they are aware of the alternatives and know the risks and benefits
- they understand how the decision is relevant to themselves
- they know that they can refuse whatever is on offer and what the likely outcome would be
- they are able to communicate their choice.

People with a serious mental disorder do not necessarily lack the mental capacity to make valid choices, but even when they have the mental capacity to refuse treatment for their mental disorder, they may be overruled. If they are detained under mental health legislation, treatment for the mental disorder can be provided without consent and their refusal is not binding on health professionals. The criteria are set out in the Mental Health Act 1983 (England and Wales), the Mental Health (Care and Treatment) (Scotland) Act 2003 and the Mental Health (Northern Ireland) Order 1986. (The law in Northern Ireland is undergoing review, but in the interim, existing legislation needs to be followed.) The mental health legislation is complex and is not our focus here, but the respective codes of practice for these pieces of legislation provide detailed guidance.[1]

This chapter sets out the law and ethics for the treatment of adults who cannot decide for themselves but do not necessarily meet the criteria for compulsory treatment without consent. In England and Wales the relevant legislation is the Mental Capacity Act 2005 (MCA). In Scotland it is the Adults with Incapacity (Scotland) Act 2000 (AWISA). In Northern Ireland, at the time of writing, decisions are still made under the common law.

In some instances, patients with impaired capacity could either be treated under the mental health or the capacity legislation. In England, the court has ruled that where the grounds for compulsory treatment under the Mental Health Act are met, this Act has primacy and should be used in preference to relying on the MCA.[2]

Common questions asked about the care of adults who lack capacity

- Who should assess a patient's capacity? Is it better if it is a practitioner familiar to the patient, such as a GP, or does assessment generally need to be done by a specialist?

(Continued)

- How do I work out what is in the best interests of an unconscious patient whom I have never seen before and who might have had strong opinions about the treatment I propose?
- If relatives have power of attorney for a patient, can they make medical decisions as well as financial ones?
- What does an assessment of capacity involve?
- What is a certificate of incapacity and who issues it?

Some of the most difficult dilemmas arise where patients lack capacity and decisions are needed about whether continuing to provide life-prolonging treatment would be in their best interests. As with other areas of practice, this involves identifying all relevant information, including the principles established in the law and professional guidelines, considering the issue from the perspective of all relevant parties and weighing up the various options. The fact that the court will ultimately make the decision in some cases (see, e.g. the case of *Re M*) does not absolve health professionals from making difficult ethical judgements. The information provided in this chapter is intended to assist with the evidence-gathering exercise that forms a crucial part of ethical decision making.

The law concerning treatment and non-treatment of adults lacking capacity to consent

General legal principles across the UK

The law varies across the UK, but some fundamental principles apply throughout. These include

- the presumption that all adults have capacity unless there is evidence to the contrary
- people can make unwise choices if they have capacity to make that particular decision
- actions on behalf of incapacitated adults should be the less restrictive option and should maximise their freedom
- decisions should be based on patients' best interests and what would benefit them
- if the patient made an advance refusal, which is valid and applicable to the current situation, this is legally binding.

England and Wales

The MCA covers England and Wales and provides a legal framework for making decisions and choices on behalf of incapacitated people aged 16 and over. Health professionals working with such patients need to be familiar with the Act and with its code of practice, which provides detailed guidance.[3] The first step must be to establish that the person lacks capacity to make the decision in question or is unable to communicate it, as a result of an 'impairment of, or disturbance in the functioning of, the mind or brain'.[4] Patients cannot be treated as unable to decide until all practicable steps to help them to do so have been unsuccessful. If this is the case, all subsequent decisions must be based on an assessment of that person's best interests. The MCA states that an action or intervention in connection with the patient's care or treatment is lawful (and health professionals have protection from liability) so long as the decision maker has a *reasonable belief* that the patient lacks capacity to consent and that the decision is in that person's best interests. It applies to treatment and also to ancillary procedures, such as taking a person to hospital. With specific safeguards, the Act also permits incapacitated adults to be enrolled in certain forms of research which may not be directly in their best interests.

Scotland

In the absence of evidence to the contrary, the AWISA also assumes that people aged 16 or over have capacity to make valid decisions. Health professionals working with incapacitated adults should be familiar with the Act and its code of practice.[5] Any intervention in the affairs of an incapacitated adult must be intended to benefit that person and the health professional proposing it should be satisfied that the desired benefit cannot reasonably be achieved by other less restrictive means. Patients should be encouraged to participate in the decision if possible, and their known past and present wishes must be taken into consideration. In non-emergency situations, or where there is a proxy decision maker, a certificate of incapacity must be issued in order to provide care or treatment. A welfare attorney or a welfare guardian can also give consent to treatment on behalf of the incapacitated adult.

Certificate of incapacity and the general authority to treat

Except for emergencies (and some treatment under mental health legislation) incapacitated adults can only be treated in Scotland once a certificate of incapacity has been issued. This is usually made out by the health professional proposing the treatment and provides a general authority to treat. Doctors, dentists, optometrists and nurses can issue a certificate for care in their specific areas, once trained in accordance with the regulations.[6] A medical examination can require a certificate but, if non-invasive, does not necessarily do so, although it should be considered if the patient is unwilling to be examined.[7] The certificate sets out the nature of the patient's incapacity, what treatment is proposed and the length of time the authority remains valid. Even where the patient has a proxy with welfare powers, an incapacity certificate must still be issued before treatment is given, except in emergencies. The general authority to treat cannot be used when it is known that a proxy has been appointed. The Public Guardian keeps a list of registered proxies appointed under the Act.

The patient's capacity should be periodically reviewed and, if appropriate, the certificate renewed particularly if new treatment options are available. When long-term care is needed, a separate certificate is not essential for each intervention. For complex and ongoing care, it may be appropriate to complete the certificate in terms of a treatment plan (examples are given in the code of practice[8]). This can set out treatment that it is reasonable to anticipate in the future, bearing in mind that the patient may be able to consent to some interventions. All adults are entitled to basic care which includes the provision of food and fluids orally, mobility support, basic hygiene and pain control. These may need to be included in the plan.[9] Treatment plans cannot authorise treatments, such as serious surgery, where written consent would be required if the adult retained capacity. In these circumstances a separate certificate of capacity must be issued.

Common law in Northern Ireland

Legislation is still being developed in Northern Ireland, where legislative reform was first proposed in 2007[10] and some policy proposals were suggested. These included the need for a single piece of legislation encompassing both mental capacity and mental health provisions for adults (aged 16 or over) and reflecting the four principles of autonomy, justice, benefit and avoidance of harm. If and when it emerges, the legislation is likely to echo principles already embodied in the English, Welsh and Scottish law, including provisions for adults, when they have capacity, to nominate an attorney to make later decisions when their capacity is lost.

In the meantime, treatment for incapacitated adults is regulated by common law. All adults are presumed to have capacity and their choices are not invalid merely because they seem unwise. When adults lack capacity, no one else has the power to consent to medical treatment on their behalf, but treatment can be provided if it is necessary and in the patient's best interests. The doctrine of necessity emerged from the need to give lawful emergency treatment to adults who were unconscious and unable to consent. In such cases, health professionals are justified in providing treatment that is immediately necessary to preserve life or to prevent a serious deterioration in the patient's condition, unless there is a valid and applicable advance refusal. (See Chapter 3.)

Assessing patients' capacity

People make choices all the time, ranging from relatively trivial decisions to others involving life-changing implications. All adults are legally assumed to be able to do this without interference, even if some of their choices seem bizarre or risky. The fact that an individual makes decisions that others would consider eccentric does not mean that the individual lacks capacity – it is the capacity to make the decision, not the nature of the decision itself, that is relevant (although bizarre decisions that appear out of character for the individual may raise questions about the individual's capacity that need further investigation). When, for example, after several highly dangerous and unsuccessful expeditions, the explorer Shackleton sought volunteers for another risky venture (describing it as 'hazardous journey, small wages, bitter cold, long months of complete darkness, constant danger and safe return doubtful'[11]), 5,000 applied without apparently raising questions about his, or their, judgement.

Major decisions generally have serious consequences, which need to be taken into account. An assessment of mental capacity is required when evidence suggests that people cannot understand that a particular choice has consequences, or are unable to envisage or weigh up the outcome, or are unable to see how it relates to themselves. Writing a will leaving all your money to yourself, for example, would suggest that you have not understood the nature of death or of wills.

What is mental capacity?

Capacity is the ability to do something. Mental capacity refers to a person's ability to make decisions that may have legal consequences. It could relate to making a will, agreeing to a contract, getting married or authorising or refusing medical treatment. Doctors can be asked to assess a patient's mental capacity to do any of these things. They need to be clear about the particular decision that is in question and know the relevant legal test for it.[12]

How is it assessed?

While all adults are legally assumed to have the ability to make choices on their own behalf, highly controversial or dangerous decisions, by people who are vulnerable in some way, can require more evidence of decision-making ability. The law recognises this by setting tests of capacity that must be applied, in relation to each particular decision, according to the gravity of the choice to be made. As a crude generalisation, if all the medical experts recommend a proven and necessary treatment that offers clear benefits, without side effects or drawbacks, the capacity of a patient who accepts treatment is unlikely to be questioned (unless there is a specific reason why capacity is in doubt). If they refused it however, when all the other indicators suggest that they would normally want to preserve their health, that refusal would probably trigger more discussion and might raise questions about capacity that need to be further explored. Obviously, health professionals are not always aware of patients' views and values when life-saving treatment is refused, which is why it is important to approach any assessment of capacity in an individualised way.

What factors indicate capacity?

Some fundamental principles are agreed as indicating that people have mental capacity. These are reflected in the codes of practice for the legislation in England and Wales[3] and Scotland[13] and are also the basis for the common law test of capacity in Northern Ireland, which was developed in the case of *Re C*[14]. The fact that people are deluded about some quite important things in their life does not necessarily mean they lack capacity to make decisions. In the *Re C* case, for example, the patient contradicted the opinion of all his doctors, believing that he himself was a world-famous clinician. In this he was mistaken since he had no medical knowledge, but his refusal to accept his doctors' recommendation was held to be a valid choice, which he had the capacity to make. When patients are unconscious, their lack of capacity is obvious but, in most other circumstances, they are likely to be able to make some decisions.

Valid refusal of treatment by a mentally ill patient: *Re C*

C had paranoid schizophrenia and was detained in Broadmoor high-security hospital. He developed gangrene in his leg but refused to agree to an amputation, which doctors considered essential to save his life. C said that he would rather die with two feet than live with one. His decision was questioned as he was clearly deluded about some things, including his belief that he had an international career in medicine. The case went to court,

(Continued)

which upheld C's decision. It emphasised that the fact that people have a mental illness does not automatically mean they lack capacity to make decisions about medical treatment. Patients who have capacity (i.e. who can understand, believe, retain and weigh the necessary information) can make their own decisions to refuse treatment, even if those decisions appear irrational to the doctor or may place the patient's health or their life at risk. The court concluded that the medical evidence failed to demonstrate that C's schizophrenia affected his decision-making ability in respect of an issue of treatment unrelated to the schizophrenia. He could therefore still make a valid decision about amputation, as long as he could understand and retain the relevant information and, in his own way, believe it. The hospital was not entitled to amputate his leg without his express written consent, nor could it do so in the future, even if his mental capacity deteriorated, as he had made his views very clear.[14]

What factors indicate impaired capacity?

Health professionals must be careful to avoid discriminatory judgements based on factors such as age, history or disability, but patients' behaviour can be among the indicators of impaired capacity, as can their mood disorders, delusions and other abnormalities of thought. Disjointed flow of speech or conversations which move in a disordered way between random topics can also indicate abnormal thought processes. None of these things necessarily mean that the person cannot make valid choices, nor does the existence of a diagnosed mental disorder or learning disability. Such factors emphasise the importance of an individualised approach, combined with a focus on the particular question to be decided. In Scotland, the code of practice accompanying the legislation makes clear that people should not be seen as lacking capacity solely because they have a psychotic illness, dementia, communication problems, brain injury or physical disability.[15]

In England and Wales, the Mental Capacity Act says that when patients have 'an impairment of, or a disturbance in the functioning of, the mind or brain', they lack capacity if, as a result of that impairment or disturbance, they are unable to understand information relevant to the decision, retain it and weigh it up, or if they are unable to communicate their choice.[16] Similar provisions are set out in the Scottish legislation, which defines adults as lacking capacity when incapable of making, communicating or understanding decisions, or remembering their decisions, by reason of mental disorder or of inability to communicate because of physical disability or neurological impairment.[17] In contrast with the judgment in the *Re C* case, another court decision highlighted how people may be incapable of making a valid choice, even if they understand what is at stake but their thinking is dominated by fear or some other overwhelming emotion (both of these cases were heard before the MCA, and its statutory test of capacity, came into effect).

Refusal of treatment due to phobia: *MB*

MB was 40 weeks pregnant, with a fetus in the breech position, but she refused a caesarean section due to her fear of needles. The Court of Appeal considered whether she had the capacity to make a valid refusal and concluded that her needle phobia dominated her mind and made her unable to consider anything else. She was found to lack capacity to refuse treatment. As a consequence, it was lawful for the doctors to administer anaesthetic in an emergency, if they believed that would be in MB's best interests. The court also said that MB was more likely to suffer significant long-term harm from death or injury to the baby than from receiving the anaesthetic against her wishes. It was likely, therefore, that should an anaesthetic become necessary, it would be in her best interests to administer it.[18]

In most cases, decisions about mental capacity to consent to treatment are made by the clinician in charge of the patient's care. When there are serious doubts or disputes about an individual's capacity that cannot be resolved by obtaining another expert opinion, legal advice should be sought. It may ultimately require a court judgment to resolve the issue. (Some instances in which courts must be consulted are mentioned later in the chapter.)

Fluctuating capacity

A person's capacity to make decisions can fluctuate for a number of reasons, such as the existence of a bipolar disorder or the effects of medication. When patients have fluctuating capacity, they may be particularly vulnerable to coercion or pressure from other people. This can have very important implications if treatment is required or legal decisions need to be made. Health professionals need to try and ascertain if the patient's choice is a voluntary one. An intermittent state of capacity is known in law as a 'lucid interval' and obviously, when possible, significant decisions should be considered in such periods. Any legal agreement made when the patient lacks capacity may be void and of no effect. If legal decisions are made during a lucid interval, they may be valid, but medical evidence of capacity is likely to be needed to show the person had capacity on that particular occasion.[19] Fluctuating capacity presents particular challenges for treatment, especially if options need to be considered urgently and cannot be deferred until the patient's condition improves. Assessment of the patient needs to be carried out at the time the decision is needed but when capacity is impaired at that time, and a decision can be delayed until it improves, it should be. Unless it is an emergency and an immediate decision is required, all reasonable efforts should be made to enhance the patient's decision-making capacity. If the decision cannot be deferred, the usual principles of best interests (in England, Wales and Northern Ireland) or providing benefit to incapacitated patients (in Scotland) apply.

Who should assess capacity and when?

Other than in emergencies when it is not possible to get consent, health professionals need to be sure that the patient consents to examination or treatment. In cases of doubt about the person's capacity to consent, an assessment is needed. It may be an informal conversation with a doctor, such as a GP, who knows the patient. When there is uncertainty about capacity and the decision is a complex one or has serious consequences for the patient or for other people, a formal assessment is advisable, perhaps involving a psychiatrist or a psychologist. Assessment should not be rushed and the professional carrying it out should have background information about the patient's medical history and about the decision for which the patient is being assessed. The practitioner proposing the treatment is generally responsible for ensuring that the patient's capacity has been assessed, although the task of actually doing the assessing can be delegated or referred to someone else.

Health professionals should encourage patients to make all the decisions they can. This may involve talking to them when they are at their best, including, if possible, when they are in a supportive, familiar environment. Information should be given in a way most suitable to their ability to grasp and remember it, possibly including visual aids. All assessments must be focused on how the individual is now (as opposed to just their medical history) and are made on the basis of the decision in question at the time it needs to be made.

Sometimes people whose capacity is in doubt are unwilling to be assessed. For stroke patients, for example, damage to the brain's language areas can make verbal communication difficult and they can have considerable trouble organising their thoughts, with the result they may strongly object to being asked even innocuous questions.[20] Patients cannot be forced to cooperate but in the absence of assessment, the choices they make may be challenged. In England and Wales, advice can be sought from the Office of the Public Guardian[21]. Separate arrangements exist in Scotland where the Office of the Public Guardian (Scotland) provides a range of guidance.[21] In Northern Ireland, the Official Solicitor provides legal representation for people who lack capacity and may be able to provide advice.

Providing care and treatment for adults lacking mental capacity

Best interests and benefit for patients

When adults have been assessed as lacking mental capacity to make a valid choice about the options on offer, decisions need to be made on the basis of an assessment of what would be in their best interests. Not only is this reflected in ethics guidance but also in the law in England, Wales and Northern Ireland. In Scotland, the law refers to *benefit* rather than best interests, but the intention is similar (the details are set out in the section on the law). Assessing where people's best interests lie, or what would benefit them, means looking at several factors including the circumstances of the case. It involves more than just an assessment of what would be best clinically and includes consideration of the individual's wishes and values, where they can be identified. Although taking account of previous wishes, it is not a 'substituted judgment test'; it is not the decision the individual would make, if able to do so, but rather what is objectively in the individual's best interests, taking account of his or her current circumstances. Wherever possible, reasonable efforts should be made to discuss the matter in question with the incapacitated adult. If patients have made an advance request or refusal, that needs to be taken into consideration and may be legally binding (see Chapter 3). Other points to consider are whether the person is likely to regain mental capacity and, if so, whether the decision can be postponed.

For many patients, a crucial part of assessing their best interests involves getting opinions from the people close to them, such as relatives, partners, friends or carers. Clearly, patient confidentiality needs to be borne in mind and any disclosures by health professionals about the patient's condition need to be justifiable in terms of the patient's best interests (this is discussed further in Chapter 6). If someone has been legally nominated to act as a proxy decision maker for the patient, that person needs to be involved in all decisions and may be legally entitled to make the decision on the patient's behalf.

The MCA and its code of practice provides advice about common factors to be taken into account for a best interests assessment. In Scotland, the task is to identify what would benefit the person, and the code of practice accompanying the legislation provides some similar general guidance about assessment of the patient's wishes, needs and risks.[22]

Best interests checklist

In England and Wales, the MCA sets out a checklist of factors which must be taken into account in determining what decision is in the best

(Continued)

interests of those who lack capacity to make the decisions themselves. When making a 'best interests' assessment, the following questions should be considered:

- have all reasonable steps been taken to encourage the individual to participate in the decision?
- is the decision discriminatory? (Is it based on age, appearance, condition or behaviour?)
- have the things been considered that the person would have taken into account if making the decision?
- have the person's past and present wishes, feelings, beliefs and values been considered?
- is the person likely to regain capacity and, if so, can the decision be delayed?
- are there less restrictive options that would achieve the same goal?
- is it clear that the decision is not motivated by a desire to bring about the person's death?
- have other people who may be able to provide information about the person's best interests been consulted?

Exceptions to best interests

There are broadly two circumstances when the best interests or benefit principle can lawfully be set to one side. One concerns the situation in which the patient has previously made an advance refusal of medical treatment. If it meets the criteria for validity and is applicable to the current situation and the treatment being proposed, the refusal is legally binding even if others think that it is against the patient's best interests or could result in that individual's death (see Chapter 3). In such cases, the patient is deemed to have made a competent anticipatory choice regardless of what might be in his or her clinical best interests. Secondly, an exception to the best interests criteria can occur when incapacitated adults are enrolled in certain forms of research.

Involving people close to the patient

Relatives and partners often assume that they are the obvious decision makers, but they are only legally entitled to say what should happen if they have been formally appointed to do so (see the section on legal proxies). Otherwise, responsibility for making treatment decisions usually rests with the clinician in overall charge of the patient's care, who – in consultation with other members of the healthcare team and those close to the patient – assesses what would be in that person's best interests (benefit in Scotland).

Legislation throughout the UK positively requires that the views of people close to the patient be taken into account, bearing in mind the duty of confidentiality, and any previous wishes of the patient about disclosure of information. The code of practice in Scotland specifically advises that the views of the following people should be sought:

- the nearest relative and primary carer
- any guardian or attorney with powers relating to the decision
- any person whom the sheriff has directed should be consulted and
- anyone who has identified himself or herself as having an interest in the welfare of the adult or the decision in question.[23]

Best interests and covert medication

Covert medication for adults with capacity is unethical and unlawful throughout the UK, but it can be acceptable as a last resort for patients lacking capacity. The Scottish code of practice specifically addresses this issue, stating that it may be permissible in some instances, primarily to avoid a risk of harm to the patient, when all other reasonable options have been explored.[5] Useful general guidance is available from the Mental Welfare Commission for Scotland[24]. The decision to administer medicine covertly to someone who cannot consent should be taken by the clinician with overall responsibility for the patient's care, in consultation with the team. The reasons justifying it should be recorded in the patient's care plan and reviewed, if it is likely to recur. It should not become routine or done for reasons of convenience. In making the decision, consideration should be given to whether there are feasible alternatives that are more respectful of the individual's choice. Consideration should also be given to the fact that changing the way that medication is administered can alter its benefits and risks. Giving it to patients in a crushed form, for example, may not be consistent with the product licence.

The role of proxy decision makers

Power of attorney in England and Wales

The legal powers transferred by giving someone power of attorney can vary and so attention needs to be given to the specific wording of each legal document. For patients' families, there can at times be confusion about what they are entitled to decide on the patient's behalf, when they have acquired power of attorney. They usually know whether it means that they can deal with the patient's financial affairs but are sometimes unclear as to whether they can also make personal welfare or treatment decisions. This confusion is partly due to there being two different types of lasting powers of attorney: powers that deal with decisions relating to property and affairs, and powers relating to health and welfare decisions. It is important that decision makers recognise that property and affairs powers of attorney cannot be used to make health and welfare decisions.

The power to make health and welfare decisions

The MCA made provision for adults (aged 18 and over) with capacity to nominate someone (an attorney) with legal authority to make a wider range of decisions on their behalf. This is called giving someone lasting power of attorney (LPA). If patients (donors) wish to nominate a person (or persons) to make decisions about medical treatment and financial matters, they must make two LPAs, one for each type of decision. Enduring powers of attorney, made before the MCA came into force, do not apply to health and welfare decisions.

An LPA dealing with health and personal welfare can only be used once the donor lacks the capacity to make the decision in question. In order to be valid a specific form must be used, which sets out the circumstances under which the appointed attorney has authority.[25] Donors must certify that they understand the purpose of nominating someone to make decisions for them when they lose capacity and attorneys also sign the document, indicating that they understand the duties involved, including the responsibility to act in the donor's best interests. A third party (called a certificate provider) confirms that the donor understands the nature and purpose of the LPA and that no fraud or pressure has been used to influence the donor. Registered healthcare professionals can be certificate providers and, GPs in particular, may find they are asked by patients to fulfil this role, but they need to be aware of the risks of coercion (see the case example of Mr and Mrs D referred to later in this chapter). Before a health and welfare LPA can be used, the patient must be assessed as lacking the capacity to make the decision in question and the LPA must be registered with the Office of the Public Guardian. Until it is registered, the attorney is unable lawfully to make decisions on the patient's behalf. A register of LPAs is kept by the Office of the Public Guardian.

The attorney's decision-making powers depend on the wording of the LPA and donors can include specific restrictions, so health professionals need to check it carefully. Attorneys can only make treatment decisions when the donor lacks capacity. They cannot refuse life-sustaining treatment on the donor's behalf unless this is expressly stated in the LPA document. No patient or attorney can insist on treatment that the clinical team thinks inappropriate. Attorneys must follow the guidance in the code of practice[26] and act in the best interests of the donor.

Disputes arising in relation to LPAs

Disagreements sometimes arise about whether patients retain the capacity to make a specific decision or whether a proposed intervention is in their best interests. In such cases, the code of practice[27] advises obtaining a second opinion and perhaps involving an advocate or mediator. If this is unsuccessful, application can be made to the courts to rule on cases of serious doubt or dispute.

Court-appointed deputies (England and Wales)

In England and Wales, the Court of Protection can appoint deputies as substitute decision makers for incapacitated adults who have not appointed an attorney under an LPA. Deputies generally make decisions about property and financial affairs but, in some cases, are appointed to make health decisions. This is rare as generally healthcare decisions can be made in the best interests of patients lacking capacity without the need for formal authorisation. A deputy may be appointed, however, when an ongoing series of complex or controversial decisions is needed. In most cases, the deputy is a family member or someone who knows the patient well, but someone independent of the family may be appointed if there have been serious family disputes, the healthcare needs are complex or there is nobody available within the family to take on the role. The scope of deputies' decision-making powers is set out in the court order appointing them, and deputies must always act in the patient's best interests and abide by the guidance in the code of practice. Deputies are not empowered to refuse consent to life-sustaining treatment on the patient's behalf. Such decisions must be referred to the court.

Independent mental capacity advocates (IMCAs) (England and Wales)

The MCA established a statutory advocacy service in England and Wales. Its purpose is to support vulnerable adults who lack capacity and who do not have anyone close to them who can provide support or whom it would be appropriate to consult. An IMCA represents the patient in discussions about life-changing decisions or serious treatment options. IMCAs cannot make decisions on the patient's behalf but can question those which do not appear to be in the patient's best interests. They are entitled to examine relevant patient records and to talk to the incapacitated person and to others well placed to know that person's wishes. They can also get a second medical opinion for the patient.

The role of IMCAs in decisions to withhold or withdraw serious medical treatment

If an adult lacks capacity and has nobody with whom it is appropriate to consult, an IMCA must be appointed when an NHS organisation proposes to provide, withhold or withdraw 'serious medical treatment'.[28] This includes cases where a fine balance exists between the benefits of the treatment and its burdens and risks, or where several choices exist and none is obviously best for the patient. Interventions involving important consequences for the patient also fall into the category of serious medical treatment. Examples include chemotherapy, major surgery, abortion, sterilization, and withholding or stopping clinically assisted nutrition and hydration.

There is no duty to instruct an IMCA when an urgent decision is needed or if the patient is detained under mental health legislation. IMCAs provide reports to the NHS body or local authority responsible for the individual's care and these must be taken into account before a decision is made.

The role of IMCAs in decisions about where patients should live

IMCAs are involved when patients need to go into hospital for more than 28 days or a care home for more than 8 weeks.[29] They can be involved in reviews of accommodation or checking the safeguarding adult procedures (in safeguarding cases IMCAs may be appointed whether or not family members or friends are involved). They may also be involved in cases where the Deprivation of Liberty Safeguards (DOLS) are applied. They cannot get involved if the patient previously nominated someone else to be consulted and that person is willing to assist, or if the patient has previously appointed an attorney under an LPA or where the Court of Protection has appointed a deputy to act on the patient's behalf in relation to his or her health or welfare.

Attorneys and guardians in Scotland

As far as possible, health professionals are obliged to take account of the views of people close to the incapacitated adult. The consent of any legal proxy with welfare powers should also be sought unless emergency treatment is needed. Proxies include guardians, welfare attorneys or people authorised under an intervention order. These can be individuals, professionals or social workers. Attorneys are nominated by patients with capacity, but the power is only transferred when the donor loses capacity. Powers of attorney must be registered with the Office of the Public Guardian (Scotland), which also provides information about setting them up.[30] Problems can arise when people who have capacity but are vulnerable to pressure are unduly influenced to grant someone else power of attorney. Safeguards designed for incapacitated adults are not activated because such patients have capacity.

Case example – need for safeguards on powers of attorney

Mr and Mrs D met at a school for people with special needs and married in 1982. They had support from Mr D's father and when he died, Mr D's brother Mr E took over. He arranged for the couple to give him power of attorney and they signed the relevant forms in the presence of his solicitor, even though they did not understand the extent of the power that they were giving away. Mr D was unable to read and his wife's reading skills were limited. The solicitor did not advise them properly or suggest they have legal advice of their own. Their GP was also later criticised for not taking enough care when signing the certificates of capacity that accompany the documents.

In 2008, when Mrs D had angry outbursts, she was referred to mental health services and social work services also became involved, as reports emerged of conflict between her and Mr E. Mrs D complained that he bullied and physically abused her, and it was noticed that he was also making welfare decisions which the Ds could have made themselves. The local authority and the Office of the Public Guardian were asked to look into Mr E's actions as attorney, but they believed that the Ds had enough capacity to take action themselves. The sheriff could have been requested to have the attorney removed or supervised, but it was left up to the couple, who were completely under Mr E's influence, to revoke his powers. Evidence showed that they were both afraid of Mr E and under pressure from him to continue. He exercised considerable control over their lives. Eventually, with help from another family member and an independent advocate, they revoked the power of attorney.

The Ds' psychiatrist and the Mental Welfare Commission for Scotland again asked the Office of the Public Guardian to investigate what had occurred, but the response was that the Ds should instruct a solicitor themselves. In its critical report of various professionals involved in the case, the Mental Welfare Commission concluded that the local authority should have intervened much earlier. 'It was wrong to rely on the couple to act to protect their own interests when there was so much evidence that they were unable to do so without considerable support'.[31] Once the power of attorney was removed, the Ds lost their fear of making decisions and of being punished by E and were able to live a freer life.

In the wake of the case of Mr and Mrs D, the Mental Welfare Commission called on the Scottish Government to revise the guidance and codes of practice relating to how doctors assess adults' capacity, especially whether the person is capable of taking the action needed. More detailed advice should also be available for doctors and lawyers (in addition to the BMA and General Medical Council's [GMC] guidance) when the certifying forms about power of attorney are completed. Particular safeguards need to be considered when the person granting the power of attorney has not personally initiated the process[31].

Under the AWISA, provision is made for an intervention order from a sheriff to deal with an incapacitated adult's financial, property or personal welfare. One-off health and welfare decisions can then be made by a 'welfare guardian', given power by the sheriff to decide about the patient's medical treatment. Doctors have responsibility for providing reports of incapacity in relation to applications for intervention orders or guardianship. At least two such reports are needed for each application. In a case where the cause of incapacity is mental disorder, one of these reports must be made by a medical practitioner approved for the purpose of Section 22 of the Mental Health (Care and Treatment) (Scotland) Act 2003.

Resolving disputes (Scotland)

In most cases, there is broad consensus about the care of an incapacitated adult. Once a certificate of incapacity is issued, treatment is given on the basis of a proxy's consent or, in the absence of a proxy, under the general authority to treat. If disputes arise, discussion can usually help proxies and relatives to understand the clinical reasoning. The legislation established a procedure for those cases where agreement cannot be reached. If, for example, a proxy requests treatment that health professionals consider to be inappropriate, the proxy can ask for a second opinion or use the NHS complaints procedure. If health professionals propose something to which the proxy objects, they should obtain a second opinion from a doctor nominated by the Mental Welfare Commission. The nominated practitioner must consult the proxy or other interested adult. If the nominated doctor agrees with the treatment, it can go ahead, despite the proxy's objection, unless an application has been made to the Court of Session. Where the nominated practitioner disagrees with the proposed treatment, health professionals can apply to the Court of Session for a ruling. Legal advice should be sought before approaching the court. Any person with an interest in the incapacitated person's welfare can challenge a decision by appealing via the sheriff to the Court of Session. This could be a treating doctor, another member of the clinical team, a proxy decision maker or someone close to the patient. While an appeal is pending, only emergency or essential treatment can be provided.

Decisions needing special safeguards

Giving treatment with serious implications

Some treatments are seen as so serious that they require special safeguards before they can be given to adults lacking capacity to consent. An example is when the proposed treatment has not been thoroughly tested and proven efficacious for the patient's condition. People with capacity can weigh up the options and may decide to take a risk on experimental treatment, especially when they have run out of other alternatives, but there need to be safeguards when the individual cannot do that. In very serious situations without other options there may be a justification for exposing incapacitated people to some risk if there is a reasonable chance of benefit. It is essential that the patient (where possible), families and the health team give careful consideration to all the evidence. Even when the prospect of success may be relatively low, the value of attempting a new treatment may be high for the patient. Care is needed not to overstate the possible benefits unless there is evidence to support them. Very sick people should not be exposed to experimental treatment if there is significant doubt about either the likelihood of success or the value of attempting it. In any case of doubt, legal advice should be sought and the courts may need to be involved.

Giving experimental treatment: *Simms*

In 2002, the High Court was asked to decide whether it would be lawful to provide treatment that had not been tested on humans to two patients with variant Creutzfeldt-Jakob disease (vCJD). Both patients, aged 18 and 16, lacked capacity to make the decision, but their parents argued that it would be in their interests to try the therapy. It involved intraventricular administration of pentosan polysulphate, which had been tested in Japan on rodents and dogs infected with scrapie. Although not expected to provide a cure, it was hoped that the treatment would improve the patients' lives. The judge agreed that the concept of *benefit* included the possibility of patients' improvement from their present state, or a continuation of that present state without deterioration for a longer period than might otherwise occur, or the prolongation of life for a longer period. Given the possibility of some benefit and the lack of other alternatives, it was held that this treatment would be in the best interests of both patients and it could lawfully be provided.[32] Eighteen-year-old Jonathan Simms became the first victim of vCJD to be given the drug pentosan polysulphate, by direct infusion into his brain in 2002. This produced some small but significant improvements. In 2009, he was the longest recorded survivor in the world. He was occasionally able to try speaking and could swallow. He stopped experiencing uncontrollable jerking movements linked with his disease and was free from the chest infections he previously suffered. He died in March 2011.[33]

Some other treatments which are hazardous or irreversible also require that an application be made to the courts in each case before they can be carried out on an adult lacking capacity. In England and Wales, the MCA code of practice says that the following decisions require court approval:

- proposals to withdraw or withhold clinically assisted nutrition and hydration from patients in a vegetative state
- cases involving organ or bone marrow donation by people lacking the capacity to consent
- proposals for non-therapeutic sterilisation
- cases of doubt about whether a particular treatment is in a person's best interests
- cases involving ethical dilemmas in untested areas.[34]

Court of Protection Practice Direction 9E has confirmed that an application should be made to the court where 'serious medical treatment' is proposed and gives examples of such treatment. In addition to those listed above, this includes certain terminations of pregnancy and treatment or procedures where a degree of force may be needed to restrain the person lacking capacity. The Practice Direction confirms that this list is not exhaustive and whether or not a procedure is regarded as 'serious medical treatment' will depend on the circumstances and the consequences for the patient. It talks about cases where there is 'a fine balance' between the benefits of treatments and its burdens and risks, where there is a finely balanced choice of treatment or where proposed treatment would be likely to involve serious consequences. It also requires court approval for the withholding or withdrawal of clinically assisted nutrition and hydration from patients in a minimally conscious state as well as patients in a vegetative state as referred to in the MCA code of practice.

Bone marrow donation: *Re Y*

A dying patient asked the court to authorise a bone marrow transplant from her mentally incapacitated sister, Y. As Y could not consent, the bone marrow donation could only proceed if it were shown to be somehow in Y's best interests. The mother of both women (the dying patient and Y) was also in poor health and would have to take on additional responsibilities if the sister died. The net effect of the death would be that Y received less care from her mother. The judge made a declaration that it would be lawful for the transplant to go ahead but said that it was a finely balanced decision, depending on three facts. Firstly, the donation procedure was low risk. Secondly, although Y could not consent, there was no evidence that she objected, and thirdly, there was some plausible benefit for Y, if her sister survived. Y's relationship with her sister was also likely to improve due to her sister's gratitude.[35]

Withholding treatment with serious implications

Treatment is only withdrawn or withheld if it cannot provide benefit, or if the patient has refused it. All decisions are made on the basis of patients' best interests or (in Scotland) to benefit them. Efforts need to be made to ascertain patients' former views, which may not give the whole answer but are among the factors to be considered. Relatives are normally consulted. If patients have made a valid advance decision refusing treatment, that is legally binding if it matches the current circumstances (see Chapter 3). Any other kind of advance care plan needs to be taken into account and any proxy decision makers consulted. (See also the sections on proxies and consulting those close to the patient.) Depending upon the treatment under consideration, a dietician, speech therapist, psychologist or physiotherapist may need to be involved. Relatives and people close to an incapacitated person should be kept informed, particularly when treatments are withdrawn from someone who is dying. The Liverpool Care Pathway for the Dying Patient[36] recommends explaining to families the plan of care when treatment is to be withdrawn.

Taking legal advice and involving the courts

Legal advice is needed if there is disagreement between the treating team and the family or if there is doubt about the patient's capacity, prognosis or best interests. Although some disagreements need to go to court, many can be resolved without a full court hearing, but it is always advisable to get a legal opinion. In some circumstances, it is obligatory to obtain a court ruling before withholding or withdrawing life-prolonging treatment, such as withdrawing artificial nutrition and hydration from patients in a vegetative or minimally conscious state. When cases are heard in court, the primary motive of the decision to withhold or withdraw treatment must be that the treatment is not beneficial or is too burdensome and not in the patient's best interests. The onus to prove this is on the person who wants treatment withdrawn or withheld. Although predictable that the patient's death will result, that must not be the motive behind the doctor's decision or the court's judgment.[37]

The Official Solicitor (England and Wales)

The Office of the Official Solicitor is an independent body, appointed by government to ensure that the interests of patients who are vulnerable by reason of a lack of mental capacity are protected. The Official Solicitor's role includes acting as

- last resort litigation friend, and in some cases solicitor, for adults who lack mental capacity, in a wide range of court proceedings
- advocate to the court, providing advice and assistance to the court, and making enquiries on behalf of the court

- last resort administrator of estates and trustee
- last resort property and affairs deputy in relation to Court of Protection clients.

The Official Solicitor is likely to be appointed to act on behalf of patients lacking capacity in any court proceedings relating to the provision or withdrawal of medical treatment.

Withholding or withdrawing life-sustaining treatment

Among the most difficult decisions health professionals make are those related to the withdrawal or withholding of life-sustaining treatment from patients lacking capacity. The BMA publishes detailed advice on this,[38] as does the GMC.[39] This guidance aims to provide a framework within which these difficult decisions can be made, taking account of the individual factors of the case and the views of all those involved. A valid and applicable advance decision should be followed, although it is important to remember that an advance decision does not apply to life-sustaining treatment unless it is in writing, contains a statement to the effect that it is to apply even if life is at risk, and is signed and witnessed. Relatives and other people close to the patient should be involved, but their views are not necessarily determinative, unless they have been formally appointed to act as proxy decision makers for the patient and the LPA contains express provision for the attorney to make decisions concerning life-prolonging treatment.

Considerations before withdrawing or withholding life-sustaining treatment include

- the person's known wishes, including any written statements made when the person had capacity
- clinical judgement about the effectiveness or otherwise of the proposed treatment
- the likelihood of the person experiencing severe unmanageable pain or suffering
- the level of awareness individuals have of their existence and surroundings
- the likelihood and extent of any degree of improvement if treatment is provided
- whether the invasiveness, risks and side effects of the treatment are justified in the circumstances
- the views of any appointed healthcare proxy or welfare attorney
- the views of people close to the person, especially close relatives, partners and carers, about what the individual is likely to see as beneficial.

Clinically assisted nutrition and hydration

Oral nutrition and hydration – by any method of putting food or liquid into a person's mouth – is offered to all patients, unless the risks outweigh the benefits. If they cannot cope with oral feeding or it does not meet their nutritional needs, clinically assisted nutrition is usually given by nasogastric tube, percutaneous endoscopic gastrostomy (PEG) or total parenteral nutrition. Although nutrition and hydration are often classed together, in any decision to withdraw treatment, they should be assessed separately and reviewed in relation to the patient's needs. Guidance from the GMC and the BMA, mentioned above, should be consulted as part of the process of making these decisions.

Relatives may request the withdrawal of clinically assisted nutrition and hydration from incapacitated patients who are not actually dying but are in an irrecoverable condition. The law relating to this was established by the case of Tony Bland (see later in text), in which it was held that it would not be unlawful to withdraw clinically assisted nutrition and hydration (referred to then as 'artificial nutrition and hydration') even though the patient was not dying and this would lead to his death. It was subsequently confirmed that when withdrawing or withholding clinically assisted nutrition and hydration is in a patient's best interests, there is no breach of the patient's rights under Article 2 of the European Convention on Human Rights (the right to life). When people are not near death, safeguards must be in place to ensure that appropriate consideration is given to their individual circumstances and interests. In England, Wales and Northern Ireland, a court declaration is required to remove clinically assisted nutrition and hydration from a patient in a vegetative state or a minimally conscious state. This might not apply if the patient had documented a specific, formal advance refusal or possibly if the patient had appointed an attorney to make the decision but legal advice should be sought in such cases.

Withdrawal of artificial nutrition and hydration: *Bland*

Tony Bland was 17 years old when he was involved in the Hillsborough football stadium disaster in April 1989. His lungs were crushed and punctured and the supply of oxygen to his brain was interrupted. He suffered catastrophic and irreversible damage to the higher centres of the brain, leaving him in a persistent vegetative state (PVS). Tony Bland could breathe unaided but he had no cognitive function. He was unable to see, hear, taste, smell, speak or communicate in any way, or feel pain. Being unable to swallow, Tony Bland was fed by a nasogastric tube. In 1992 an application was submitted to the court for a declaration that it would be lawful to withdraw all life-sustaining treatment, including artificial nutrition and hydration. The application had the support of Tony Bland's family, the consultant in
(Continued)

charge of his care and two independent doctors. In approving the application the House of Lords was satisfied that there was no therapeutic, medical or other benefit to Tony Bland in continuing to maintain his nutrition and hydration by artificial means. It was also held that the provision of feeding by means of a nasogastric tube was 'medical treatment'.[40]

When patients lack capacity, clinically assisted nutrition and hydration are provided when in their best interests. If the patient is not dying, has not made a prior refusal of clinically assisted feeding and could survive for a considerable time if so fed, non-provision of nutrition and hydration can be very controversial. In 2011, the English Court of Protection ruled that it would be unlawful to withdraw clinically assisted nutrition and hydration from a woman in a minimally conscious state because she had not made a formal advance refusal to that effect. (See the *Re M* case described in Chapter 3.) The judgment made clear that the default position in such cases would be to preserve life.[41] Relatives of the patient said that before her incapacitating illness, she had said several times that she would not want to be kept alive in the kind of situation in which she eventually ended up. As there was no documentary evidence of her wishes nor of the degree to which she had considered them, any decisions made on the patient's behalf needed to be in her best interests. This case was considered to be significantly different from the Tony Bland case because the patient could feel pain and respond in a limited way to external stimulae.

Some people regard clinically assisted feeding as essential care which should be continued. Judgments in legal cases in England and Scotland[42] classified artificial nutrition and hydration as medical treatments which can be withheld or withdrawn in some circumstances. It is also established in common law that decisions not to insert a feeding tube, or not to reinsert it if it becomes dislodged, are medical decisions which are taken after assessment of the individual circumstances of the case. The GMC's guidance requires that a second clinical opinion is sought before clinically assisted nutrition or hydration is withheld or withdrawn from a person who is not imminently dying.[43] This opinion should be sought from a senior clinician (medical or nursing) who has experience of the person's condition and who is not directly involved in the individual's care. This is to ensure that, in this most sensitive area, the person's interests have been thoroughly assessed. Given that the Practice Direction from the Court of Protection states that the withdrawal of clinically assisted nutrition and hydration from patients in a vegetative state or minimally conscious state should be referred to the court, legal advice should be sought in these cases. In Scotland, the withdrawal of clinically assisted feeding does not necessarily require a court declaration, but doctors who have the court's authority are not liable to prosecution.[44] They might be if they do not seek authority from the Court of Session.

Safeguards for participation in research

Other areas where special safeguards are needed are research and innovative therapy. Wherever possible, consenting adults with capacity should be the ones involved but, for conditions involving a degree of mental impairment, some research needs to be done with people who have that condition. Many people with impaired capacity can give valid consent or refusal, if the issues are explained carefully. Special rules apply when they cannot consent personally.

Checklist for involving incapacitated people in research

- Individuals should be positively involved in decision making to the maximum of their ability.
- If apparently unwilling, they should not be included in research or experimental treatment.
- Any advance refusal made by the individual when competent must be respected.
- Extra safeguards must be in place when participants cannot consent.
- Incapacitated people can only be involved if the research cannot be done with people who can consent.
- The research must relate to the participant's condition.
- The expectation should be that participating involves no risks, or the benefits to the participant are expected to outweigh any risk of harm.
- Information for proxy decision makers must be as detailed as for people consenting or refusing personally.

Dementia research

Dementia is a growing problem requiring more research, including on the effectiveness and transferability of different models of care and support, but explaining that to patients with dementia is challenging. Even more so is describing the distinction between treatments which might benefit them and those which are only expected to benefit future patients. Where possible, consent or refusal should be discussed when individuals are at their best. Some detailed guidance is available from the Nuffield Council on Bioethics, which also covers the option of proxy consent by a relative or welfare attorney.[45] It notes, however, that some people have particular concerns about a proxy's ability to second-guess the wishes of a person with dementia. The PREDICT project[46] also looked at the involvement of older people in research when they might have cognitive or communication problems. It recommends specific training for researchers undertaking trials with an older population so that extra time and support are given to the participants.

Emergency research

Research in the context of emergency care is also challenging. Usually, there is no time to contact families or proxy decision makers if the patient is unconscious or unable to communicate. In 2004, the UK implemented the Medicines for Human Use (Clinical Trials) Regulations, which cover clinical trials of investigational medicinal products (CTIMPs). The Regulations required that consent for participation in research be provided in advance of the incapacitated person being involved, but this made it impossible to research drugs for conditions such as cardiac arrest. It was widely agreed that for emergency research, some exception to the requirement for prior proxy consent was needed. In 2006, the regulations were amended to allow CTIMPs on incapacitated adults in emergency situations without prior consent, as long as a research ethics committee (REC) agreement had been obtained. Proxy consent is still needed for continuing participation in the trial of emergency measures but in the absence of such consent at the start, patients can be initially entered. All trial protocols – including those for emergency care – should be scrutinised by RECs, which consider whether the exception should apply to individual emergency trial protocols. The amendment applied to CTIMPs in emergency situations throughout the UK.

Control, restraint and deprivation of liberty

Safeguards are also needed for activities which have the effect of limiting an incapacitated patient's freedom. Incapacitated adults may be a risk to themselves or others, so that the issue of protection comes up, but this also generally involves the use of control or restraint. Wherever possible, the issues need to be discussed with the individuals concerned, who should be given support to make their own decisions if they can. Some measures may not be recognised as deliberately limiting people's freedom but still have that effect. For example, retaining mobility in later life is an important facet of well-being and independence and a variety of aids exist to help older people remain active. Removal of such aids in residential and in-patient settings can limit people's liberty and form an unacceptable measure of restraint.

The deliberate use of restraint should be a last resort and proportionate in terms of the likelihood and seriousness of the risk to be managed. The minimum amount should be used to achieve the objective and it should be clear that the patient would be at risk of harm, if left unrestrained. Decisions involving restraint should be documented in the medical record, including the reason, type and duration of its use. Physically restricting someone's ability to move is the most obvious form of restraint, but the definition also includes the threat of force to make someone do something they would resist.[47] Restraint can be overt, such as locked doors, or it can be covert and indirect, such as exit doors that are too heavy to open easily or the use of low chairs from which older people find it difficult to move. It can be psychological, such as forbidding people to do certain things or browbeating them to do as they are told. It can also be chemical, involving sedation or the over-medication of patients,[48] especially older people in care homes or in hospitals.[24]

Case example – powers of restraint

ZH was an autistic young man who was unable to communicate by speech. He suffered from epilepsy and learning difficulties. When aged 16 in 2008, he was taken to a swimming pool by his school, with the help of a classroom assistant, SB. ZH was fixated by the pool and refused to leave when the other pupils left. SB remained with him. The pool manager wanted him removed and called the police, who attempted to take hold of him, but ZH fell in the pool and had to be helped out by lifeguards. He struggled and was restrained by five policemen. Handcuffs and leg restraints were used but were removed when ZH was moved to a cage in a police van and calmed down. When the case went to court, it was claimed that he suffered psychological trauma, which made his epilepsy worse. Proceedings were brought against the police for assault, battery, breach of his human rights, false imprisonment and disability discrimination. The court agreed that force had been used and the police should have first consulted SB and other carers to find out what was in his best interests. They had not acted in accordance with the Mental Capacity Act provisions on the use of restraint of incapacitated people. The court said it was not enough for the police to have acted in good faith. ZH was awarded £28,250 in damages. The case was seen as having particular implications for staff in emergency services and other professionals who come into contact with incapacitated patients. This case is an important one for anyone working with incapacitated individuals where restraint is used. It confirms that when staff restrain incapacitated individuals, they must be aware of the Mental Capacity Act's provisions and be able to demonstrate that the restraint is necessary to prevent harm to the individual, is proportionate to the likelihood and seriousness of harm, and is in the individual's best interests.[49] In January 2013, the police were appealing the judgment.

In separate cases, the Court of Appeal noted that the Mental Capacity Act only applies to people who lack capacity due to an impairment of, or disturbance in, the functioning of the mind or brain. It also confirmed, however, that, in the absence of any express provision, the courts' inherent jurisdiction could be used in cases where the MCA is not applicable because the lack of capacity, or inability to consent, arises for some other reason.[50]

One of the more complex areas of the law in England and Wales involving adults lacking capacity relates to the distinction between restraint and treatment that amounts to a deprivation of liberty. It was initially raised in relation to the *Bournewood* case.

Deprivation of liberty: *Bournewood*

HL had profound learning disabilities and lived in Bournewood Hospital for over 30 years. In 1994, he started living in the community with carers, Mr and Mrs E, but in July 1997, he became agitated at a day centre and was taken to the Accident and Emergency Department of Bournewood Hospital under sedation. HL was compliant and did not resist admission, so doctors chose to admit him informally rather than using compulsory powers under the Mental Health Act. He did not attempt to leave the hospital, but his carers were not allowed to visit him, as it was anticipated that he would try to leave with them. They sought a judicial review of the decision by the Bournewood Community and Mental Health NHS Trust to keep HL in hospital.

In the High Court, it was noted that HL had not been prevented from leaving as he had not tried to do so, but the Court of Appeal said that the trust had been wrong in assuming that he could be kept as an inpatient without his consent as long as he did not object. The court held that, if it was necessary to detain HL, the Mental Health Act 1983 should have been invoked. Not only had the trust misinterpreted the Act but so had many other institutions, and many other patients had also been unlawfully detained, without the safeguards of the Act. The case went to the House of Lords, which considered that using the mental health legislation in every case was likely to stigmatise informal patients and have severe resource implications. A majority of the Lords concluded that HL had *not* been detained in the sense of being falsely imprisoned because he had not actually been stopped from leaving and, even if he had been, it would have been justified under the common law of necessity.

Although HL went back into the care of Mr and Mrs E in December 1997, the case was pursued at the European Court of Human Rights for a declaration that HL had been deprived of his liberty unlawfully in the meaning of Article 5 of the European Convention on Human Rights (ECHR). The European Court found that HL had been detained and that the common law doctrine of necessity did not provide the requisite safeguards for informal detention of compliant but incapacitated patients. It said that

- HL had been deprived of his liberty contrary to Article 5;
- the detention was arbitrary and not in accordance with a procedure prescribed by law;
- the lack of a procedure under which the lawfulness of his detention could be reviewed did not comply with Article 5(4) of the ECHR.[51]

Following the ruling of the European court, the UK government consulted widely about its potential consequences, including the implication that compliant but incapacitated adults in care homes and hospitals are effectively deprived of their liberty in the meaning of the Convention. This consultation resulted in the amendment of the MCA to introduce the 'DOLS', which was intended to plug the so-called 'Bournewood gap' in the law in England and Wales. They provide a mechanism, with safeguards for the patient, by which deprivation of an incapacitated individual's liberty can be authorised.

Deprivation of Liberty Safeguards

Health professionals working with incapacitated adults should be familiar with the DOLS procedures and able to recognise what constitutes a deprivation of liberty. The safeguards require that legal authorisation be obtained before incapacitated adults can be cared for in a hospital or care home in conditions which amount to a deprivation of their liberty. An application for authorisation must be made to an appropriate supervisory body.

England and Wales

Guidance on deprivation of liberty for England and Wales is available in the DOLS code of practice.[52] In England, the appropriate supervisory body to give authorisation for people's liberty to be restricted in an individual case is usually the commissioning body or local authority. In Wales, it is either the National Assembly or a Local Health Board. When the application is made, the supervisory body initiates a series of assessments, which can take up to 21 days to complete. When authorisation is needed urgently because people are already deprived of their liberty, the care home or hospital can issue an urgent authorisation lasting 7 days. This provides a breathing space during which a standard authorisation must then be sought. Further detailed information on applying the safeguards is available in the code of practice.

Scotland

In Scotland too, where the circumstances of care for an incapacitated adult amount to deprivation of liberty, an order is required to ensure that it is in accordance with a procedure prescribed by law. Detailed advice on this is provided in the code of practice for the AWISA.[53] This emphasises that consideration must be given as to whether any proposed care intervention would amount to a deprivation of liberty under Article 5 of the European Convention on Human Rights. It sets out, in an annex, a list of factors to consider in assessing whether patients are, or are likely to be, deprived of their liberty. Guidance is also available from the Mental Welfare Commission for Scotland.[54] This notes that people can have their liberty infringed in various locations, as well as in secure facilities. They may be limited in their own home or by being under 24-hour escort or being restricted within a defined area. This could possibly include restrictions in a care home. In such cases, legal advice should be sought.

Northern Ireland

In Northern Ireland, interim guidance about the care of incapacitated adults who might be deprived of their liberty was issued in 2010, pending the introduction of new mental health and mental capacity legislation.[55] This guidance points out that until new legislation is enacted, depriving incapacitated adults of their liberty is unlawful and suggests the use of mental health powers instead, including guardianship. It recognised that heath and social care professionals need to continue looking after incapacitated patients while ensuring that they are not arbitrarily deprived of their liberty.

The difference between protection, restraint and deprivation of liberty

Protective measures sound reassuringly benign, whereas *restraint* conjures up a more controversial image. Although it would be useful to draw a clear distinction between them, in reality it is hard to do so and the borderline is often fluid. Despite the benign impression, protective measures can be unfairly or disproportionately restrictive of patients' activity. Bedrails, for example, are installed as a protective measure to stop people from accidentally falling out of bed, but they are a form of restraint if used deliberately to prevent people getting out of bed. An important distinction is that the aim of restraint (whether or not it is overt) is to restrict liberty, whereas protective measures are designed to manage risk without depriving individuals of their liberty. Consideration needs to be given to whether less restrictive measures could be effective in protecting vulnerable people. Patients with dementia, for example, may display aggression, inappropriate behaviour and wandering. Focusing on the individual needs and circumstances of each case can defuse some problems; aggressive behaviour is often the result of anxiety and fear in patients with cognitive impairment. Adjusting routines to suit patients' needs and discussing their preference rather than imposing routines on them can reduce anxiety. Addressing the underlying causes of difficult behaviour and providing personalised support can reduce the need for protective measures that constitute restraint in many cases.

The difference between restraint and deprivation of liberty depends on the circumstances but is primarily a matter of degree and intensity. A deprivation of liberty without proper authority is unlawful. The DOLS code of practice suggests that factors likely to be relevant when assessing whether the circumstances of care amount to a deprivation of liberty include the following:

- use of restraint or sedation to admit a person who is resisting to an institution
- when staff have complete control over a person for a significant period
- when staff control assessments, treatment, contacts and residence
- cases where the person is not allowed to live elsewhere nor be released into the care of others unless the staff agree
- when requests by carers for a person to be discharged are refused
- when the person is unable to maintain social contacts because of the restrictions imposed.

Since the DOLS code of practice was prepared, the meaning of deprivation of liberty has been the subject of various (and sometimes conflicting) court judgments.[56]

A last word on caring for adults who lack capacity

Assessing that patients lack capacity is a very serious matter. Their choices and freedoms are likely to be curtailed as a result and so it is important that, whenever possible, they are assessed when at their best and the assessments are repeated, if there is evidence of improvement. Some decisions cannot wait for such opportunities. Choices then have to be made on an assessment of what would be in the patient's best interests (or benefit in Scotland). As discussed in the chapter, however, measures taken with the aim of protecting patients can result in legal action if any restrictions amount to a disproportionate deprivation of their liberty. Cases, such as that of ZH discussed earlier, illustrate the dangers for emergency services, other care providers and patients, if attention is not first given to assessing where the patient's best interests lie.

Among the most difficult decisions of all are those involving the withdrawing or withholding of life-prolonging treatment. The very detailed advice issued by the GMC and the BMA, mentioned earlier in the chapter, should be consulted. If a valid advance decision has been made, specifying a refusal of some or all treatment, it is binding on health professionals. In the majority of cases, however, patients have not done this. Discussion about best interests and benefit then needs to involve the health team, people close to the patient and any nominated proxy decision makers or people with a power of attorney that extends to welfare issues. If agreement fails to be reached, the courts are likely to be involved.

References

1 Department of Health (1983) *Code of Practice for the Mental Health Act*, DH, London; Scottish Government (2003) *Code of Practice for the Mental Health (Care and Treatment)(Scotland) Act 2003*, SEHD, Edinburgh; Department of Health and Social Services (1992) *Mental Health (Northern Ireland) Order 1986: Code of Practice*, HMSO, Belfast.

2 *GJ v The Foundation Trust and Ors* [2009] EWHC 2972 (Fam), para 58.

3 Department for Constitutional Affairs (2007) *Mental Capacity Act Code of Practice*, The Stationery Office, London.

4 Mental Capacity Act 2005, s 2(1).

5 Scottish Executive (2010) *Adults with Incapacity (Scotland) Act 2000. Code of Practice for Practitioners Authorised to Carry Out Medical Treatment or Research under Part 5 of the Act*, 3rd edn, SG/2010/57, SEHD, Edinburgh, para 2.60.

6 Adults with Incapacity (Requirements for Signing Medical Treatment Certificates) (Scotland) Regulations 2007.

7 Scottish Executive (2010) *Adults with Incapacity (Scotland) Act 2000. Code of Practice for Practitioners Authorised to Carry Out Medical Treatment or Research under Part 5 of the Act*, 3rd edn, SG/2010/57, SEHD, Edinburgh, para 1.35.

8 Scottish Executive (2010) *Adults with Incapacity (Scotland) Act 2000. Code of Practice for Practitioners Authorised to Carry Out Medical Treatment or Research under Part 5 of the Act*, 3rd edn, SG/2010/57, SEHD, Edinburgh, annexe 5.

9 Scottish Executive (2010) *Adults with Incapacity (Scotland) Act 2000. Code of Practice for Practitioners Authorised to Carry Out Medical Treatment or Research under Part 5 of the Act*, 3rd edn, SG/2010/57, SEHD, Edinburgh, para 2.20.

10 The Bamford Review of Mental Health and Learning Disability (Northern Ireland) (2007) *A comprehensive legislative framework*, DHSSPS, Belfast.

11   From a recruiting poster by British explorer Ernest Shackleton for his 1914 Antarctica expedition.

12   Advice on assessing capacity in a range of circumstances is given in: British Medical Association, Law Society (2010) *Assessment of Mental Capacity*, 3rd edn, Law Society, London.

13   Scottish Executive (2010) *Adults with Incapacity (Scotland) Act 2000. Code of Practice for Practitioners Authorised to Carry Out Medical Treatment or Research under Part 5 of the Act*, 3rd edn, SG/2010/57, SEHD, Edinburgh, para 1.22.

14   *Re C (Adult: Refusal of Medical Treatment)* [1994] 1 All ER 819.

15   Scottish Executive (2010) *Adults with Incapacity (Scotland) Act 2000. Code of Practice for Practitioners Authorised to Carry Out Medical Treatment or Research under Part 5 of the Act*, 3rd edn, SG/2010/57, SEHD, Edinburgh, para 1.9.

16   Mental Capacity Act 2005, s 3.

17   Scottish Executive (2010) *Adults with Incapacity (Scotland) Act 2000. Code of Practice for Practitioners Authorised to Carry Out Medical Treatment or Research under Part 5 of the Act*, 3rd edn, SG/2010/57, SEHD, Edinburgh, para 1.20.

18   *Re MB (Medical Treatment)* [1997] 2 FLR 426.

19   This is discussed in more detail in: British Medical Association, Law Society (2010) *Assessment of Mental Capacity*, 3rd edn, Law Society, London, chapter 4.

20   This is discussed in: British Medical Association (2009) *The Ethics of Caring for Older People*, 2nd edn, Wiley-Blackwell, Chichester, p.36.

21   The Public Guardian (Scotland) provides advice at: http://www.publicguardian-scotland.gov.uk (accessed 8 June 2012).

22   Scottish Executive (2010) *Adults with Incapacity (Scotland) Act 2000. Code of Practice for Practitioners Authorised to Carry Out Medical Treatment or Research under Part 5 of the Act*, 3rd edn, SG/2010/57, SEHD, Edinburgh, chapter 4.

23   Scottish Executive (2010) *Adults with Incapacity (Scotland) Act 2000. Code of Practice for Practitioners Authorised to Carry Out Medical Treatment or Research under Part 5 of the Act*, 3rd edn, SG/2010/57, SEHD, Edinburgh, para 1.6.6.

24   Mental Welfare Commission for Scotland (2006) *Covert Medication: Legal and Practical Guidance*, Mental Welfare Commission for Scotland, Edinburgh.

25   LPA forms are available from the Office of the Public Guardian: http://www.publicguardian.gov.uk (accessed 11 June 2012).

26   Department for Constitutional Affairs (2007) *Mental Capacity Act Code of Practice*, The Stationery Office, London, pp.114–135.

27   Department for Constitutional Affairs (2007) *Mental Capacity Act Code of Practice*, The Stationery Office, London, pp.258–259.

28   Mental Capacity Act 2005 (Independent Mental Capacity Advocates) (General) Regulations 2006. SI 2006/1832.

29   Department for Constitutional Affairs (2007) *Mental Capacity Act Code of Practice*, The Stationery Office, London, pp.178–179.

30   See: http://www.publicguardian-scotland.gov.uk (accessed 11 June 2012).

31   Mental Welfare Commission for Scotland (2012) *Powers of Attorney and Their Safeguards: an Investigation into the Response by Statutory Services and Professionals to Concerns Raised in Respect of Mr and Mrs D*, MWCS, Edinburgh.

32   *Simms v Simms, A v A* [2002] 2 WLR 1465; [2003] 1 All ER 669.

33   Anon. (2011) Belfast man with vCJD dies after long battle. *BBC News Online* (7 Mar). Available at: http://www.bbc.co.uk/news (accessed 6 August 2012).

34   Department for Constitutional Affairs (2007) *Mental Capacity Act Code of Practice*, The Stationery Office, London, p.143.

35   *Re Y (Mental Incapacity: Bone Marrow Transplant)* [1996] 2 FLR 787.

36   The Marie Curie Palliative Care Institute Liverpool (2009) *The Liverpool Care Pathway for the Dying Patient (LCP) Core Documentation*, MCPCIL, Liverpool.

37   Mental Capacity Act, s 4(5).

38   British Medical Association (2007) *Withholding and Withdrawing Life-Prolonging Medical Treatment*, 3rd edn, Blackwell, Oxford.

39   General Medical Council (2010) *Treatment and Care towards the End of Life: Good Practice in Decision Making*, GMC, London.

40   *Airedale NHS Trust v Bland* [1993] 1 All ER 821.

41   *W v M* [2011] EWHC 2443 (Fam), para 249.

42   See, for example: *Frenchay Healthcare NHS Trust v S* [1994] 1 WLR 601; *Re D (Medical Treatment)* [1998] 1 FLR 411; *Law Hospital NHS Trust v Lord Advocate* [1996] SLT 848.

43   General Medical Council (2010) *Treatment and Care towards the End of Life: Good Practice in Decision Making*, para 121.

44   *Law Hospital NHS Trust v Lord Advocate* [1996] SLT 848.

45   Nuffield Council on Bioethics (2009) *Dementia: the Ethical Issues*, NCB, London.

46   See: http://www.predicteu.org (accessed 4 October 2012).

47   Mental Capacity Act 2005, s 6(1)–(3).

48   See, for example: House of Commons Health Committee (2004) *Elder Abuse Second Report of Session 2003–4*, The Stationery Office, London, vol. 1, para 65; Joint Committee on Human Rights (2007) *The Human Rights of Older People in Healthcare. Eighteenth Report of Session 2006–7*, The Stationery Office, London, vol. 2, evidence sessions 173 and 222.

49   Bowcott O (2012) Autistic teenager wins damages from the police after being restrained. *The Guardian* (14 Mar). Available at: http://www.guardian.co.uk (accessed 11 June 2012); RadcliffesLeBrasseur (2012) Case update – powers of restraint and the High Courts' inherent powers in relation to incapacitated individuals. *Mental Health Law Briefing* 178 (April). Available at: http://www.rlb-law.com (accessed 26 September 2012).

50   See, for example: *A Local Authority and other v DL* [2012] All ER (D) 134 Mar.

51   *HL v United Kingdom* (45508/99) [2004] 40 EHRR 761.

52   Ministry of Justice (2008) *Mental Capacity Act 2005 Deprivation of Liberty Safeguards. Code of Practice to Supplement the Main Mental Capacity Act 2005 Code of Practice*, The Stationery Office, London.

53 Scottish Executive (2010) *Adults with Incapacity (Scotland) Act 2000. Code of Practice for Practitioners Authorised to Carry Out Medical Treatment or Research under Part 5 of the Act*, 3rd edn, SG/2010/57, SEHD, Edinburgh.

54 Mental Welfare Commission for Scotland. *Autonomy, Benefit and Protection*, MWCS, Edinburgh. Available at: http://www.mwcscot.org.uk (accessed 11 June 2012).

55 Department of Health, Social Services and Public Safety (2010) *Deprivation of Liberty Safeguards (DOLS) Interim Guidance*, DHSSPS, Belfast.

56 The leading case, *Cheshire West and Chester Council v P* [2011] EWCA Civ 1257, is, at the time of writing, being appealed to the Supreme Court.

5: Treating children and young people

10 things you need to know about . . . treating children and young people

- Valid consent for the treatment of children and young people can come from people with parental responsibility, young patients themselves (if judged to be competent) or the courts.
- Parental responsibility is a legal concept that gives adults (and, in some cases, local authorities) the rights, duties, powers, responsibilities and authority that legal parents have. Not all genetic parents have it.
- Young people are presumed to be able to consent to medical treatment when aged 16. Below that, much depends on their competence (or lack of it) and on the gravity of the decision.
- In England, Wales and Northern Ireland, medical treatment to save life or prevent serious damage to health can be imposed upon competent minors (up to the age of 18) who refuse it.
- In Scotland young people become adults at the age of 16. If competent young people under that age refuse life-saving treatment, it probably cannot be given. It is advisable to get legal advice in such situations.
- Decisions for children who lack competence must be made in their best interests. Where possible, children who lack competence to decide should still be asked their opinion and this should be recorded.
- Unless there is evidence to the contrary, parents are generally best placed to judge where a child's best interests lie.
- The courts may have to be involved when people who have parental responsibility refuse treatment for children that is considered to be in the child's best interests by the health team.
- The duty of confidentiality applies to all patients, including children and young people, but this is not absolute.
- In some circumstances, there may be a duty to disclose relevant information to an appropriate authority – for example, where there is a suspicion of child abuse.

Setting the scene

Children and young people are often discussed as if they were a homogenous group. In practice, the way that decisions are made for babies or young children is vastly different from the manner in which choices are offered to a teenager. Some common factors apply in that, where possible, all young patients should be told about their care in a way they understand. They should be listened to,

---

Everyday Medical Ethics and Law, First Edition. Ann Sommerville.
© 2013 BMA Medical Ethics Department. Published 2013 by John Wiley & Sons, Ltd.

which is not the same as saying that their views necessarily prevail. Once they have sufficient understanding and intelligence to weigh up the options, their consent (or refusal) is likely to have more weight, but they should still be encouraged to take decisions with their parents.

Treating young people can sometimes present difficult ethical dilemmas. The evolving nature of young people's competence and the extent to which it is appropriate to intervene to protect them against their own harmful actions, or the actions of others, can lead to a sense of conflicting rights and duties. Doctors sometimes struggle with their wish to provide a safe environment within which young people can seek confidential help and advice, while also offering a degree of protection for young people who may not be able to defend their own interests. Knowing when and how to intervene requires careful consideration of the principles, rules and guidelines, and a weighing up of the relative benefits and harms of the various options available in each case. This chapter aims to pull together the law, principles and key ethical guidance around the treatment of young people in order to help doctors with this ethical decision-making process.

Common questions about treating children and young people

- What happens if I take a radically different view from parents about what would be best for a child? If one parent agrees with me, is that enough to proceed?
- How do I judge whether a child or young person is competent enough to make a decision alone?
- Can I insist on only seeing children with an accompanying adult?
- Whose consent do I need if I am asked to do a paternity test? Does the mother have to know?
- What should I do if I have concerns about a child's welfare but the parents refuse to let me examine him?

Consent to examination and treatment

For children and young people, consent to examination or treatment can come from people who have parental responsibility or young patients themselves, if they are competent. In England, Wales and Northern Ireland, other people who look after a child, such as grandparents or childminders, can authorise 'what is reasonable in all the circumstances of the case for the purpose of safeguarding or promoting the child's welfare',[1] which could include consenting to examination and treatment. In Scotland, the situation is slightly different; steps should be taken to ascertain the parents' views if carers bring children for treatment.[2] To preserve life, health or well-being in emergencies when nobody is available to consent, essential treatment, such as emergency life-saving surgery, can proceed without consent.

Competence to consent to or refuse treatment or examination

There is no absolute minimum age at which children and young people can legally make choices about medical treatment. Once they reach legal adulthood (aged 16 in Scotland and 18 in the rest of the UK), they are presumed able to make decisions, to consent and refuse, without interference. They may also be able to do so when they are younger. Below 16, much depends on their competence (or lack of it) and on the gravity of the decision. Criteria exist to indicate the kind of skills and understanding they need to have in order to be considered competent and able to decide validly about different things. (This is known as 'Gillick' competence and is discussed later in the chapter.) Generalisations can be made about the stage of development at which they become competent, but individuals differ significantly.

Whereas the consent to medical treatment given by competent children and young people is usually respected, their refusal is generally given less weight, particularly if serious harm would result. They have sometimes been overruled by the courts when they refuse life-prolonging treatment. Treatments that are only expected to bring minimal improvement or only a small chance of success are unlikely to be imposed if refused by young people who understand the implications.

Consent or refusal on behalf of babies and young children

This section focuses on cases where children are too young and immature to make the decision. Choices are made for them by people with legal parental responsibility, with advice from the health team. Although adults decide, this does not mean that children who are past babyhood cannot be actively involved. Where feasible, even the very young should be told about what will happen. Children who have a serious or continuing illness often have a much better understanding of treatment options than their contemporaries, based on their past experience. From an early age, they can be good at expressing their own preferences, if given encouragement to understand the options and why the treatment is important. Children of the same age also differ in their ability and willingness to participate in decisions and so it is important not to approach them with preconceptions, based on experience of other young patients.[3] Development is a continuous but uneven process, in which mental skills, confidence, and social and emotional understanding increase with experience and encouragement.

Parental responsibility

Parental responsibility is a legal concept that gives an adult all the rights, duties, powers, responsibilities and authority that parents usually have. It includes the right to consent to medical treatment that is in a child's interests. In England, Wales and Northern Ireland, parental responsibilities may be exercised until a young person reaches 18. In Scotland, only the aspect of giving guidance to the young person lasts up to 18 and all other aspects of parental responsibility cease when the young person reaches 16.

Not all genetic parents have legal parental responsibility. If they were married at the time of the child's conception or at some time later, both parents have it and keep it if they divorce or if the child is in care or custody. If the parents never married, only the mother automatically has it. Unmarried fathers who are registered on the child's birth certificate can have parental responsibility, but the law across the UK varies about timing. In England and Wales, fathers registered on birth certificates from 1 December 2003 have parental responsibility; in Northern Ireland, those registered from 15 April 2002 have it, and in Scotland those from 4 May 2006. Prior to these dates, unmarried fathers lack parental responsibility (even if named on the birth certificate) unless they make a formal parental responsibility agreement with the mother or a parental responsibility order has been made by a court. In some same-sex couples, both partners have parental responsibility for a child.[4] Parents lose parental responsibility if their child is adopted by someone else. Other people can acquire it, if appointed as the child's guardian by a court or by having a residence order made in their favour. A local authority acquires parental responsibility (shared with the parents) while a child is the subject of a care order. When there is doubt about who has parental responsibility (and therefore has access to the child's record and is entitled to give consent for the child), further enquiries should be made. The BMA has detailed guidance on parental responsibility.[5]

Best interests

Decisions for children too young to be judged competent must be made in their best interests. In Chapter 4, we discussed how adults' best interests are more wide-ranging than just finding the optimal clinical outcome. Respect must be given to the person's known wishes and values, which can be very idiosyncratic. For children too, assessing their best interests means looking beyond the strictly clinical aspects, especially as the child develops his or her own views.[6] Parents are generally best placed to judge where their child's best interests lie but exceptions can arise. Loving parents who are Jehovah's Witnesses, for example, can believe it is in their child's best interests to refuse blood, but the courts (which also have a duty to decide in the child's best interests) may disagree.

In order to assess the child's best interests in a given scenario, parents need the same sort of information as if they were choosing for themselves (see Chapter 3). They are assumed to be the best judge of their child's interests, but, ideally, choices should be made in partnership with the health team. When serious differences of opinion cannot be resolved by lesser means, it is ultimately the courts which rule on where the child's best interests lie.[7] Parents are not generally allowed to select treatment that health professionals consider inappropriate or contrary to the child's interests, unless the courts agree with the parents' viewpoint. The following cases indicate how the courts have taken a different tack, depending on the circumstances of each case.

Parents requesting treatment considered inappropriate: *Re C*

C was 16 months old and suffered from spinal muscular atrophy, which causes severe emaciation and disability. She was kept alive by intermittent positive pressure ventilation, but doctors did not believe that continuing this was in her interests and asked the High Court to allow its withdrawal. They also proposed that resuscitation should not be attempted if C suffered respiratory relapse as they thought that continuing treatment would cause her increasing distress and medical complications. C's doctors told the court that her death was being delayed but without any possibility of significant alleviation of her condition. C's parents disagreed. They were orthodox Jews whose religious beliefs centred on the importance of prolonging life. C's mother argued that allowing C to die would result in punishment by God. While sympathising with the parents, the judge agreed that resuscitation and ventilation should be withheld and palliative care provided to 'ease the suffering of this little girl to allow her life to end peacefully'.[8]

Court decisions do not inevitably support the medical viewpoint. In the superficially similar case of *Re MB*, for example, the High Court agreed with the parents against the unanimous view of the medical team, which supported the withdrawal of ventilation.

Courts insisting on continuing treatment for a young child: *MB*

MB was 18 months old and also had spinal muscular atrophy. Like C, he was unable to breathe unaided and was kept alive by positive pressure ventilation. His condition would inevitably deteriorate and the regular interventions he needed caused him distress and pain. The medical team took

(Continued)

the view that continuing ventilation was contrary to MB's best interests. His parents argued that the child was also able to experience pleasure from, for example, being with his family, watching certain DVDs or listening to music. The judge in this case rejected the arguments of the healthcare team and agreed with the parents that MB gained pleasure from touch, sight and sounds, and this was not outweighed by the discomfort, distress or pain that he felt. Treatment could not be withdrawn as the court ruled it would not be in the child's interests.[9]

Decisions to stop life-prolonging treatment can be psychologically more difficult to make for children than for adults. The outcome of continuing it can also be less predictable, as was shown by the case of Charlotte Wyatt. This highlighted the difficulty of accurately assessing prognosis in seriously ill young children and the importance of keeping treatment decisions under review.

The unpredictability of prognosis in some young children: *Charlotte Wyatt*

In 2003, Charlotte Wyatt was born prematurely, at 26 weeks' gestation. Her organs were underdeveloped and she suffered brain damage that left her blind and deaf, as well as having chronic respiratory and kidney problems. A long legal battle developed around the treatment that should be provided. Doctors thought that she felt pain but doubted that she would experience pleasure. In 2004, they anticipated that she would succumb to respiratory failure and argued in court that artificial ventilation would not be in her best interests. They thought that, even if it were provided, she only had a small chance (around 5%) of surviving another year. The judge overruled Charlottes' parents, who wanted assurances that treatment would continue. He agreed with the medical team that further invasive and aggressive treatment should not be provided.[10]

Charlotte's condition did not deteriorate as expected. In fact, it had actually improved and so her parents asked that the court judgment opposing more treatment be stayed while more investigations took place. The judge refused,[11] but the parents applied again to the courts. Not only had Charlotte survived longer than expected, she also seemed able to respond to noise and no longer needed constant sedation. Despite these improvements, the judge considered that there had been no change in her underlying condition and again refused the parents who again appealed against this decision. Their appeal was dismissed.[12]

By 2005, Charlotte had been able to leave hospital and go home a couple of times, so the court agreed to rescind the earlier declaration.[13] In the following months, however, Charlotte developed a viral infection. She was likely to need intubation and ventilation, which doctors considered would not be in her best interests. Again the matter went to court, which agreed with the medical team and issued another declaration that it would be lawful to withhold intubation and ventilation.[14] Again, against medical expectations, Charlotte's condition improved. In 2006, she was still in hospital.[15] By 2007, she was in foster care because her parents, having separated, were unable to care for such a disabled child.[16]

Disagreements between people with parental responsibility

When parents disagree about treatment, health professionals are usually reluctant to override the views of one of them, even though legally, for most procedures, they only need consent from one person who has parental responsibility. Further discussion of the pros and cons of the treatment should clarify where the child's interests lie and may resolve the objection but, if not, the clinician in charge has to decide whether to go ahead on the basis of having legal authorisation from one parent. The onus is then on the parent who opposes treatment to take legal steps to stop it. If the dispute is over an irreversible, controversial, elective procedure, such as non-therapeutic male infant circumcision, doctors must not proceed without the authority of a court.[17]

Refusal by people with parental responsibility

The courts may also have to be involved when parents (or other people who have parental responsibility) refuse treatment for children. Judges are obliged to put the child's welfare first[18] and almost invariably rule that serious treatment should be given, when there is a good chance of it benefitting the child, but there are exceptions.

Parental refusal: *Re T*

In an unusual case, the courts agreed to go along with parents' refusal of treatment, even though that appeared contrary to the child's interests. Most cases going to court would not have this result, but it indicates the weight some judges give to parents' views when parents are experts on the issue in question. C was the child of health professionals and when he was 3 weeks old, he had major surgery, which was unsuccessful. He suffered from biliary atresia and, without a liver transplant, was not expected to survive to the age of 3, but his mother, who was his main carer as his father worked abroad, was opposed to further surgery. She did not want to expose C to pain and distress. Despite her objection, C was referred to a hospital for a transplant, but when a liver became available, C and his mother could not be contacted. When they returned to England from overseas, C's mother continued to oppose the operation. The local authority asked the court to rule that a transplant would be in C's best interests and authorise the surgery, but the Court of Appeal disagreed. It recognised that the child's welfare depended to a great extent on his mother and was apparently influenced by the fact that the parents were experienced health professionals and therefore well able to weigh up the pros and cons of surgery. Lord Justice Waite considered that it would not be in C's best interests to override them, even though a transplant had a good chance of success. He said that when there was genuine scope for disagreement about the child's interests, the court would generally be influenced by what the parents wanted.[19] C's mother later changed her mind and permitted the transplant to go ahead.

Involving older children in decisions

During the passage from childhood to adolescence, people begin to gain the maturity that eventually allows them to take responsibility for their own lives. As soon as they are able to participate in decisions, children should be encouraged to do so. While they may be unable to make big decisions, they should have a say about small ones, such as whether to stand or sit on a parent's lap for vaccination, for example. Information needs to be given simply and in a way they can grasp it. Some may not want to know the details or, when very serious treatment is needed, parents may try to insist on secrecy in order to protect the child from painful facts.[20] This delicate situation needs careful handling and much depends on the individual circumstances, but some research suggests that many children prefer to be told rather than be left in the dark.[21] The BMA and the General Medical Council (GMC) generally favour the sharing of information if the child seems willing to know it, unless revealing it would cause serious harm.[22] Children should not be considered unable to participate merely because they seem reluctant at one stage. They may be more willing later. Questions should be answered as frankly and as sensitively as possible, including when there is uncertainty.

The law throughout the UK stresses that children's views should be heard in decisions that affect them. This is not the same as saying that decisions are left up to them, especially if they refuse medical treatment and may lack full understanding about the implications. Their anxieties may be focused more on the immediate rather than the long-term effects of the proposed intervention but, in any case, they should have opportunities to talk about what frightens them and, where possible, obtain reassurance.

GMC guidance on effective communication between doctors and children and young people

The GMC advises doctors to

- 'involve children and young people in discussions about their care
- be honest and open with them and their parents, while respecting confidentiality
- listen to and respect their views about their health, and respond to their concerns and preferences
- explain things using language or other forms of communication they can understand
- consider how you and they use non-verbal communication, and the surroundings in which you meet them

(Continued)

- give them opportunities to ask questions, and answer these honestly and to the best of your ability
- do all you can to make open and truthful discussion possible, taking into account that this can be helped or hindered by the involvement of parents or other people
- give them the same time and respect that you would give to adult patients'.[23]

Unaccompanied minors

When children or young people make an appointment or turn up to a clinic without an adult, they should be seen. The GMC advises doctors to make it clear that they are willing to see them on their own if that is what they want, rather than implying that they must invariably come with an adult.[24] Much depends on the reason why the child prefers to come alone and this can usually only be clarified by talking about it. (See also, e.g. the section on child protection.)

Whether or not the child or young person can actually be treated depends on the assessment of competence and the kind of treatment sought. If patients lack the competence to make a valid choice, health professionals need the consent of someone else legally entitled to provide it before any treatment can proceed (unless treatment is required immediately 'to save the life of, or prevent serious deterioration in the health of, a child or young person'[25]). The advantage of young patients having the support of an adult should be discussed, even though the patient may reject that idea. The reasons may then need to be explored. If serious and continuing treatment is needed, clearly it may be essential to involve parents or someone with parental authority, but this should be with the young person's agreement, if competent (see also the section on *Gillick*). If tests are arranged, such as for pregnancy or sexually transmitted infection, some advance agreement should also be made about how the results will be collected, if they are not to be sent to the patient at the parents' home address.

Confidentiality

Some people think that doctors' duty of confidentiality only applies when patients are adults. This is not the case; the duty of confidentiality applies to all patients (see Chapter 6). In exceptional circumstances where disclosure is justified, the confidentiality of any patient of any age can be overridden. Even when doctors consider a child too immature to consent in a valid way to the treatment requested, the BMA thinks that confidentiality about the consultation should still generally be maintained if a child does not want a parent to be informed. Dilemmas arise if a child asks for something like contraceptive advice or needs to be tested for sexually transmitted infections when she is underage and therefore considered legally unable to consent to sexual intercourse. Further discussion with the patient is needed if it seems possible that she is at risk of abuse or exploitation. Depending on the circumstances, child protection concerns may arise, and in these cases, doctors must respond appropriately. Confidentiality issues are covered in more detail in Chapter 6.

Assessing competence in children and young people

As children develop, the degree to which they are involved in decisions should increase until, as young adults, they become fully responsible for deciding for themselves. Whether or not they are ready to do this at a particular time depends on an assessment of their competence.[26] As with the assessment of adults' capacity (see Chapter 4), attention needs to focus on the specific decision that has to be made at that time. This *functional* approach looks at the nature, complexity and implications of the decision so that the graver the impact of the choice, the greater the evidence of competence needed. All patients are competent to consent to medical treatment if they understand its nature and purpose, can retain the information and weigh it in the balance to arrive at a decision. Competence can fluctuate due to factors, such as the patient's medical condition, medication or mood. In these cases, where possible, doctors should attempt to promote competence, for example, by delaying a discussion until a time when the patient's competence is optimal.

Assessment should take account of factors, such as the child's cognitive development and ability to understand the choices, as well as the ability to balance the risks and benefits of the particular options, including the option of no treatment. Structured tests of cognitive development can provide general information but may not be sufficiently task-specific for this. Some abilities develop more through experience rather than just reflecting the patient's general stage of cognitive development. Assessment should involve gauging whether the patient understands what the illness means, the need for treatment for it and what that involves, including the expected outcome, as well as the implications of not having it. These abilities might be demonstrated through talking about the illness and about hopes and fears for the future. Some judgements can be based on how patients answer questions or on the type of questions that they themselves ask. Information must be retained for long enough to make an informed decision, but the fact that a child is reluctant to engage with the conversation or is bored by it is not itself evidence of incompetence.

Competence to consent

Once they reach 16, patients are presumed to be competent to consent to medical treatment, unless the contrary is shown.[27] Younger people who have sufficient understanding and intelligence to comprehend fully what is proposed can also give valid consent to treatment, regardless of their age[28] but, whenever feasible, they should be encouraged to involve their parents. If they refuse to involve them, treatment can proceed, even against parents' wishes or without their knowledge, if the young person is competent to decide and cannot be persuaded to include them.

Consent by people under 16: *Gillick*

When the Department of Health and Social Security published guidance saying that doctors were not acting unlawfully in prescribing contraceptives for under-16s, provided that they acted in good faith, Mrs Gillick challenged it. She took her local health authority to court when it refused to assure her that her five daughters under 16 would not be given contraception, without her consent. She argued that parents had to be consulted because a minor's consent was legally ineffective and inconsistent with parental rights. The case went through the courts and Mrs Gillick's view was rejected by the House of Lords. The majority opinion was that the relevant test was whether the girl or young woman had sufficient understanding and intelligence to enable her to grasp fully what was proposed. If she had, a doctor would not be acting unlawfully in giving advice and treatment.[29]

To be valid, consent must be based on competence, information and voluntariness. The requirements can be broken down into several fundamental points, which stem from the *Gillick* judgment:

- the ability to understand that there is a choice and that choices have consequences
- the ability to weigh the information in the balance and arrive at a decision
- a willingness to make a choice (including choosing to let someone else decide)
- an understanding of the nature and purpose of the proposed procedure
- an understanding of its risks and side effects
- an understanding of the alternatives and their risks
- freedom from undue pressure.

The general term used to refer to young people under 16 who meet the legal criteria to make medical decisions is 'Gillick competence'.

After the judgment in the *Gillick* case, specific guidance was issued for doctors considering providing contraception to those under the age of 16. These are known as 'the Fraser guidelines' (after one of the judges in the case, Lord Fraser). Before providing contraception to young people, health professionals must

- consider whether the patient understands the potential risks and benefits of the treatment
- consider whether the patient understands the advice given
- discuss with the patient the value of parental support
- take into account whether the patient is likely to have sexual intercourse without contraception
- assess whether the patient's physical or mental health or both are likely to suffer if the patient does not receive contraceptive advice or treatment
- consider whether the patient's best interests would require the provision of contraceptive advice or treatment or both without parental consent.

It is important for young people who are seeking contraceptive advice to be aware that, although the doctor is obliged to discuss the value of parental support, they are entitled to confidentiality (see Chapter 6).

Case example – requests for contraception by underage patients

In many of the queries raised with the BMA, the core issue centres on whether or not young women can be given contraceptives without their parents' knowledge. Although the *Gillick* case made clear that people with competence under the age of 16 can lawfully be provided with them, the issue of whether, say, a patient aged 13 or 14 can be given the pill often poses dilemmas. Following the *Gillick* judgment, it is clear that the answer depends on the maturity and understanding of the patient. Following the Fraser guidelines, doctors need to consider whether she can understand their advice, including about the risks and benefits of taking the pill. The value of having the support of parents needs to be raised and, if the patient objects, the reasons need to be explored while reassuring her that her confidentiality will be respected (unless there is good reason to think otherwise). The voluntariness of the decision may also need to be talked about, especially if the young person seems to be under pressure from a boyfriend or a peer group, and in some cases, child protection issues may be raised. Consideration also needs to be given to whether she is likely to have sex without contraception and whether her best interests require that it be provided, without parental consent.

Requests for contraception by very young children will always raise concerns. Doctors should usually share information about sexual activity involving children under 13 with child protection services. Any decision not to share this information should be discussed with a named or designated doctor for child protection, and the reasons for the decision not to share recorded.[30]

Competence to refuse

The bar is generally set higher when it comes to assessing a child or young person's competence to refuse important treatment. When refusal cases go to court (not all do), a higher level of evidence of competence is needed where a young patient wants to decline life-saving treatment. Their views can conflict with other people's opinions about their best interests. Parents and health professionals are then torn between respecting their wishes and protecting young patients from the adverse effects of their inexperience. This raises questions of who is best able to judge, and at what stage, what is in an individual's interests. In Chapter 3 and Chapter 4, we have discussed how, for all patients, including adults, autonomy has some limits and this is also true of young people. Both law and ethics stress that the views of children and young people must be heard. In some cases, however, their views alone do not determine what eventually happens.

Young person's refusal of a heart transplant: *Re M*

When M was 15, she refused to have a heart transplant when her own heart was failing. Her mother gave legal consent on her behalf, but health professionals were unwilling to proceed without M's agreement. She said she did not want to die but neither did she wish to have the transplant because this would make her feel different from other people. She was able to explain her ambivalence quite clearly, saying

'I understand what a heart transplant means, procedure explained . . . checkups . . . tablets for the rest of your life. I feel depressed about that. I am only 15 and don't want to take tablets for the rest of my life . . . I don't want to die. It's hard to take it all in . . . If I had children . . . I would not let them die . . . I don't want to die, but I would rather die than have the transplant . . . I would feel different with someone else's heart, that's a good enough reason not to have a heart transplant, even if it saved my life'.[31]

The case was heard in the High Court, and after listening to her views, Mr Justice Johnson decided that M was not capable of making the decision herself and he authorised the operation to go ahead despite her reluctance. 'Events have overtaken her so swiftly that she has not been able to come to terms with her situation', he said.[32] Once that decision had been made on her behalf, M agreed to comply with treatment.

Consent and refusal by competent young people

Consent

As has already been made clear, once the competence of young people has been established, they can consent to treatment on their own behalf, regardless of age. Consent has been described in terms of 'key holders' protecting health professionals from litigation. In England, Wales and Northern Ireland only one key holder is needed to authorise treatment, so that either the competent young person or a person with parental responsibility can do this. In Scotland, the law is slightly different as to whether a parent's consent is enough when a competent young person refuses.

Refusal

Refusal is a different matter to consent in most of the UK where courts have been more reluctant to accept the refusal of minors, even when they are competent. The general trend in England and Wales is for young people's choices to have more weight when they match what health professionals propose. The same is true in Northern Ireland. In these regions of the UK, refusals which jeopardise young people's health can be overridden by a court. Thus, in England, Wales and Northern Ireland, the law is clear that medical treatment to save life or prevent serious damage to health can be imposed upon competent minors who refuse it; this includes 16–18 year olds who are presumed competent.

The power to override a young person's competent refusal: Re W

W was 16 and living in a specialist adolescent residential unit under local authority care. She had anorexia nervosa to such a serious degree that the authority wanted to transfer her to a specialist hospital. W refused. She preferred to stay in the residential unit and said that she would cure herself. An application was made to the court for the authority to move W and give her medical treatment without her consent if necessary. The judge in the Family Division of the High Court concluded that W was competent to refuse treatment but that, even so, the court had the power to override such a refusal when that was in her best interests. W appealed against the decision, but when her condition deteriorated, the Court of Appeal made an emergency order for her to be taken to a specialist hospital and treated. It ruled that the Family Division judge had been wrong to conclude that W was competent because a desire not to be treated was symptomatic of her illness rather than an expression of choice. It also confirmed that courts have the power to override the refusal of competent minors, including those aged 16 and over.[33]

In practice, when young people refuse important or essential treatment, all possibilities of a compromise solution should be explored before resorting to legal process, including involving independent advocates, where appropriate. Where the young person is a Jehovah's Witness refusing a blood transfusion, for example, efforts should be made to accommodate the individual's beliefs, including using any other feasible alternatives to blood or referral to a specialist centre where techniques such as bloodless surgery are practised. If such efforts fail, legal advice should be sought and the courts may need to be involved.

Overriding a young person's refusal of a blood transfusion: *P*

P was a 16-year-old Jehovah's Witness with an inherited condition called hypermobility syndrome, the symptoms of which include a tendency to bleed because of the fragility of the patient's blood vessels. The patient was admitted to hospital suffering from what appeared to be a ruptured aorta, and both the patient and his parents expressed their objection to any treatment using blood or blood products. The doctors acceded to these views because the operation that would be necessary to cure what was then a suspected ruptured aorta was dangerous and likely to be unsuccessful; a blood transfusion was therefore considered futile. The crisis passed but the problem was unresolved. The doctors envisaged that a similar crisis may occur in which the use of blood products could become necessary to save P's life. The hospital asked the court to authorise the use of blood products, despite P's objections, should this become necessary.

There was no suggestion in the judgment that P lacked competence to make the decision or that he was not fully aware of the consequences of his decision. Mr Justice Johnson said there were 'weighty and compelling reasons' not to make the order but, nonetheless, looking at P's best interests, in the widest sense, 'medical, religious, social, whatever they be', 'P's "best interests" in those widest senses will be met if I make an order in the terms sought by the NHS Trust with the addition of . . . "unless no other form of treatment is available" '.[34]

Mr Justice Johnson was mindful of the court's responsibility to ensure so far as it can that children survive to adulthood. He referred to a statement by Nolan LJ in *Re W* that 'In general terms the present state of the law is that an individual who has reached the age of 18 is free to do with his life what he wishes, but it is the duty of the court to ensure so far as it can that children survive to attain that age'.[33]

Ultimately, whether or not cases go to court for resolution depends on the gravity or urgency of the situation and the likelihood of the treatment being successful. It seems unlikely, for example, that chemotherapy would be given against a competent young person's wishes if it had been tried before without making any significant improvement. In the case of Hannah Jones,[35] a decision was made not to involve the courts, despite the grave implications of this young person's refusal of treatment. As the case did not go to court, it should not be seen as a precedent for future problems of this kind. If in doubt, legal advice should always be sought.

Case example – Hannah Jones's refusal of a heart transplant

When aged four, Hannah Jones was diagnosed with leukaemia and spent much of her childhood undergoing treatment which led to her heart being damaged. A heart transplant was proposed when she was 12, but Hannah refused it and her parents supported her choice. Herefordshire Primary Care Trust (PCT) sought legal advice on whether to take the issue to court but decided against that when it was advised that Hannah was competent to make the decision. The PCT's chief executive wrote to Hannah's parents, explaining that it would be inappropriate to seek a court order obliging Hannah to have the transplant when she understood what was at stake and knew that she could die as a result of her refusal. A year later, following a change in her condition, Hannah consented to a heart transplant.

In Scotland, young people become adults at the age of 16. If competent young people under that age refuse life-saving treatment, it probably cannot be given. This is based on a legal case in which the sheriff ruled that competent children of any age can consent to, *or refuse*, treatment. Some commentators see this as more logical than the situation in the rest of the UK where the bar is set higher for refusal than for consent.[36] Again, it is advisable to get legal advice in such situations, as the Scottish courts have not made a definitive ruling on the matter.

A young person's refusal of treatment in Scotland: *Houston*

An application was made to the Glasgow Sheriff's Court regarding a 15-year-old patient with psychotic symptoms who refused to stay in hospital and declined treatment. His doctors believed him competent to make these decisions and thought he understood the implications. They also thought that the right to consent or refuse were of equal validity, so that a young person's competent refusal could not be overridden by his mother's consent. Therefore, treatment without his consent could only be given under Section 18 of the Mental Health (Scotland) Act 1984, which permits detention, if approved by a sheriff. The doctors wanted to avoid invoking this because of the stigma attached to a detention order. As the patient's mother was willing to consent to his treatment, some thought that the proposed order was unnecessary. The sheriff saw the matter differently and said that competent young people could not be overruled by parents. Logic, he said, demanded that a competent young person's decision took precedence over that of a parent and, in his view, the Age of Legal Capacity (Scotland) Act covered refusal as well as consent to treatment. The sheriff granted the detention order with the observation that, despite the stigma, the patient's serious illness and its treatment were the paramount considerations in this case.[37]

This judgment is taken by some to suggest that a competent young person's refusal cannot be overridden, but this legal point has not been finally settled. As there was an alternative way of dealing with the matter, the sheriff was able to bypass the issue of defining the Scottish court's powers to override a competent refusal. In future cases such as this, legal advice should be sought.

Research involving children and young people

Parental consent or refusal for children and babies

Pharmaceutical products have to be specifically designed for children, which means that some young patients and babies participate in research on new drugs. If they did not, treatment for this age group would stagnate and unproven remedies would be perpetuated, but children are obviously a very vulnerable population. Neonates and premature babies can be seen as the most vulnerable of all. Protocols involving them require particularly thorough scrutiny from ethics committees and investigators. For clinical trials of investigational medicinal products, consent for participation by babies or young children is given by people with parental responsibility. They need clear and candid explanations of the purposes, risks, and expected benefits of the research. Parents may also need independent support when making decisions. It has been suggested that a 'cultural mediator' could usefully be involved in seeking consent from families of a different cultural background to that of the researcher.[38] Particular attention needs to be given to parents being clearly told which procedures are standard care and which are specific to research. Much of the research on babies and young children involves relatively routine things such as the taking of blood samples. Where these are additional to the blood tests required for the child's own medical treatment, it is important that those with parental responsibility are fully aware of that and know that they can refuse such procedures without any detriment to the child's treatment.

In some situations, parents may disagree with each other about whether a young child should be included in research or experimental therapy. The reasons for a parent's hesitation need to be taken very seriously, even if the other parent consents. The Medical Research Council says that if agreement cannot be reached, the child should not be involved in the research study, unless a treatment option that the child specifically needs is only available as part of the research programme. In such a scenario, every effort should be made to overcome the disagreement without the need to go to court.[39]

The GMC publishes advice on the involvement of children in research, stressing that either the potential therapeutic benefits for them (if they are patients) should outweigh the foreseeable risks or the research should be only minimal risk (such as asking questions) and not be against their best interests.[40] The Royal College of Paediatrics and Child Health (RCPCH) publishes detailed guidance, pointing out that since children are not small adults, they have an additional, unique set of interests. Research involving them should not only meet the minimum standards set for research on adults but also take account of children's special interests and perspective. Researchers need to bear in mind that many children are easily bewildered and unable to express their needs. 'Potentially with many decades ahead of them, they are likely to experience, in their development and education, the most lasting benefits or harms from research'.[41]

Assent from children who lack competence

Wherever possible, children should still be included in the discussion about participation, even if they cannot understand what the research involves. Seeking agreement from children who lack competence is sometimes called *assent* rather than *consent*, which reflects a positive agreement by people who do understand. *Assent* is more passive and refers to the patient's acquiescence. Children who cannot consent may still be able to assent, indicating a lack of any objection. Assent is contentious as it is sometimes unclear whether children agree to participate or are simply complying with what they are asked to do. A child's assent needs to be backed up by properly informed consent from someone with parental responsibility. If children do not assent or show real unwillingness to participate, this should generally be respected, without reasons having to be given. They should be able to withdraw from the research, unless that would be detrimental to their health.

Consent or refusal by competent children and young people

Competent children should be consulted before being involved in research. Their agreement needs to be voluntary and based on adequate knowledge and understanding of the key information. The *Gillick* case[42] established the common law (in England, Wales and Northern Ireland) but in the past, it was queried whether the legal principles relating to minors' consent to medical treatment applied equally to their consent to participate in medical research. Light was shed on this by the Medicines for Human Use (Clinical Trials) Regulations, which define a minor as someone under the age of 16 and stipulate that, for under-16s, consent for research participation is also needed from parents or the patient's legal representative.[43] So even when competent under-16s consent, it is also necessary to obtain consent from someone with parental responsibility. The explicit wish of a competent child or young person to refuse participation or to be withdrawn must be taken seriously and, in most cases, should be respected.

Emergency research involving children and babies

In 2007, the Medicines and Healthcare products Regulatory Agency consulted on whether the same rules applying to emergency research on incapacitated adults without prior consent (see Chapter 4) should be extended to children in emergency situations. The proposal was to allow a child to be entered into an emergency research trial, without consent by parents or guardians, as long as a research ethics committee had studied the protocol and given approval. In 2008, the Medicines for Human Use (Clinical Trials) and Blood Safety and Quality Amendment was passed, enabling children to take part in emergency care trials when there would be no time to seek parental consent first.

Availability of research and trial data

It is unethical to replicate trials unnecessarily in any patient group and so information gained in any trial should be made available to other researchers and the public. Systematic registration of paediatric trials and publication of results, including unfavourable ones, should take place and the public should be able to access an international database to ensure against replication.

Consent and refusal in exceptional circumstances

Male infant circumcision

Circumcision when there is a clear clinical need is uncontroversial, but in the absence of clinical indications, it can give rise to dilemmas. A spectrum of views exists within society and the medical profession about whether it is a beneficial, neutral or harmful procedure, and whether it should be carried out on children incapable of deciding for themselves. The medical harms or benefits have not been unequivocally proven except to the extent that there are clear risks of harm, if it is done inexpertly. The onus is on parents to say why circumcision is in their child's best interests. The BMA[44] and the GMC[45] note that consent for it should be given by both parents and it has been described by the courts as an important and irreversible decision that should not be taken against the wishes of one parent.[46] If parents disagree about the procedure, the parent arguing for circumcision can try to get a court order authorising it. When a child has only one parent, obviously that person can decide.

Circumcision and a child's best interests: *Re J*

J was a 5-year-old boy who lived with his mother, a non-practising Christian. His father, a non-practising Muslim, wanted him to be circumcised. Asked to decide whether J should be circumcised, the Court of Appeal considered all the factors relevant to J's upbringing and concluded that J should not be circumcised because of three key facts:

- he was not, and was not likely to be, brought up in the Muslim religion
- he was not likely to have such a degree of involvement with Muslims as to justify circumcising him for social reasons
- as a result of these factors, the 'small but definite medical and psychological risks' of circumcision outweighed the benefits of the procedure.[46]

Children capable of expressing a view should be involved in the decision and have their wishes taken into account. Further detailed advice is available in the BMA's guidance note.

Serious difference of opinion between parents and health professionals

Disagreements can usually be resolved through the offer of a second opinion or mediation but in some cases where this has not proved possible, it may be necessary to seek a court declaration. Health professionals should not be deterred from seeking a legal ruling because of the risk of appearing confrontational, as legal review can be the fairest way of deciding what is in the child's interests. The case of *Glass v United Kingdom* highlighted the need to involve the courts as soon as possible when there is a dispute that cannot be resolved, rather than wait until the situation becomes an emergency. Other than in an emergency situation, treatment must not be provided for a child or young person who lacks competence without the consent of someone with parental responsibility or the court.

Involving the court: *Glass*

David Glass was severely mentally and physically disabled, requiring 24-hour care. After surgery to alleviate an upper respiratory tract obstruction, when he was 12 years old, he became critically ill and was put on a ventilator. Doctors thought he was dying. His condition improved briefly and he returned

(Continued)

home but was readmitted a few days later when doctors proposed to use morphine to alleviate his distress. His mother refused, believing it would compromise his chance of recovery. She also made clear that she wanted David resuscitated if his heart stopped. Relations between the family and the healthcare team broke down, to the extent that some members of the family were prosecuted for attacking hospital staff. Although the doctor managing David's care noted the possible need for a court order in such cases of total disagreement, no order was sought and the morphine was provided without consent.

The Glass family argued that the hospital should have involved the courts when the dispute arose to clarify whether, despite his mother's objections, the treatment proposed was in David's best interests and that the doctors were wrong in believing the urgency of the case made that unnecessary. Although dismissed by the UK courts, the European Court of Human Rights took a different view. It said that David's Article 8 right to privacy under the European Convention on Human Rights, and in particular his right to physical integrity, had been breached. As it had been clear that there was a dispute over treatment before the situation reached crisis point, the UK courts should have been used to settle the dispute before an emergency situation arose.[47] In March 2004, the European Court awarded Carol Glass and her son David compensation on the grounds that doctors treated David contrary to his mother's wishes, without a court order.

Paternity testing

Consent to testing

Health professionals are sometimes asked to carry out a paternity test to verify whether or not a child is the genetic offspring of the assumed father. Testing can be done using a blood sample, a few hair follicles or a mouth swab, but consent is required. It is a criminal offence in the UK to have human material for DNA analysis and paternity testing, without consent.[48] If they are competent and understand what is at stake, children and young people can consent themselves to testing or people with parental responsibility can also give consent on their behalf (in England, Wales and Northern Ireland). In Scotland, someone with parental responsibility can only give consent for children who are not competent.

Refusal of testing

If competent young people refuse testing, it may not be in their best interests to proceed, regardless of the views of the adults. If the person with parental responsibility in England, Wales and Northern Ireland refuses to consent to the testing of a person under 16, it can still go ahead if a court considers that it would be in the child's best interests.

Testing and best interests

Health professionals should only agree to participate in a test when it is in the best interests of the child or young person, and each case needs to be considered on its merits. In some cases, the certainty of knowing is likely to be better for the child than an unresolved suspicion, but tests are sometimes requested without thought being given to the impact of the result on all concerned. Health professionals should ask why the test is requested and whether the implications for family relationships have been considered.

Tests which do not involve testing the mother's DNA should only take place if the mother consents to the child being tested, or the father has parental responsibility, or if a court considers the test to be in the child's best interests and authorises testing of the child on that basis. Legally, where the assumed father has parental responsibility for the child, such testing could be undertaken without the mother's knowledge. The BMA has published guidance about paternity testing,[49] which says that where doctors are consulted, they should encourage those seeking testing to discuss their plans with the child's mother and the BMA advises doctors not to become involved if that advice is rejected. Irrespective of the outcome, confidentiality must be respected and no information about the discussion should be passed to the mother or the child without the man's consent.

Advance decision making

In England, Wales and Northern Ireland, where a young person's contemporaneous refusal of treatment may not be determinative, it follows that advance decisions refusing treatment made by young people cannot be legally binding on health professionals. In Scotland, where there is more uncertainty, legal advice should be sought.

In England and Wales, 16–17 year olds are specifically excluded from those parts of the Mental Capacity Act that refer to advance refusals of medical treatment (see Chapter 3).[50] In Scotland, young people are considered adults at 16 and so would be covered by the Adults with Incapacity (Scotland) Act (see Chapter 3).

Using restraint to provide treatment

Restraint is rarely used but can be an option of last resort, for example, in situations where an essential treatment has been authorised by a court but it is impossible to persuade the young person to cooperate.[51] Any form of restriction of liberty should be used only when unavoidable to give essential treatment or to prevent children from hurting themselves. It should be the minimum necessary to achieve that aim. Legal advice should be sought when treatment involves restraint. Treatment plans should include safeguards to ensure that restraint is used as little as possible after the child and parents have been informed why it is needed. Any use of restraint should be recorded in the medical records and subject to clinical audit and review by external agencies. The child or young person may also record his or her own account and response in the records of the incident.

Refusal of medical or psychiatric examination under the Children Act 1989

In certain circumstances, competent children and young people have a legal right to refuse to be examined medically or to have a psychiatric examination or other assessment. The courts can ask for an examination in order to make an interim care, supervision, child protection or emergency protection order, but if children are 'of sufficient understanding to make an informed decision', they can refuse.[52] This provision of the Children Act and its equivalents in other UK jurisdictions is often quoted out of context, giving the erroneous impression that the Act gives young people a general statutory right to refuse any examination for care or treatment. On the contrary, the provisions apply only in the limited cases described earlier. Even in these cases, the High Court in England and Wales has dealt with competent young people refusing examination under the Children Act in the same way as other refusals by competent young people, by overriding their statutory right to refuse.[53] This approach is controversial, and doctors faced with a competent young person refusing examination in such circumstances should seek legal advice. This is particularly necessary in Scotland, where there is likely to be less scope for overriding a competent young person's wishes. Legal advice should be sought if a court order is required swiftly from a judge over the phone.

Child protection

When children or young people are suspected of being at risk of significant harm, their interests override those of parents or carers. Health professionals working with them should be able to identify signs of maltreatment and neglect, and know how to respond appropriately.[54] This is not always straightforward and it is often an extremely difficult judgement call to decide when a suspicion of neglect or abuse warrants urgent action, especially when the medical evidence could be open to interpretation.

In cases where parents are suspects, there can be great reluctance to involve them in any discussion, but where possible, they should be informed about what is going on and their cooperation should be sought. Sometimes, this is essential to find out what has occurred and whether or not prompt multi-agency action is needed.

Case example – judging who should act and when

In one case, the lack of communication between social services and a GP resulted in a traumatic experience for a family from overseas living in the UK. The family's youngest child attended a nursery as both parents worked and took turns in collecting her. A nursery worker taking the child to the lavatory noticed a rash on the girl's genital area and told the father to take the child to the doctor. His English was not good and he did not realise that this was an instruction, not a suggestion. He replied that the family already had medicine for the rash. The nursery staff did not raise the issue with either parent again but when the child was not taken promptly to the doctor, they reported their suspicions that the parents were neglecting or abusing the child to social services who immediately asked for the family's records. The GP released the records, without question or comment and no one informed the parents. A police officer and social worker subsequently went to the family's home. They told the parents that they were under investigation and the child could be taken into care. Now mistrustful of the GP, the parents consulted a paediatrician who examined the child and noted that she did have a slight rash over parts of her body. His report was highly critical of the way the case had been escalated without evidence or discussion. Medical records showed that the child was prone to asthma, eczema and allergies. The GP had seen her regularly and prescribed treatment for these since it was not unusual for her to have an allergic reaction to a new washing powder or bath product. The paediatrician said the GP could have been more proactive in questioning why the records of a family he knew quite well were demanded and should have drawn attention to the documented history of allergic reactions.

The GMC[55] and BMA[56] have produced guidance on safeguarding children and young people. There is also Intercollegiate guidance[57] and individual Royal College guidance[58] – for example, from the Royal College of General Practitioners (RCGP) and the RCPCH. Among other difficulties, these acknowledge the dilemmas that can arise in assessing evidence which is often incomplete or contradictory. In some cases, such as the high-profile tragedies summarised later, the evidence is unambiguous, but professionals can still be unclear about whose obligation it is to ensure that the information is documented, shared and acted upon.

Case example – Victoria Climbié

Eight-year-old Victoria Climbié died as a result of abuse and neglect. She came from the Ivory Coast to live with her aunt in the UK. When she was registered with a GP, the practice was told that she had no health problems, but a neighbour reported concerns about the child's treatment to social services. Evidence of abuse grew after the aunt's boyfriend moved in. Victoria was seen in hospital and found to have injuries that appeared to be non-accidental. She was admitted overnight, and the police and social services were informed. A week later, she was admitted to a second hospital with a severe scald. During her stay, evidence of deliberate physical harm was again noted, but she was returned to her aunt. Her contact with the outside world became sporadic, although she was seen by professionals on several occasions without anything untoward being noticed. The aunt told a social worker that her boyfriend was sexually harming Victoria and was advised to move away from him but later retracted the allegations. Victoria had no further contact with professionals until she was admitted to hospital before her death. Post-mortem examination showed death by hypothermia and malnourishment. Marks on her body showed that she had been tied up and beaten by sharp and blunt instruments. The pathologist said that it was the worst case of deliberate harm to a child that he had ever seen.[59]

Lord Laming's report into Victoria Climbié's death said that protecting her would have 'required nothing more than basic good practice'.[60] Gross system failures were identified, with individuals and agencies failing to act. Information was known but not documented in health records, or was recorded but not shared. Investigations were deferred or assumed to have been carried out by somebody else. Necessary action was identified but was not carried out. Of the Inquiry's 108 recommendations, 27 related specifically to health care, focusing on enquiring about the child's living conditions and social circumstances at registration, improving communication, ensuring that concerns are acted upon, keeping records and attributing clear responsibility for child protection to a single hospital consultant. The Laming Inquiry also recommended that no child about whom there are such concerns should be discharged from hospital without the permission of a senior doctor. Documented plans should be drawn up for the future care of children in such cases. The report's recommendations were reflected in legislation in England and Wales in the Children Act 2004. Despite the impetus for change following his report, Lord Laming was called upon to carry out a further review following the death of Baby P.

Case example – Baby P

Peter Connelly (known at the time as Baby P) was 17 months old when he died in August 2007. His mother, her partner and a lodger were found guilty
(Continued)

of causing or allowing his death. Baby P had previously had contact with health professionals numerous times as a result of non-accidental injuries, resulting in hospital admissions. He was on a child protection register and was the subject of a multi-agency child protection plan involving social services, health services and the police. His mother was arrested twice as a result of Baby P's injuries. Despite this level of professional attention and concern, his post-mortem examination revealed 22 injuries, including a broken back and ribs, as well as signs of many lesser assaults.[61] The GMC subsequently suspended a GP who had seen Baby P 14 times before his death. A consultant paediatrician who had allegedly failed to fully examine Baby P when he was brought in for a developmental check relinquished her registration.

The second Lord Laming report was published in 2009[62] and highlighted how reforms proposed by the earlier report had still not been implemented. It identified a disproportionate focus on meeting targets rather than on managing risks. Recommendations relevant to health included the following:

- systems should be installed and training undertaken so that healthcare staff know if a child has recently presented at any accident and emergency department and is the subject of a child protection plan. When cause for concern arises, contact should be made with other professionals and further medical examinations carried out. No child should be discharged while concerns remain
- all adult mental health, adult drug and alcohol services should have referral processes which prioritise the protection of children. These should include automatic referral where domestic violence or drug or alcohol abuse may put a child at risk of abuse or neglect
- the Department of Health should promote the statutory duty of all GP providers to comply with child protection legislation. It should ensure that they have the skills and training to do this and take steps to raise the level of expertise in child protection within GP practices.

In addition to these, the RCGP also recommends that GPs flag whenever maltreatment is considered using the code 'child is cause for concern'.[63]

Another review of the Baby P case was published by the Care Quality Commission.[64] This also highlighted problems such as poor communication, shortage of staff, lack of training, absence of child protection supervision, lack of awareness of child protection procedures and inadequate governance.[65] As a result of these cases, renewed emphasis was placed on child protection training for health professionals as well as for social workers. All health professionals need to be aware of and follow best practice guidelines, including those from bodies such as the Royal Colleges,[66] health departments[67] and the GMC.[55]

Confidentiality and disclosure of information about abuse or neglect

Patients are entitled to confidentiality but this is not an absolute rule. When child maltreatment is considered or suspected, information sharing and action to protect the victim are essential. If children or young people are competent, they should ideally be involved in the decision to disclose information to the police or child protection agencies. If they cannot be persuaded to agree voluntarily to disclosure, but urgent action is needed, it needs to be explained to them why the disclosure is essential, especially if other young people may be at risk. Without information sharing, it may be impossible to protect the victim or take action against the abuser. In all cases, health professionals' primary responsibility and duty is to safeguard vulnerable patients and act in the child's best interests, but they must also weigh up whether a specific disclosure is justifiable on public interest grounds (see Chapter 6).

Where health professionals believe children or young people who are not competent are at risk, and those with parental responsibility refuse to share relevant information with other health professionals or agencies, disclosure may take place in the public interest without consent. Parents should usually be informed of the information and the reasons for disclosure in advance.

In some cases, vulnerable young people who suffer abuse are willing and anxious to be rescued but their experiences are not believed. This was shown in 2012 by a high-profile trial of nine men from Rochdale who were found guilty of having sexually exploited a number of victims, including a 13 year old who became pregnant and had an abortion. One of the 15-year-old victims had given videotaped testimony to the police in late 2008, but no case was brought at that time as she was seen as an unreliable witness, although her evidence was later central to the trial. Police described 47 of the victims of abuse as being from 'chaotic and council house backgrounds',[68] the implication being that their stories were unbelievable. The case involved repeated rapes and exploitation of young women which focused the media spotlight on the small percentage of abuse that is ever disclosed to the police and large number of cases that, once reported, still never go to trial.[69]

Best practice in child protection

- In all cases, a doctor's primary responsibility is to protect the well-being of the child or children concerned. Where a child is at risk of serious

(Continued)

harm, the interests of the child override those of parents or carers. Never delay taking emergency action.

- All doctors working with children, parents and other adults in contact with children should know when to suspect or consider maltreatment,[70] that is, to be able to recognise, and know how to act upon, signs that a child may be at risk of abuse or neglect, both in a home environment and in residential and other institutions.
- Any doctor seeing a child who raises their concerns must make a record in the medical notes and should ensure follow-on care. In particular, children should not be discharged from hospital without a full examination if there are concerns.
- Efforts should be made to include children and young people in decisions which closely affect them. The views and wishes of children should therefore be listened to and respected according to their competence and the level of their understanding. In some cases translation services suitable for young people may be needed.
- Wherever possible, the involvement and support of those who have parental responsibility for, or regular care of, a child should be encouraged, in so far as this is in keeping with promoting the best interests of the child or children concerned. Older children and young people may have their own views about parental involvement.
- When concerns about deliberate harm or neglect to children or young people have been raised, doctors must keep clear, accurate, comprehensive and contemporaneous notes. These must include a future care plan and identify the individual with lead responsibility.
- All doctors working with children, parents and other adults in contact with children must be familiar with relevant local child protection procedures and must know how to deal promptly and professionally with any child protection concerns raised during their practice.
- All doctors working with children, parents and other adults in contact with children should understand the role of the named and designated professionals and know how to contact them for specialist child protection advice.
- All children and young people health teams should have access to a paediatrician with child protection experience and skills (of at least level 3 safeguarding competencies) available to provide immediate advice and subsequent assessment, if necessary. The requirement is for advice, clinical assessment and the timely provision of an appropriate medical opinion, supported with a written report.[71]
- All doctors working directly with children should ensure that safeguarding and promoting their welfare forms an integral part of all stages of the care they offer. Where doctors have patients who are parents or carers, they must also consider the potential impact of health conditions in those adults on the children in their care.
- Wherever a doctor sees a child and neglect or maltreatment is considered or suspected, and so the child may be at risk, he or she should ensure that systems are in place to ensure follow-up care.
- As full a picture as possible of the circumstances of a child at risk must be drawn up.
- Where a child presents at hospital, enquiries should be made about any previous admissions.
- Where a child is admitted to hospital, a named consultant should be given overall responsibility for the child protection aspects of the case.

(Continued)

- Any child admitted to hospital about whom there are concerns about deliberate harm should receive a thorough examination within 24 hours unless it would compromise the child's care or well-being.
- Where a child at risk is to be discharged from hospital, a documented plan for the future care of the child should be drawn up.
- A child at risk should not be discharged from hospital without being registered at an identified GP.
- All professionals must be clear about their own responsibilities, and which professional has overall responsibility for the child protection aspects of a child's care.

Advisory services and involving the courts

Legal cases involving children are brought for a variety of reasons, many of which have been mentioned in the case examples earlier in the chapter. Children and young people can also be subject to an application for care or supervision proceedings by social services, or an application may be made for them to be adopted. The family courts are also involved when parents who are separating or divorcing do not agree on arrangements for their children. In such circumstances, the organisation, Cafcass,[72] has the role of ensuring children's interests are considered. It represents the child and advises the family courts in England on what it believes to be the best option for the child in individual cases. Children have a right to have their views communicated to the court either directly, through Cafcass or through legal representatives. Judges are also encouraged to permit older children to instruct lawyers directly.[73] Cafcass' website provides a brief overview of the law about children in the sort of cases in which Cafcass is involved, but it cannot provide specific legal advice unless it has been appointed to be a child's legal representative.

Equivalent organisations can be found in the devolved nations:

- Northern Ireland Guardian Ad Litem Agency[74]
- Cafcass Cymru[75]
- The Scottish Children's Reporter[76] and Children's Hearings Department of the Scottish Executive.[77]

In England, Wales and Northern Ireland, courts can authorise treatment on behalf of patients under 18, even when they are competent to decide for themselves. Courts can also override a refusal of treatment by a child or by parents. Scottish courts have the same powers to authorise treatment on behalf of under-16s who lack competence, but it is unclear whether they can override a decision of a competent child. Throughout the UK, courts cannot compel doctors to treat contrary to their professional judgement.

A last word on treating children and young people

The treatment and protection of children and young people can often be part of a difficult balancing act, in which health professionals try simultaneously to respect patients' autonomy and encourage them to take responsibility for their own health while also trying to steer them away from pitfalls that could have a lasting, damaging effect on their lives. When there is evidence, for example, of young people drinking to excess, taking drugs or getting involved in exploitative relationships, the first step is usually to try to engage them in discussion about the risks they are taking and look for workable solutions to help them. They may agree to information being shared with parents or other trusted adults who could help them. If the family is very dysfunctional, the situation can be even more complicated as parental support and assistance is unlikely to be readily available and other agencies may need to be involved. While every situation has to be carefully considered, the courts have shown themselves ready to intervene if the autonomous choices of children and young people could be seriously damaging for them. Health professionals also have responsibilities to intervene, without delay, where they suspect a child may be at risk.

References

1   Children Act 1989, s 3(5); Children (Northern Ireland) Order 1995, s 6(5).
2   Children (Scotland) Act 1995, s 5(1)(b).
3   For discussion of children's abilities and willingness to participate in decisions see: Alderson P. (1993) *Children's Consent to Surgery*, Open University Press, Buckingham.
4   Civil Partnership Act 2004.
5   British Medical Association (2008) *Parental Responsibility: Guidance from the British Medical Association*, BMA, London.
6   General Medical Council (2007) *0–18 Years: Guidance for All Doctors*, GMC, London, paras 12–13.
7   British Medical Association (2010) *Children and Young People Toolkit*, BMA, London, card 6 'Disputes'.
8   *Re C (a Minor) (Medical Treatment)*, sub nom *Re C (a Minor) (Withdrawal of Lifesaving Treatment)* [1998] 1 FLR 384:389.
9   *An NHS Trust v MB* [2006] 2 FLR 319.

10 *Portsmouth NHS Trust v Wyatt* [2005] 1 FLR 21.

11 *Portsmouth NHS Trust v Wyatt* [2005] EWHC 117.

12 *Portsmouth NHS Trust v Wyatt* [2005] 2 FLR 480.

13 *Portsmouth NHS Trust v Wyatt* [2005] 1 FLR 554.

14 *Portsmouth NHS Trust v Wyatt* [21 October 2005] (unreported).

15 Anon. (2006) Disabled Charlotte to be fostered. *BBC News Online* (Oct 16). Available at: http://www.bbc.co.uk/news (accessed 6 June 2012).

16 The last posting on the http://www.savecharlotte.com website dates from December 2007 and said that Charlotte's condition was continuing to improve (accessed 2 October 2012).

17 *Re C (Welfare of Child: Immunisation)* [2003] 2 FLR 1095 CA. *Re J (a Minor) (Prohibited Steps Order: Circumcision), sub noms Re J (Child's Religious Upbringing and Circumcision)*; *Re J (Specific Issue Orders: Muslim Upbringing and Circumcision)* [2000] 1 FLR 571.

18 Children Act 1989, s 1(1); Children (Northern Ireland) Order 1995, art 3(1); Children (Scotland) Act 1995, s 16(1).

19 *Re T (a Minor) (Wardship: Medical Treatment)* [1997] 1 FLR 502:514.

20 Young B, Dixon-Woods M, Windridge KC, *et al.* (2003) Managing communication with young people who have a potentially life threatening chronic illness: qualitative study of patients and parents. *BMJ* **326**, 305–308.

21 Leveton M, American Academy of Paediatrics Committee on Bioethics (2008) Communicating with children and families: from everyday interactions to skill in conveying distressing information. *Pediatrics* **121**, e1441–1460.

22 General Medical Council (2007) *0–18 Years: Guidance for All Doctors*, GMC, London, para 20.

23 General Medical Council (2007) *0–18 Years: Guidance for All Doctors*, GMC, London, para 14.

24 General Medical Council (2007) *0–18 Years: Guidance for All Doctors*, GMC, London, para 15.

25 General Medical Council (2007) *0–18 Years: Guidance for All Doctors*, GMC, London, para 22.

26 For detailed advice about assessing competence see: British Medical Association (2001) *Consent, Rights and Choices in Health Care for Children and Young People*, BMJ Books, London.

27 Family Law Reform Act 1969, s 8(1); Age of Majority Act (Northern Ireland) 1969, art 4(1); Age of Legal Capacity (Scotland) Act 1991, s 1(1)(b).

28 *Gillick v West Norfolk and Wisbech AHA* [1985] 3 All ER 402; R *(on the application of Axon) v Secretary of State for Health* [2006] 2 WLR 1130; Age of Legal Capacity (Scotland) Act 1991, s 2(4).

29 *Gillick v Wisbech and West Norfolk AHA* [1985] 3 All ER 402.

30 General Medical Council (2007) *0–18 Years: Guidance for All Doctors*, GMC, London, para 67.

31 *Re M (Child: Refusal of Medical Treatment)* [1999] 2 FLR 1097:1100C-D.

32 *Re M (Child: Refusal of Medical Treatment)* [1999] 2 FLR 1097:1100G.

33 *Re W (a Minor) (Medical Treatment: Court's Jurisdiction)* [1992] 4 All ER 627.

34   *P (Medical Treatment: Best Interests)* [2004] 2 FLR 1117, para 12.

35   Dyer C. (2008) Trust decides against action to force girl to undergo transplant. *BMJ* **337**, a2480. (See also correction *BMJ* **337**, a2659).

36   Thomson JM. (2002) *Family Law in Scotland*, 4th edn, E Butterworths/Law Society of Scotland, Edinburgh, pp.189–190; Wilkinson AB, Norrie KM. (1999) *The Law Relating to Parent and Child in Scotland*, 2nd edn, Green, Edinburgh; Sutherland EE. (1999) *Child and Family Law*, Clark, Edinburgh, para 3.71.

37   *Houston (Applicant)* [1996] 32 BMLR 93. Children (Scotland) Act 1995, s15(5)(b).

38   European Commission (2006) *Ethical Considerations for Clinical Trials Performed in Children*, European Commission, Brussells.

39   Medical Research Council (2004) *Medical Research Involving Children*, MRC, London, p.28.

40   General Medical Council (2007) *0–18 Years: Guidance for Doctors*, GMC, London, para 37.

41   Royal College of Paediatrics and Child Health (2000) *Guidelines for the Ethical Conduct of Medical Research Involving Children*, RCPCH, London, p.177.

42   *Gillick v West Norfolk and Wisbech AHA* [1986] AC 112; [1985] 3 WLR 830; [1985] 3 All ER 402, HL.

43   Medicines for Human Use (Clinical Trials) Regulations 2004, schedule 1, part 1(2).

44   British Medical Association (2006) *The Law and Ethics of Male Circumcision – Guidance for Doctors*, BMA, London.

45   General Medical Council (2008) *Personal Beliefs and Medical Practice*, GMC, London, paras 12–16.

46   *Re J (a Minor) (Prohibited Steps Order: Circumcision) sub noms Re J (Child's Religious Upbringing and Circumcision); Re J (Specific Issue Orders: Muslim Upbringing and Circumcision)* [2000] 1 FLR 571.

47   *Glass v United Kingdom* (61827/00) [2004] ECHR 103 (9 March 2004).

48   Human Tissue Act 2004, s 45.

49   British Medical Association (2009) *Paternity Testing, Guidance from the BMA Ethics Department*, BMA, London.

50   For more details, see: Department for Constitutional Affairs (2007) *Mental Capacity Act 2005 Code of Practice*, The Stationery Office, London, chapter 12.

51   Royal College of Nursing (2003) *Restraining, Holding Still and Containing Children and Young People: Guidance for Nursing Staff*, RCN, London.

52   Children Act 1989, s 38(6); Children (Northern Ireland) Order 1995, art 57(6); Children (Scotland) Act 1995, s 90. The Scottish legislation gives competent young people the right to refuse to submit to medical or psychiatric examination or other assessment that has been directed by the court or a children's hearing for the purpose of a supervision requirement, assessment, protection or place of safety order.

53   *South Glamorgan CC v B sub nom South Glamorgan CC v W and B* [1993] FLR 574.

54   National Collaborating Centre for Women's and Children's Health (2009) *When to Suspect Child Maltreatment*, RCOG Press, London.

55   General Medical Council (2012) *Protecting Children and Young People: the Responsibilities of All Doctors*, GMC, London.

56 British Medical Association (2009) *Child Protection – a Toolkit for Doctors*, BMA, London.

57 Intercollegiate document (2010) *Safeguarding Children and Young People: Roles and Competences for Health Care Staff*, RCPCH, London.

58 Royal College of General Practitioners (2009) *Safeguarding Children and Young People: a Toolkit for General Practice*, RCGP, London; Royal College of Paediatrics and Child Health (2006) *Child Protection Companion*, RCPCH, London.

59 The Victoria Climbié Inquiry (2003) *Report of an Inquiry by Lord Laming*, The Stationery Office, London.

60 The Victoria Climbié Inquiry (2003) *Report of an Inquiry by Lord Laming*, The Stationery Office, London, para 1.16.

61 *R v (B)(The boyfriend of Baby Peter's mother)(C)(Baby Peter's mother) and Jason Owen*. Sentencing remarks, Central Criminal Court, 22 May 2009, para 2.

62 Lord Laming (2009) *The Protection of Children in England: a Progress Report*, The Stationery Office, London.

63 Royal College of General Practitioners (2011) *RCGP Recommendations for Recording Concerns about Child Maltreatment in Primary Care*, RCGP, London. Available at: http://www.clininf.eu/childmaltreatment (accessed 26 September 2012).

64 Care Quality Commission (2009) *Review of the Involvement and Action Taken by Health Bodies in Relation to the Case of Baby P*, CQC, London.

65 Care Quality Commission (2009) *Review of the Involvement and Action Taken by Health Bodies in Relation to the Case of Baby P*, CQC, London, p.25.

66 Intercollegiate Document (2010) *Safeguarding Children and Young People: Roles and Competences for Health Care Staff*, RCPCH, London; Royal College of General Practitioners (2009) *Safeguarding Children and Young People: a Toolkit for General Practice*, RCGP, London; Royal College of Paediatrics and Child Health (2006) *Child Protection Companion*, RCPCH, London.

67 Department of Health, Home Office, Department for Education and Employment (2010) *Working Together to Safeguard Children. A Guide to Inter-agency Working to Safeguard and Promote the Welfare of Children*, The Stationery Office, London; Department of Health (2006) *What to Do if You Are Worried a Child Is Being Abused*, DH, London; Welsh Assembly Government (2007) *Safeguarding Children: Working Together under the Children Act 2004*, WAG, Cardiff; Scottish Executive Health Department (2003) *Protecting Children. A Shared Responsibility. Guidance for Health Professionals in Scotland*, SEHD, Edinburgh; Department of Health, Social Services and Public Safety (2003) *Co-operating to Safeguard Children*, DHSSPS, Belfast.

68 Martinson J. (2012) The great silent crime. *The Guardian* supplement (May 10), p.7.

69 According to NSPCC research published after the trial, only 34 percent of sexually abused children tell anyone about it and the Crown Prosecution Service said that of 17,000 reported cases of sexual offences involving children, only 4,000 went to court in 2011. Data reported in *The Guardian*, 10 May 2012, p.6.

70 National Institute for Health and Clinical Excellence (2009) *When to Suspect Child Maltreatment (CG89)*, NICE, London.

71 Royal College of Paediatrics and Child Health (2011) *Facing the Future: Standards for Paediatric Services*, RCPCH, London, standard 10.

72   See: http://www.cafcass.gov.uk (accessed 7 June 2012).

73   *Mabon v Mabon and Others* [2005] EWCA Civ 634.

74   See: http://www.nigala.hscni.net (accessed 22 January 2013).

75   See: http://www.new.wales.gov.uk/cafcasscymru (accessed 7 June 2012).

76   See: http://www.scra.gov.uk (accessed 7 June 2012).

77   See: http://www.chscotland.gov.uk (accessed 7 June 2012).

6: Patient confidentiality

10 things you need to know about . . . confidentiality

- Confidentiality is a key facet of the trust between health professionals and their patients.
- Anything that health professionals learn about a patient in the course of their professional duties is confidential.
- All patients, including children, are entitled to confidentiality, but that right is not absolute.
- The duty of confidentiality extends beyond death.
- Information may be shared, but this requires the patient's consent or some legal authority or the disclosure must be justified in the public interest.
- Patients are usually considered to have given their implied consent to information being shared as part of the delivery of their health care, but an explanation of this should be readily available to patients.
- While identifiable patient information is confidential, anonymous data can be used more freely.
- Anonymous information must be used for purposes other than direct patient care unless a lawful justification for disclosure exists.
- Disclosure without consent or a reasonable justification can result in complaints to the General Medical Council (GMC) or a fine by the Information Commissioner.
- Applying the 'least principle' (the least amount of information, used by the least number of people necessary for the purpose) can reduce the risk of a breach of confidentiality.

Setting the scene

By far the most common enquiries to the BMA's Ethics Department concern aspects of patient confidentiality or of record keeping (see Chapter 7 on the management of health records). While the basic rules seem straightforward, applying them to complex situations or society's changing expectations is not. Doctors' duty to keep information confidential has a very long history and is seen as a cornerstone of their relationship with patients, but confidentiality

Everyday Medical Ethics and Law, First Edition. Ann Sommerville.
© 2013 BMA Medical Ethics Department. Published 2013 by John Wiley & Sons, Ltd.

remains a topic of significant debate. This is principally about how doctors can maintain a confidential relationship with their patients while allowing health information to be used to support the management and improvement of the NHS. In many questions raised with the BMA, the doctor is unsure whether consent is required for the sharing of information for a particular purpose or, in more complex cases, doctors must judge whether the particular circumstances justify disclosure in the public interest. Legal rules, principles and guidelines can help to set out the framework within which the decision is made, but doctors are still required to weigh up the conflicting interests, consider the various options and the views and interests of all parties in order to reach a judgment. The information contained in this chapter is intended to inform that process.

Common enquiries about confidentiality

- Should there be automatic disclosure to the police if a crime has occurred?
- Once patients have died, can their relatives have all their information?
- What are the rules about confidentiality when adults lack mental capacity?
- Can patients stop me sending a report to an insurer, if they previously agreed?
- Is it OK to leave a bland message for patients on their answerphone?
- Do I need patients' agreement to use their information for financial or clinical audit?
- Are there any limits on what I share with social services when discharging patients who need social support?
- Do I need patients' permission to tell the police when they have been beaten up?

Patients provide information, often very sensitive information, to their doctors on the basis of consent and within a relationship of trust.

Medical information should remain confidential unless disclosure is justified by

- patient consent (either implied or express)
- a legal authority (e.g. a legal requirement to report certain diseases or a court order to disclose information)
- the public interest, such as where failure to disclose would result in death or serious harm.

The duty of confidentiality extends beyond death.

The GMC advises that all disclosures of identifiable information should be the minimum necessary to achieve the objective, so that where possible, anonymised or coded patient information should be used when disclosure is not about giving the patient care. It also urges health professionals to keep up to date with all relevant legal requirements,[1] which is an increasingly challenging task (the BMA's website aims to offer such up-to-date information). In situations where healthcare professionals are unsure about whether or not a particular disclosure is appropriate, advice can be sought from a number of sources, including professional bodies like the BMA or Caldicott guardians, who are senior NHS staff appointed to protect the confidentiality of patient information.

Inappropriate sharing of information is likely to damage the trust which is so fundamental to the doctor–patient relationship and could, over time, lead to patients being reluctant to provide relevant information because of fears their confidentiality will not be respected. Equally, however, patients expect that appropriate information will be made available promptly to other health professionals providing their care. In addition, the use of patient information for research and planning purposes can lead to significant benefits for both the individual patient and the overall provision of care. It is important that these benefits are not lost because of overly restrictive limits on the use of information but also that patients are always aware of how their information might be used. For example, it is often the case that the use of anonymisation or aggregation would allow beneficial access to health information without compromising confidentiality. Where identifiable patient information is needed, however, there must be a clear legal justification for disclosure.

With changes to the NHS and the increasing use of electronic health records, the need for an appropriate balance between the protection of patient information and the sharing of information to improve patient care will continue to be debated. Currently, strong differences of opinion coexist about where boundaries should be drawn in this area.[2] The reality is that patients are generally unaware of how their personal information is shared and used.[3] While many probably have no objection to it being used for purposes such as research, they still like to be asked.

What is confidential?

Any information a health professional learns in the context of providing care to patients is confidential. This includes details such as patients' NHS number, the name of the doctor they see and the clinics they attend, as well as any treatments recommended. It is sometimes argued that many patients do not feel strongly about these kinds of details but would want assurances that anything particularly *sensitive* in their history would be protected. The obvious problem with this approach is that while we may all agree on the most likely areas of sensitivity (such as issues around mental health, sexuality, paternity, pregnancy, abortion), massive scope remains for disagreement about other details in individual cases. In law all health information is regarded as 'sensitive' and must be protected from inappropriate disclosure. Some electronic record systems allow certain pieces of information to be hidden or have access restrictions in place at the request of the patient (see Chapter 7).

Identifiable data

Health or background social information which identifies a living person is confidential. Doctors are expected to safeguard all identifiable patient information obtained as part of their professional activity[4] and this can include social details about patients' family or relationships. Clinical information about a named person's diagnosis or treatment obviously falls within the definition of identifiable material, as do identifiable images of patients such as photos, X-rays or videos. Audiotapes can also fall within the scope of confidential material. Any information linked to a patient's name, address, full postcode or date of birth has the potential to identify them. This means that electronic communications, such as faxes about treatment appointments or operations, also need to be kept securely. Some information might identify an individual only when linked with other information. For example, even if all obvious identifiers are removed, the fact that patients have a rare disease or unusual drug treatment or a particular genetic make-up can render them identifiable in some circumstances. Statistical analyses which have very small numbers within a small population can do the same. A breach of confidentiality does not occur if patients know the extent of disclosure and to whom it will be made, and agree to it.

Anonymised data

Patient information can be used more freely, without consent, if it is effectively anonymised. This raises the question of what counts as effective anonymisation. True anonymisation is a permanent process. Some argue it is impossible to achieve it when using detailed information about an individual as there will always be some identifiable factor, even if only patients themselves or people close to them recognise it. Removal of obvious details such as the patient's name, date of birth, NHS number and postcode can still leave material identifiable in some circumstances, but information is generally accepted as anonymous, once those details are separated from clinical or administrative data. Wherever possible, information that has had these details removed (often referred to as de-identified data) should be used for purposes not directly connected with the care of the patient. It must be borne in mind, however, that rare diseases and other exceptional factors may still allow individuals to be identified and any combination of details increases the chances of that happening. The risk of re-identification depends on several factors such as the actual content of the information and the availability of other information that could be used to reveal identity. At the time of writing the Information Commissioner was in the process of producing a code of practice on anonymisation which will provide guidance on how information can be successfully anonymised and how to assess the risks of identification. Information about this will be included on the BMA's website. Information on the role of the Health and Social Care Information Centre in anonymising data is provided later in this chapter.

While their consent is not essential for the use of anonymised data, patients should generally have access to material explaining what is involved. Legally, the duty of confidentiality is lifted when data are effectively anonymised.[5] This was clarified in a legal case concerning the sale of prescribing data.

The use of anonymised data: *Source Informatics*

Source Informatics was the name of an American company which sought information about doctors' prescribing habits to sell on to pharmaceutical companies. Access to the prescribing data would allow the drug companies to market their products more effectively. Source Informatics was interested in the identity of the prescribing doctors and in knowing what they prescribed but was uninterested in the identity of the patients. It proposed that pharmacists should collect anonymous data by computer and pass it to Source Informatics for a fee. The Department of Health published guidance, saying this was a breach of confidentiality and the judge at first instance upheld that view. Source Informatics appealed against the decision, which was overturned in the Court of Appeal. This held that confidentiality was not breached as long as patients' identities were protected. The Department of Health's guidance was withdrawn.[5]

Pseudonymised data

Reversible anonymisation is sometimes called pseudonymisation or 'key coding' of data. It is described as being similar to anonymisation because the holder of the information cannot reasonably identify someone from it, but differs, because the original provider of the information can do so. The provider can keep a way of identifying individuals, by attaching codes or other unique references to their details. 'Pseudonymisation allows information about the same individual to be linked in a way that true anonymisation does not'.[6] The process involves replacing patient identifiers (name, address, NHS number) with a pseudonym that allows the data to be reconstructed when required. It is useful in some kinds of research, where the patient's identity is irrelevant for much of the project but researchers need to be able to distinguish between individuals or to link data at a later stage. For professionals who have access to both the pseudonymised data and the means to reconstitute them, the information must be treated as identifiable but for those without the means of reversing the process, the information is anonymous and patient consent is not required. Legally, the pseudonymised information may still fall within the Data Protection Act's definition of 'personal data' and use of the information should comply with the requirements of the legislation. Although this point has not been tested in court, the Information Commissioner advises NHS bodies and clinicians to apply the Act in these circumstances. As there remains a small risk of re-identification of pseudonymised data, additional safeguards are required, such as contractual obligations to link data only with the permission of the original data controller and not to disclose the data to third parties where there is a possibility of re-identification.

Keeping information secure

Sometimes, breaches of confidentiality occur inadvertently or as a result of poor practice rather than deliberate disclosures. Health professionals have a responsibility to ensure that health information is kept securely and is protected from unauthorised access.

Case examples – breaches of confidentiality

In 2009, the GMC found a GP guilty of deficient professional performance for breaching confidentiality after he dictated a referral letter in the reception area of the surgery. Other patients were waiting to be seen and could over-hear the details, which included the procedure requested and a summary of the patient's family medical history. The GMC imposed conditions on the GP's registration for 12 months.[7]

In 2011, a medical practice in Durham sent discharge letters about two patients, by fax, to the wrong number. The staff member failed to notice the incorrect number when forwarding information about the patients' surgery. The recipient reported the incident and destroyed the faxes. The practice agreed to use faxes only in exceptional cases in future and send most electronic discharge letters by secure mail. It also programmed regularly used numbers into the fax machine to minimise future errors.[8]

Steps should be taken to ensure that information is kept securely, for example, by ensuring that doors and filing cabinets are locked and that information sent or kept electronically is encrypted and password protected.

Case examples – failure to keep data secure

In September 2011, the Information Commissioner's Office (ICO) required two NHS facilities to tighten up their data security after they lost sensitive patient information.

A medical student, on a placement at the University Hospital of South Manchester's burns unit, copied the data of 87 patients onto a personal USB stick for research and then lost it. The trust had wrongly assumed that the student had data protection training and, ironically, had provided an encrypted memory stick for the student to carry out an audit. At the end of the placement the student copied the data from the encrypted stick on to a personal one, which was then lost. The trust was told to ensure all students had security training in future.

In the second case, a laptop was stolen from the home of an ambulance service staff member who had emailed confidential data to a personal, unencrypted laptop in order to work from home. The ICO was critical in both cases that agreed policies and procedures were still not being implemented. He said that 'health workers who wouldn't dream of discussing patient information openly with friends, continue to put information on unencrypted memory sticks . . . Complying with the law need not be a day-to-day burden if effective measures are built in and become second nature'.[8]

Informing patients about possible uses of their health information

Professional and regulatory bodies, such as the GMC, set out standards and principles which doctors and other health professionals need to observe. For doctors, the GMC stipulates that patients should have ready access to explanations about the circumstances in which their health information may be disclosed as part of their care or for local clinical audit. It should be made clear to patients that they can object to information sharing for these purposes and that their consent is required before their information is disclosed for purposes unconnected to their care, unless the law requires disclosure or it is justified in the public interest.

The NHS Care Record Guarantee sets out the legal and policy position for patients in England on how the NHS uses their information.[9] It stresses patients' rights and, among its commitments, promises patients access to their own records and controls on access by other people. It offers patients options to further limit access and sets out the provisions needed for access in an emergency or when patients become incapable of making decisions for themselves. Other similar policies and standards exist in the four nations which provide guidance for healthcare professionals to ensure that patients are fully involved with decisions about the use of their information and that information provided by patients is kept confidential.[10]

The law on confidentiality and disclosure

The law in this area of practice consists of a complex patchwork of statute and common law. It specifies some situations in which disclosure of health information is obligatory, as well as other scenarios where it is severely restricted or where judgements have to be made by health professionals about whether or not it can be justified in an individual instance.

The common law protecting confidentiality

A lot of the law protecting confidentiality is not set out in statute but has evolved through legal judgments. (The differences between statute and common law are explained in Chapter 1.) Society has an interest in maintaining a confidential health service[11] and under common law, health professionals have a legal duty to protect patient information when it is given by patients in situations where an obligation of confidence is implied, or when it is, by its nature, confidential. Most medical information falls into one, or both, of these categories. Even sensitive personal information can be disclosed, however, with the consent of the person to whom it relates. Or it can be released without consent where the law requires, or authorises, its disclosure. In addition, legal judgments have established that confidentiality may be breached when there is an overriding public interest which trumps a patient's right to confidentiality.

Data Protection Act 1998

At the time of writing, the European Commission was reforming European Union (EU) data protection legislation to provide a stronger framework for data use. In the long term, this will have a knock-on effect on UK law.[12] In the meantime, the Data Protection Act 1998 regulates the use and disclosure of identifiable information about living people throughout the UK. Its provisions are overseen by the Information Commissioner whose role is to enforce the Act. The ICO can impose sanctions on people or organisations that breach the Act, which can result in heavy fines.[13] The legislation is based on eight principles. These require that data must be fairly and lawfully processed for specific purposes, which means that patients have rights to be informed about how identifiable information about them will be used. Information cannot be used in ways that are incompatible with the purposes for which it was given. The data must be accurate, relevant, secure, not excessive and cannot be kept for longer than necessary. Processing must respect data subjects' rights and their information cannot be transferred abroad without adequate protection.[14]

Case example – retention of information

A GP, who was approaching retirement, asked the BMA's ethics department for advice about the use of patient information. He was planning to download the contact details of his patients to his laptop and then wanted to use this information, after his retirement, to send them literature about a private health screening company he would be working with. He was advised that this would breach the Data Protection Act and that he should not retain any patient information – including names and addresses – when he was no longer involved in the patients' care or treatment.

Although health professionals need to be aware of the Data Protection Act, and specifically the principles mentioned above, in practical terms it is the professional code of medical confidentiality, underpinned by the common law, that generally governs the use and sharing of health information. This requires that identifiable patient information is shared only with consent, where there is a relevant legal authority or an overriding public interest.

Health professionals also need to be aware of the statutory rights afforded to patients, to have access to information about themselves and to have inaccurate information corrected. This is covered in Chapter 7.

Health and Social Care Act 2012 (England)

The Health and Social Care Act 2012 established an NHS Information Centre for Health and Social Care (HSCIC) in England, to carry out the functions of an 'honest broker' so that information from medical records can be used for the benefit of the health service. This means the HSCIC can collect data from a range of healthcare providers, linking them where relevant, and carry out de-identification processes in a secure, central environment (a 'safe haven') which has safeguards in place to protect the confidentiality of the data it holds. The data will be made available in a de-identified format to those who require it to pursue research and improvements to health care. The HSCIC will also publish some of the information it collects and will have a role in quality assuring the information.[15]

Under the Act, the Secretary of State for Health and selected NHS organisations can mandate the HSCIC to collect identifiable data from healthcare providers when necessary for their functions. Healthcare providers must comply with such requests from the HSCIC. Among the bodies entitled to ask for identifiable data are the NHS Commissioning Board, the Care Quality Commission (CQC), Monitor (the independent regulator of NHS foundation trusts) and the National Institute for Health and Clinical Excellence (NICE). Identifiable data cannot actually leave the HSCIC unless there is an existing legal basis for the disclosure to these bodies. All data collection under the Act must also comply with the statutory code of practice.[16] The Act also created a National Information Governance Committee, replacing the National Information Governance Board , which will function within the CQC until 2015. (For information about developments after that, see the BMA website.)

The NHS Future Forum and the review of information governance

In 2011, during the passage through Parliament of the (then) Health and Social Care Bill, the Government took time to reflect on its modernisation plans for the NHS. It established an independent advisory panel called the NHS Future Forum to listen to the concerns that people had about the Bill and report back to the Prime Minister. How patient information was being used in the NHS was one of the issues considered. It recommended that a review of the information governance rules be carried out, with the aim of ensuring an appropriate balance between the protection of patient information and the sharing of it to improve patient care. In February 2012, it was announced that Dame Fiona Caldicott would lead the review, scheduled to report in early 2013. As part of this review, consideration would be given to information governance within the new NHS organisational structures, including the changes needed for the transition from paper to electronic records and the use of health information for commissioning. Changes to the existing statutory provisions may also result from the review. Information about the practical impact of any recommendations arising from this review will be included on the BMA website.

Statutory disclosures

Some disclosure of health information is legally required, regardless of patient consent, although patients should usually be made aware of it. Statutory reporting normally only obliges the release of some specific facts, not large tracts of patient history.

Examples of statutory obligations to disclose information

- Designed to monitor and control the spread of infectious diseases, various pieces of public health legislation oblige health professionals to report notifiable diseases. The identity, sex and address of patients suspected of having such conditions, including food poisoning, must be submitted to the relevant authority.[17] In England and Wales, this obligation includes reporting on patients who have undergone some form of contamination which could be harmful to others.[18]
- Doctors carrying out a termination of pregnancy are required under the Abortion Regulations 1991 (in England, Wales and Scotland) to notify the Chief Medical Officer.[19]
- Industrial injuries and accidents fall under the Reporting of Injuries, Diseases and Dangerous Occurrences Regulations 1995 (UK-wide). These require the notification of any death, major injury or accident that results in a patient missing work for more than 3 days. They also cover certain diseases.[20]

As part of the requirements of registration with the CQC, English NHS trusts must report serious patient safety incidents, deaths or events that may indicate risks to ongoing compliance with registration requirements.[21]

Statutory restrictions on disclosure

The law restricts what can be disclosed by health professionals when information is perceived as highly sensitive.

Examples of statutory restrictions on disclosure

- Transsexuals who have taken steps to live permanently in their acquired gender can apply for legal recognition of it under the Gender Recognition Act 2004. The legislation is UK-wide. Under it, an offence is committed if 'protected information', acquired in an official capacity, is disclosed. This includes information about peoples' applications for gender recognition and their gender history, after they have changed gender under the Act.[22]
- Information that could identify a patient examined or treated for any sexually transmitted disease, including HIV, is severely restricted under the NHS (Venereal Disease) Regulations 1974. Disclosure is permitted to a doctor in connection with the patient's treatment and for the prevention of the spread of the disease. In England and Wales, this obligation extends to all employees of trusts or commissioning bodies under the Sexually Transmitted Diseases Directions 2000. Different interpretations of the Regulations and Directions exist, but the GMC has issued advice on them, taking the view that they do not preclude disclosure if it would otherwise be lawful at common law, for example, with the patient's consent or in the public interest without consent.[23]

(Continued)

- The Human Fertilisation and Embryology Act 1990 (as amended) protects the confidentiality of the information held by clinics and the Human Fertilisation and Embryology Authority (HFEA). Information can only be accessed by staff working in licensed centres, staff or members of the HFEA, the patient to whom the information relates and another licensed centre needing it to carry out its licensed functions. In certain circumstances, the Registrar General or a court may also have access. Patients can consent to the disclosure of their own information and disclosure can occur in medical emergencies and for specific formal proceedings.[24] Disclosure of information identifying the patient to another party without consent is a criminal offence. The Human Fertilisation and Embryology Act 2008 amended the 1990 Act to permit some information protected under the Act to be disclosed for research purposes. This was given effect through the Human Fertilisation and Embryology (Disclosure of Information for Research Purposes) Regulations 2010.

Human Rights Act 1998 (UK-wide)

Human rights law affects medical practice in a variety of ways (see Chapter 1). Among other provisions, it guarantees a right to 'respect for private and family life'. This right is not an absolute right and can be set aside in certain circumstances, such as when it is essential to do so in the interests of national security and public safety, or to prevent crime and disorder. Overall, this legislation reinforces the common law duty of confidentiality. Its message is that privacy is important, but confidentiality may be breached, exceptionally, when it conflicts with other significant interests.

Confidentiality and the Human Rights Act: *Campbell*

Model Naomi Campbell was photographed leaving a Narcotics Anonymous meeting. When the photos were published in the *Mirror* newspaper, she brought a claim for breach of confidence, engaging the Article 8 right to private and family life. She asked the court to recognise the private nature of the information and to rule that her privacy had been breached. She did not challenge the disclosure of the fact she was a drug addict, but she challenged the disclosure of information about the location of her narcotics meetings. The photographs, she argued, formed part of this information. The publisher of the photos, Mirror Group Newspaper (MGN), was found liable and appealed. The Court of Appeal reversed the earlier decision, saying that the photos could be published since they were peripheral to the story about her addiction and treatment. Naomi Campbell then appealed to the House of Lords, which held that MGN was liable. Two judges disagreed, arguing that since she did not challenge the *Mirror* publishing that she was a drug addict receiving treatment, printing the photos was within the editors' discretion. Three other judges were not persuaded by this argument and

(Continued)

said that the photos added something of real significance. One, Lord Hope, said that a duty of confidence arises wherever the defendant knows, or ought to know, that claimants can reasonably expect their privacy to be protected. The Lords engaged in a balancing test. The first step was to assess whether Naomi Campbell had a reasonable expectation of privacy (Article 8) and, if she did, would that interfere with the newspaper's freedom of expression (Article 10). They held that Naomi Campbell's right to privacy outweighed MGN's right to freedom of expression.[25]

NHS Act 2006 (England and Wales)

Under the NHS Act 2006 (Section 251), the Secretary of State for Health can make regulations which allow the common law duty of confidentiality to be set aside, if anonymised data are insufficient and seeking patient consent is impracticable for certain purposes. The regulations are set out in the Health Service (Control of Patient Information) Regulations 2002 and can only be used to support 'medical purposes' that are in the interests of patients or the wider public. These purposes include medical research and some essential NHS activities needing identifiable data. Prior to the regulations, there was no secure legal basis for disclosures of data without consent to support cancer registries, or for communicable disease surveillance by the Health Protection Agency. For disclosures to disease registries (other than cancer registries), doctors should check if Section 251 approval has been given – this information is available on the National Information Governance Board for Health and Social Care (NIGB) website.[26]

Responsibility for administering powers under Section 251 was given to NIGB, which delegated them to an Ethics and Confidentiality Committee (ECC). NIGB produced guidance on the ECC approval process and the data protection and public interest considerations, which needed to be taken into account when applications were assessed. These required that the Data Protection Act's principles on fair processing and use of minimal information were observed and that consideration be given to how the proposed research would serve the public good and whether individuals might be harmed by disclosure. The reasons for not seeking patient consent and whether other information sources would suffice also had to be considered.[27] The Health and Social Care Act 2012 abolished NIGB and created a National Information Governance Committee to replace it. The ECC was due to continue its current work until March 2013 when it was intended that the Health Research Authority would take over this role. (Up-to-date information can be found on the BMA's website).

Although the Section 251 powers were originally intended as a transitional measure, while consent or anonymisation procedures were developed, it has become clear that either they or some comparable statutory powers are necessary in the longer term.

Comparable arrangements in Northern Ireland

Northern Ireland's Privacy Advisory Committee can advise on some of the same considerations as described above for England and Wales, but it lacks statutory powers. It cannot lawfully authorise disclosures of identifiable data without consent. Discussions are ongoing about the need to introduce a new legislative framework for information governance in Northern Ireland.

Comparable arrangements in Scotland

In Scotland, patient information is brought together and managed at a national level by the Information Services Division (ISD), which is part of NHS National Services Scotland. A Privacy Advisory Committee provides advice to the Caldicott Guardian for the ISD on the use of personal health information for research.[28] This does not have statutory powers and so disclosures of identifiable data without consent have to rely on a public interest justification.

Computer Misuse Act 1990 (UK-wide)

This Act makes it illegal to access computer material without prior authority. It legislates against the use of another person's ID and password without authority in order to use, alter or delete data.

Use of patient information for purposes directly related to care

Consent by patients with capacity

Most patients understand and accept that information must be shared within the healthcare team in order to provide care. This might include sharing information among the healthcare team in order to deliver care, record keeping (see Chapter 7) and local clinical audit. In order to rely on implied consent, however, the GMC states that information must be 'readily available to patients explaining that unless they object, personal information about them will be shared within the healthcare team'.[29] In practical terms the concept of 'no surprises' is a helpful one to bear in mind when considering whether disclosure related to the provision of care would be appropriate – would the patient be surprised to learn that this information is being shared with this person for this purpose?

All professionals who have access to people's personal health information must have training in confidentiality and security issues and should be subject to contractual obligations to preserve confidentiality.

Case example – information fraudulently requested

A doctor's receptionist in one practice phoned another GP practice pretending to be a hospital employee to find out what medication her sister-in-law was on. She also got her sister-in-law's GP to fax sensitive information about the sister-in-law to her at the surgery where she was the receptionist. When the sister-in-law found out, she complained to her GP and the receptionist was prosecuted under the Data Protection Act. She was given a 2-year conditional discharge and ordered to pay the costs of the prosecution. The Information Commissioner criticised the way she had used her 'insider knowledge of the healthcare system to blag this information in an act that she believed would go undetected'.[30] He said that there would always be an audit trail.

Even where adequate safeguards are in place to prevent inappropriate access to information, some patients may object to some details about their care being shared. For example, some patients do not wish their GP to be informed of an episode of secondary care. If that is their wish, then their refusal should be respected, but they need to know what impact this will have on the future care they receive. It may mean that the health team has to curtail the range of procedures it offers if the outcome might be in jeopardy due to the patient's decision. Patients also need to know whether there are other options. In all cases, disclosures should be kept to the minimum necessary to achieve the purpose. When receiving a patient referral, a consultant needs to know information relevant to the episode of care but does not need access to the patient's full medical history.

There are some cases where, even though information sharing is directly related to the patient's care, additional legal restrictions on disclosure to other health professionals apply. Examples include information related to sexually transmitted infections and restrictions under the Gender Recognition Act 2004. In cases such as these, where explicit consent is required to share information, the individual must actively agree to sharing information and the patient's inaction or failure to object cannot be relied upon.

Sharing information with other health professionals

In the past, there was often an erroneous assumption that health professionals could share information between themselves at will, even when unconnected with the provision of patient care. This was based on the theory that, since they each have a strong duty of confidentiality, they could talk freely about patients among themselves, as long as they did not allow the conversation to go beyond their professional circle. Now, the emphasis is clearly on only sharing the minimum of information essential for the provision of a safe standard of care to patients, unless patients specifically authorise some other arrangement. In other words, information should be shared on the basis of a clear 'need to know' in order to provide care. If health professionals, or other staff who are uninvolved in a patient's care, ask for that patient's details without good reason, the request should be refused unless the patient has given express consent or there is some other justification for disclosure.

Case example – inappropriate discussion

A doctor and dentist were found guilty of breaching confidentiality after informally discussing a patient they had both treated. The subject came up during a round of golf, in which the doctor disclosed the fact that a patient had undergone an abortion. This disclosure was completely inappropriate and was not something that the dentist needed to know. He exacerbated the situation by passing on the gossip to his wife, who told someone else until it eventually came back to the patient. Both the doctor and dentist were found guilty of serious professional misconduct and were suspended from their professional registers.[31]

Patients generally understand that essential information is shared with other health professionals looking after them, on a 'need to know' basis. As discussed above, information should be readily available to patients, which explains how their information is used and disclosed for the provision of their care, and what they can do if they object. Sometimes patients think sharing should be automatic and are frustrated if asked to go over the same details to different health professionals. This is sometimes 'a major annoyance for patients, who feel that they should not constantly have to repeat the same information about themselves as they pass through the treatment pathway'.[3] Equally, there may be some patients who do not want information which is particularly sensitive to them to be disclosed outside of their GP practice, for example. Multidisciplinary care places emphasis on seamless, integrated planning and partnership working,[32] requiring routine information sharing among a variety of care pro-viders. Patients generally expect this but, if they do not already know about it, the manner in which information is shared must be explained to them so that they have a chance to object. The way in which the information is shared should obviously be secure.

Sharing information with relatives, parents and patients' friends

When patients have capacity, their consent should be sought before informa-tion is shared with their relatives and friends, even though patients in hospital often assume that people who ring up or visit are automatically kept in the picture. In Chapter 5 we have discussed the fact that children and young people who are competent are entitled to confidentiality and that competence is a matter of their maturity and understanding rather than just chronological age. Nevertheless, from the age of 12 or so, young people are generally expected to be competent to consent to the release of information.[33] In Scotland, anyone aged 12 or over is legally presumed to have such competence.[34] Unless there are convincing reasons to the contrary, a young person's refusal to permit dis-closure to parents or guardians should be respected but, depending on the nature of the examination or treatment, the reasons may need to be explored further. (See the sections on 'Gillick competence' and child protection in Chapter 5.) Reasonable efforts should be made to persuade the young person to involve his or her parents.

Sharing information for social care

Patients should know when health and social care providers are working together on their behalf and know that they can say if they see any aspect of the information disclosure as problematic. Subject to the provisos that they know about the information sharing and have no objection, implied consent is sufficient when the information directly contributes to the patient's care or to the local clinical audit of that care when undertaken by the team that provided care or those working to support them.[35] The main consideration is that patients are aware that information from the health service is used in their social care. If they object, they need to know about any detrimental effect non-disclosure will have for their care. In 2010, a Common Assessment Framework was piloted in England for the sharing of information across health and social care. It provided a model for how health and relevant information from social care records could be integrated into shared records for multi-agency use, with patient consent.[36]

Leaving phone messages for patients and texting them

Predictably, many routine problems about confidentiality occur when there is a mismatch of expectation between health professionals and patients about the ways information is used or communicated back. It is surprising how commonly some basic queries crop up, such as whether messages about appointments or test results can be left on patients' home answering machines. It is often unclear what the patient expects, but this needs to have been discussed in advance. If it has not been, a cautious approach is recommended so that, even if clinical information is omitted, no message is left without prior agreement with the patient. GMC's guidelines require that patient information is effectively protected at all times[37] and, in some situations, the mere fact of a telephone call from a clinic or hospital can raise questions with parents or partners with whom the patient has not discussed anything. Increasingly, other routine measures are used to minimise missed appointments, such as texting patients to remind them. This too should be agreed with the patient in advance.

When adults lack capacity

Patients with mental impairments or learning disabilities should not be assumed to lack capacity to consent to disclosure of their information (or to refuse it). Patients who lack capacity are still owed a duty of confidentiality. An assessment has to be made about whether the proposed sharing of information would be in their best interests (in England, Wales and Northern Ireland) or would benefit them (in Scotland). Clearly, it is important that appropriate information is shared with other health and social care providers so that patients' care is managed in as supportive and seamless a way as possible, but information should be released on a 'need to know' basis in order to facilitate their care. In England and Wales, the Mental Capacity Act also permits information sharing with other people where it is in an incapacitated person's best interests. Usually, this means sharing relevant information with their carers, or near relatives, as long as it is not contrary to the patient's known wishes. The general duties owed to adults who lack capacity are discussed in detail in Chapter 4.

Sharing information to invoke a Lasting Power of Attorney (LPA)

In England and Wales, patients' relatives may need information if seeking to invoke an LPA, in order to manage either a patient's property or personal welfare (see Chapter 4). Although this can sometimes be a straightforward decision to disclose in the patient's best interests, in some cases there is ambiguity about capacity and the patient refuses to be assessed. Unless there is evidence to the contrary, in the patient's record or from other sources, adults' capacity is presumed. If possible, health professionals need to talk to the patient to try and assess whether that person has capacity and can validly object to disclosure.[38]

Sharing information with other proxy decision makers

When someone has been formally appointed to make decisions on behalf of an incapacitated patient, clearly it is essential for that person to have access to all the relevant information necessary for them to fulfil that role.

England and Wales: Under the Mental Capacity Act 2005, welfare attorneys and court-appointed deputies can make decisions about the health and welfare of an incapacitated adult. If no relatives or friends are available, the Act requires an Independent Mental Capacity Advocate (IMCA) to be appointed and consulted about all decisions about 'serious medical treatment'. Such attorneys, deputies or IMCAs need to have essential information (but not necessarily the whole patient record) to ensure that the patient's interests are protected (see Chapter 4).

Scotland: Under the Adults with Incapacity (Scotland) Act 2000, while they have mental capacity, people over 16 can appoint a welfare attorney to make health and personal welfare decisions for them later, if they become incapacitated. The Court of Session can also appoint a deputy to make these decisions. The same principles as those in England and Wales apply in that information should only be disclosed in order to benefit the patient.

Northern Ireland: In the absence of specific legislation, information should only be disclosed in accordance with the common law, in the patient's best interests.

Information sharing when children lack competence

In most cases, parents consent to a child's treatment when the child is young and not yet competent. They need to be kept informed of the treatment options for their child's illness or injury (see Chapter 5). People with parental responsibility can also consent, on the child's behalf, for the sharing of information with other people who provide some aspect of care.

Occasionally, children or young people ask for a drug or treatment without understanding the implications. The most typical example is a request for contraception by a young woman, judged to lack the competence to consent to it or to sexual activity. She may insist that her parents are not told about her request and this should generally be respected, unless there are strong reasons not to do so (such as when abuse or exploitation is suspected). Young people should always be encouraged to involve their parents in decisions about treatment and to talk to them as frankly as they can, but they cannot be forced to do so. In some cases, however, the risks of harm to patients stemming from their lifestyle mean that the consultation needs to be disclosed to someone with parental responsibility (see Chapter 5 for an explanation of what parental responsibility involves). Attempts should first be made to try and convince young patients of the value of doing that themselves. Whenever feasible, the child should be told before any information is disclosed. This may not be practicable in some cases of child abuse or exploitation (see Chapter 5).

Uses of patient information for purposes indirectly related to care

When patients' personal information is used for health purposes not directly related to their care, this is often called a 'secondary use'. Such information is needed for a variety of functions to keep the NHS working effectively. Unless there is a specific legal provision requiring identifiable patient information to be collected, express consent is generally needed before it can be used for purposes unrelated to the patient's own care.[39] Common secondary uses include public health surveillance, financial audit, commissioning, research and teaching as well as clinical audit when undertaken by those not directly involved in the patient's care. The solution is often to anonymise the information before it is disclosed.

Secondary uses of data

Wherever feasible, the use of anonymous data should be preferred for all of these purposes but, where that is impractical and identifiable data are needed, patients must give express consent unless there is another secure legal basis under which the data can be disclosed. For example, there are specific statutory directions which permit disclosure of identifiable data to commissioning bodies in certain circumstances in order for the NHS to function effectively. Even where there is a statutory basis for disclosure without explicit consent, patients still need to know about these disclosures, why data are used and by whom. For GPs, the Information Commissioner advises that this can be achieved through the use of a combination of posters and leaflets in the surgery, verbal reminders during consultations and the inclusion of leaflets in any other letters sent to patients. He also said that simply placing a poster or a notice in a local paper is unlikely to meet the fair processing requirements of the Data Protection Act as not all patients will see it.[40] The NHS code of practice on confidentiality also emphasises the need for express consent for the use of information for secondary purposes where there is no clear legal justification.[41] The BMA has produced guidance on handling requests for disclosure for secondary purposes.[42]

Clinical audit

Some processes straddle the boundary between directly supporting individual patients' care and providing benefit to the healthcare system as a whole. Audit is one of these. Implied patient consent is sufficient for the use of data in clinical audit within the health organisation providing the patient's care. When audit is undertaken by the care team or its support staff, identifiable patient information can be used as long as patients know about it and are aware that they can object but have not done so.[43] If an external third party carries out an audit, the health team responsible for the patient's care should first anonymise the data. If this is impracticable, or if identifiable data are essential, explicit patient consent should be sought.[44] When this is not feasible, in England and Wales, it may be possible to seek approval for disclosure under Section 251 of the NHS Act.

Financial audit and other healthcare management purposes

Health records are often used for a number of standard financial and administrative purposes outside the direct provision of care. These include disclosures of information for financial audit purposes by GPs to commissioning bodies, health and social services boards (HSSBs), local health boards (LHBs) or health boards for post-payment verification (PPV) and the Quality and Outcomes Framework (QOF). These bodies may also require information for other purposes, such as the quality assurance of care.

Anonymous data are often sufficient for standard financial purposes. They should be used whenever possible, according to the GMC.[45] It says that, where practicable, information about patients should only be disclosed for financial or administrative purposes in anonymised or coded form. Otherwise, patient consent is usually needed for the use of identifiable information. It goes on to say:

> 'You must draw attention to any system that prevents you from following this guidance, and recommend change. Until changes are made, you should make sure that information is readily available to patients explaining that their personal information may be disclosed for financial, administrative and similar purposes, and what they can do if they object'.[46]

The GMC also states that clinical information should always be recorded separately from financial and administrative information.

Commissioning agencies' use of patient information

Various regulations and codes of practice provide a limited statutory basis for commissioning bodies and health boards to access GP-held information on an identifiable basis. Ideally, either anonymised data should be used or patient consent obtained, but sometimes, neither of these options is feasible. Disclosure in such cases is supported by secondary legislation and associated codes of practice.[47] Care should be taken to determine the minimum requirements and disclose only relevant information. In each case, consideration needs to be given to whether anonymisation is practicable.

Codes of practice issued by the UK health departments emphasise that commissioning bodies and health boards should only rarely need identifiable data from GPs, without patient consent. Situations when it may be lawful for GPs to disclose such data include

- NHS purposes, such as the QOF annual review process
- if the commissioning body is investigating the quality and provision of clinical care
- when data are needed for a contract, if remedial action is being considered, for example
- if the commissioning body considers there is a serious risk to patient health or safety
- in an investigation of suspected fraud or any other potential criminal activity.[48]

Looking to the future, one of the biggest changes under the Health and Social Care Act 2012 was the establishment of the NHS Commissioning Board and Clinical Commissioning Groups. The intention behind this new structure is that services will become more tailored to the needs of local populations and will be provided in 'closer to home' settings. Clearly, these commissioning organisations will need patient information to support effective commissioning and care planning. At the time of writing, it was unclear which organisations would be processing patient information within the new structures and, crucially, to what extent identifiable information would be required.[49] In most instances, anonymised information will be adequate to support commissioning activities. Where identifiable, patient information is necessary; for example, for specialist commissioning, it must be used with a secure legal basis such as consent or specific statutory authority. The Caldicott review will be considering a number of questions in relation to the legal basis for the processing of information in relation to commissioning and further information will be available on the BMA's website when these arrangements have been finalised.

Teaching

Where possible, anonymous information should be used for teaching, but where identifiable material is essential, patient consent is needed.[50] Images should be pixilated where possible and identifying details – such as names on X-rays – should be obscured. Junior doctors or other staff who are not part of the team providing care should not have access to identifiable patient information without the patient's express consent. Medical students not involved in providing care also need patient consent before they can access patients' information. If patients lack mental capacity and cannot give consent, information may be shared with students and trainees to the extent necessary for their education and training.[51] Ideally, however, information from patients who can consent should be used instead.[52] Parents, or other people with parental responsibility for a young child, can consent to the child's information being used in teaching. Once children are competent to consent or refuse, their own view should be sought.

Medical research

In Chapter 3 we discussed the importance of patients having access to relevant information before they agree to participate in research. Many research projects do not require their active involvement but do need information about their health and treatment. The degree to which identifiable patient information can be used, without patients giving express consent, is an area in which there has been considerable debate and disagreement.

Good quality research and innovation potentially benefit everyone and the NHS is committed to supporting them[53] while at the same time safeguarding confidentiality.[54] The BMA's view is that patients provide information for their own care and must be able to trust the health service with this information. From the patients' point of view, research shows that while large numbers of people support research, and are happy for their own information to be used, they still believe they should be asked.[55] In most cases, consent is required for the disclosure of identifiable data for research purposes. An exception is where the approval process set up under Section 251 of the NHS Act is used. In terms of professional guidance, the GMC also states that research can, in some cases, warrant disclosure in the public interest (and therefore would not require patient consent). To justify disclosure in the public interest, the research must depend on having identifiable information in situations where it is neither practicable to anonymise it nor to seek the subject's consent.[56] The GMC requires that a number of criteria be met before disclosure is made. These include giving consideration to the nature of the information, the use to which it will be put and how many people will have access to it. The security arrangements for research projects are also important and occasionally, the advice of an independent expert (such as a Caldicott Guardian) should be sought. Finally, attention should be given to the potential for harm or distress to patients.[57]

Any proposed medical research (whether within the NHS or not) has to be first scrutinised by a research ethics committee. Among the practical and ethical issues the committee examines are patient confidentiality, the importance of the research project and the security of data. It also takes account of the quality, comprehensiveness and comprehensibility of the information provided to research subjects in the participant information sheet. Where a research project has been scrutinised by a research ethics committee, and the necessary legal authority for disclosure is in place, there are good reasons for complying with requests for information. Many patients are very keen to participate in research and for their identifiable health information to be used for the benefit of others, and doctors should support this aim.

Debate will no doubt continue about the level and type of patient consent required for the use of identifiable information in research. Clearly, a balance is needed and, at the time of writing, this issue was under consideration by the Caldicott review on information governance, which could ultimately lead to greater clarity in this area. In the meantime, the one thing that everyone agrees on is that the public generally should be much more aware of how health information can be valuable in improving services and treatment options.

Public health

Public health surveillance and research rely on vast quantities of data, which should be anonymised wherever possible. As discussed above, the law requires the reporting of some infectious diseases. Health professionals must comply with such statutory requirements. Patients should be told about the legal obligation to disclose. In the absence of any statutory requirement, their consent should be sought for the disclosure of identifiable information. Exceptionally, if it is neither possible to seek consent nor prepare aggregated data (e.g. when dealing with rare diseases that do not become adequately anonymised on aggregation), an application may be made for disclosure under Section 251 of the NHS Act in England and Wales. The Health Service (Control of Patient Information) Regulations 2002 support communicable disease surveillance and monitoring in England and Wales. Disclosure is intended to prevent or limit the spread of diseases which pose a risk to public health. In the rest of the UK, there is no comparable legal allowance for disclosures of identifiable information without consent in these circumstances, unless the public interest justification is appropriate.

Disclosures unrelated to health care

Employment, insurance, immigration and social benefits

Individuals often request or authorise the use of their medical information for non-medical purposes. They need to understand the extent of information that will be disclosed, to whom it will be disclosed and for what purpose. Express consent is needed for such disclosures. Reports may either be written by the patient's GP, based on the medical record, or by an independent assessor on the basis of an examination.

Reports to insurers and employers

Prior to releasing information to insurers and employers, health professionals need to have sight of the subject's written consent, or authorisation from someone legally able to act on the subject's behalf. Where the report is prepared by the patient's GP, or someone else who has been involved in the patient's care, the individual has a right to see the report before it is sent (see Chapter 7).

GMC advice on disclosure of information to third parties

When preparing reports for a third party, doctors should

- be satisfied the patient has had sufficient information about the scope, purpose and likely consequences of the examination or disclosure, and the fact that relevant information cannot be concealed
- obtain or have seen written consent to the disclosure from the patient or a person properly authorised to act on the patient's behalf
- only disclose factual information that can be substantiated, presented in an unbiased manner; information should be relevant to the request and in most circumstances it is not appropriate to disclose the full medical record
- offer to show the patient, or give them a copy of, any report you write about them for insurance purposes before it is sent, unless
  - they have already indicated they do not wish to see it
  - disclosure would be likely to cause serious harm to the patient or anyone else
  - disclosure would be likely to reveal information about another person who does not consent.[58]

An electronic copy of the subject's signed form is enough if the agency requesting the information has security measures in place to prevent tampering with it. People being examined need to understand precisely what information about them will be disclosed. It should only rarely involve the person's whole past medical record, but if it does, the individual needs to know that and that they can refuse. The BMA has published joint guidance with the Association of British Insurers on best practice concerning the use of medical information in insurance.[59]

Disclosure to government departments

Government departments may request information about a patient, for example, for disability or other state benefits. The individual's consent should have first been obtained before the request for disclosure is made. Health professionals normally need to see evidence of that consent before releasing information, but they may 'accept an assurance from an officer of a government department or agency or a registered health professional acting on behalf of that patient' that the patient has consented to the disclosure.[58]

Disclosure to the driver and vehicle licensing agency (DVLA)

The BMA has an agreement with the DVLA that doctors approached by the DVLA can accept that patients have consented to the disclosure of their information on the basis of trust.[60] Sometimes, the situation is the other way around and the doctor wants to raise concerns about a patient with the DVLA. A common scenario is one in which the patient should not drive but refuses to take medical advice (see section on disclosures in the public interest).

Releasing health information to the media

Some patients publish articles or letters or put information on websites to complain about things that have gone wrong and doctors may want to respond. Doctors may also be asked to comment on the health of their celebrity patients. In all such cases the general rules of confidentiality apply. Health professionals cannot respond publicly to allegations made about their professional activities. Although this is often frustrating or distressing, the GMC warns doctors that they cannot ignore their duty of confidentiality. They must not put any information, gained in confidence, in the public domain without the patient's consent.[61] If misleading information has been reported, doctors can point that out but without disclosing any patient details (unless the patient consents).

Even when patients themselves reveal their clinical data, health professionals should not do so.

Clinical information and the media: *Ashworth*

In one high-profile case, the House of Lords ruled that a high-security hospital had an independent interest in keeping health records confidential, even if the patient had already put the information in the public domain. In September 1999, the detained murderer, Ian Brady, objected when he was transferred between wards in Ashworth Hospital and went on hunger strike. Simultaneously, he began a media campaign, giving details about his fast and complaining about his treatment. The *Daily Mirror* newspaper published an article about him which included verbatim extracts from his medical record. Ashworth issued a series of press releases, answering enquiries from the media, but also pointed out that Brady refused permission for the hospital to disclose any clinical details. In April 2000, MGN, which owned the *Daily Mirror*, was ordered by a court to disclose the source of the leak from Brady's records but refused. The journalist said that he did not know the identity of the source but assumed it to be a staff member at Ashworth. Although the information leaked from Brady's record and then published was merely a watered-down version of the material that Ian Brady had already disclosed to the media, when the case went to the House of Lords, the leak was viewed as very serious. The Lords said that any leaking of confidential information could have detrimental effects on treatment of patients and on staff morale. It could damage the doctor–patient relationship, deter patients from being truthful, and create distrust and conflict. Once confidence in the security of a database was undermined, the Lords said, the use of the database for recording sensitive information would be inhibited and this would have the effect of dissuading patients from providing information about themselves.[62]

Disclosures to identify and address poor health care

Patient complaints

When patients complain about an episode of care, the matter cannot usually be investigated without some access to their health information. They need to know this and should be told who will see the information, as well as being informed about the safeguards in place. If they refuse to allow disclosure for this purpose, the complaint may not progress, unless the information can be disclosed in the public interest. Complainants also need to know if complaints are heard in a public place and if the media have access. Some complaints systems, such as the GMC's, protect complainants' identities from the press. Patients sometimes authorise relatives or carers to complain on their behalf but, before responding, health professionals should check that the patient consents to the disclosure. Guidance on confidentiality in NHS complaints procedures is available from the health departments.[63]

Involving elected representatives

Some patients who complain also involve their Member of Parliament (MP), who argues on their behalf and requests information about the case. Disclosure to elected representatives acting on behalf of constituents is covered by secondary legislation.[64] The NHS code of practice on confidentiality advises that if MPs put in writing that they have patient agreement to disclosure, it can go ahead without further reference to the patient.[65] In some cases, however, if the disclosure is likely to upset patients, it is advisable to contact them first about it before passing the information on to the MP.[66] Only information relevant to the complaint should be disclosed and the patient should be copied into the response.

Whistle-blowing about substandard care

The crucial importance of health professionals taking steps to report substandard practice is discussed in Chapter 2 (see the sections on providing a safe service and whistle-blowing). Doctors have both an ethical and a professional duty of candour and must ensure that patient safety and quality of care are not compromised. Organisations too should foster a culture of openness and a willingness to question existing practices. Where possible, consent should be sought before any information about patients is disclosed, unless it can be effectively anonymised. Ultimately, however, if patient safety is jeopardised by poor systems, bad practice or inexperienced or sick colleagues, disclosure is likely to be justified in the public interest (see section on disclosures in the public interest).

Disclosure to agencies monitoring standards

A number of agencies can require the disclosure of information to monitor standards and detect fraud. Patients' consent is not essential for this but, where possible, patients should be made aware of the disclosure. Examples include the following:

• the NHS Counter Fraud and Security Management Service (England and Wales) can compel disclosure of information and documentation as part of its investigations into suspected fraud in the NHS.[67] Its powers extend over

NHS bodies and over people and organisations contracting with the NHS. Serious penalties may result for non-compliance with its requests for disclosure

* the CQC (England only) has powers, under the Health and Social Care Act 2008, to enter and inspect premises. It can also demand medical records, other documents and information from English NHS trusts.[68]

Disclosure requested by regulatory bodies

Regulatory bodies have statutory powers and can require information when assessing health professionals' performance. If a regulator believes that disclosure is necessary, in the interests of justice or to ensure patient safety, it should be made. The GMC, for example, is entitled to access confidential patient health records under section 35A of the Medical Act 1983. Other regulatory bodies have similar powers[69] and most have codes of practice, specifying how confidential personal information will be accessed and used. Where practicable, patients should be told about such disclosures, even if their consent is not required, unless to do so would undermine the investigation.[70]

Patients' consent should be sought, however, in any situation where their records are requested, but not required by law, or if records are needed when a healthcare professional reports concerns about a colleague to a regulatory body, unless disclosure of records is justified in the public interest.[71] If patients refuse to agree, or if it is not practicable to seek consent, anonymised information should be used where possible but, in some cases, the statutory body may insist on having identifiable data, despite patients' objections.

Disclosures related to crime prevention, detection or prosecution

Health professionals may sometimes be called upon to disclose patient information to prevent or detect crime. They, and all other citizens, have a legal duty in some limited circumstances, to report information to the police in order to prevent or detect crime. Examples include suspicions relating to possible terrorism (under the Terrorism Act 2000) and, in certain circumstances, road traffic offences (under the Road Traffic Act 1988).

Disclosure to the police and investigatory agencies

Many of the routine enquiries to the BMA concern requests from the police for access to patient records or to other confidential health information.

Doctors have the discretion to release information in situations where patient consent is unobtainable or inadvisable, if they can justify doing so in the public interest, but they are not obliged to release information unless a court order has been obtained requiring it. On the other hand, they may be criticised if they fail to act to prevent serious harm when they have relevant information about it. When a serious crime has taken place, or is foreseeable, there is likely to be an overriding public interest to disclose information if it would assist the police.[72] Evidence relevant to some serious crimes, such as murder, manslaughter, rape, and child abuse or neglect, almost invariably justifies disclosure, although decisions should be made on a case-by-case basis. As well as information being passed to the police, it may need to be given to other agencies, for example, social services. What is often difficult to assess is whether the disclosure requested would actually throw light on the situation or whether it is just part of a more vague 'fishing' exercise. What is usually needed is more detail about the nature of the crime, the type of information that the police hope to find and clarity about how that would help the investigation. Some health organisations have a specific form (a 'section 29 form'[73]) for such police requests. This requires clarification of the information needed and why it is expected to be helpful, enabling health professionals to assess whether disclosure is justified.

Case example – police request for too much information

In one case raised with the BMA, the police were investigating the death of a newborn, whose body had been found abandoned. They asked for a list of all pregnant women in the area from nearby GP practices to try and find the mother. After emphasising that this information was confidential and spelling out the criteria which justify disclosure of patients' details (consent, statutory obligation or the public interest), the BMA advised that the police request was too broad and needed to be more specific. The police had asked for the details of *all* pregnant women. The terms of the request needed to be narrowed considerably and, for example, focus on patients seeking post-partum care who could not account for the absence of a child. Although there was a strong public interest in investigating the baby's death, the police were requesting more information than was necessary or could be justified.

The Crime and Disorder Act 1998 permits, but does not oblige, the disclosure of patient information to the police, local authority or probation service.[74] Similarly, the Children Act 1989 permits disclosure to other organisations such as local authorities, social services and schools.[75] In either situation, health professionals may only disclose information when the patient has given consent or they believe there is an overriding public interest.

Gunshot and knife wounds

Gunshot and knife wounds have been highlighted as being a special consideration. In 2009, responding to a request from the Association of Chief Police Officers, the GMC advised doctors that all gunshot and knife wounds be reported to the police. Exceptions to the rule are cases where the patient's injury is very clearly accidental or the result of self-harm. Notification to the police is made on an anonymised basis so that a victim arriving at hospital is not initially identified to the police.[76] Identifying details can only be disclosed with patient consent or where it is in the public interest or the information is required by law.[77]

Domestic violence

Evidence of domestic violence can pose particularly difficult dilemmas for health professionals. Victims of domestic violence who are adult and have mental capacity can generally forbid the disclosure of their injuries to the police (but see also the sections on knife and gunshot wounds). Efforts should be made to encourage them to agree to talk to the police themselves, but they cannot be forced or pressured. Disclosure decisions generally rest with them unless other people, particularly children, are also at risk. Adults who have been assaulted by someone with whom they have a relationship often deny that the harm was deliberate rather than accidental. They may be fearful that worse things will happen to them if they talk about it. Breaching patient confidentiality in such cases can destroy patient trust and simply result in more denial of what occurred. Unless the victim has enough encouragement and support to agree to disclosure, it may not be possible.

Patients should always be made aware of the help that is available and encouraged to make use of support services. High-risk cases of domestic abuse are discussed in local Multi-Agency Risk Assessment Conferences (MARACs). Health professionals can make referrals to MARACs using the Co-ordinated Action Against Domestic Abuse (CAADA) Risk Identification Checklist, which helps referring agencies determine the level of risk.[78] Patient consent is needed for disclosure of information to MARACs. Exceptions arise if a court order or other legal requirement obliges disclosure. If other vulnerable people (children or adults who lack mental capacity) are at risk, disclosure is likely to be justified in the public interest even if the patient objects. (Disclosure in the public interest is discussed later in the chapter.)

GMC advice: disclosures to protect the patient

'It may be appropriate to encourage patients to consent to disclosures you consider necessary for their protection, and to warn them of the risks of refusing to consent; but you should usually abide by a competent adult patient's refusal to consent to disclosure, even if their decision leaves them, but nobody else, at risk of serious harm. You should do your best to provide patients with the information and support they need to make decisions in their own interests, for example, by arranging contact with agencies that support victims of domestic violence'.[79]

Abuse of vulnerable adults and minors who lack capacity

Evidence or suspicion of the abuse or neglect of a person lacking capacity (including a child) is an exceptional circumstance which usually justifies disclosure, in the public interest, to an appropriate person or agency. When health professionals have concerns about a patient lacking capacity who seems to be at risk of abuse or neglect, it is essential that action is taken. Information should be given promptly to an appropriate person or a statutory body. Protection of vulnerable people generally takes precedence over confidentiality in such circumstances. When there is doubt about whether disclosure would be in the patient's best interests, health professionals can discuss the matter anonymously with senior colleagues, Caldicott Guardians, their professional body or defence organisation. They should record their concerns, any advice sought and the actions taken to address their concerns, in the patient's medical records. All health professionals should be familiar with local safeguarding children procedures (see Chapter 5).

GMC advice: neglect or abuse of people who lack capacity

'If you believe that a patient may be a victim of neglect or physical, sexual or emotional abuse, and that they lack the capacity to consent to disclosure, you must give information promptly to an appropriate responsible person or authority, if you believe that the disclosure is in the patient's best interests or necessary to protect others from a risk of serious harm. If, for any reason, you believe that disclosure of information is not in the best interests of a neglected or abused patient, you should discuss the issues with an experienced colleague. If you decide not to disclose the information, you should document in the patient's record your discussion and the reasons for deciding not to disclose. You should be prepared to justify your decision'.[80]

Disclosure to courts and tribunals

Courts, including coroner's investigations, and some tribunals have legal powers to require disclosure without patient consent. Once they have received a court order requiring them to disclose information, health professionals have to comply with it if they think it falls within the scope of what the court needs, but they should not go beyond what has been requested. Refusal to disclose the information requested can be an offence. If health professionals think it should not be disclosed because, for example, it reveals confidential material about a third party unrelated to the case in hand, they should object to the judge or the presiding officer. Patients must also be given the opportunity to object. The courts have acknowledged the importance of confidentiality in such situations and confirmed patients' rights to make representations against disclosure.[81]

Patients' rights to object to disclosure: *TB*

A young woman of 14, known as TB, was receiving psychiatric treatment when her medical history was requested by the court in the trial of a 34-year-old man for sexual offences. The solicitors acting for the accused man issued a summons to the NHS trust to produce TB's medical records and alleged that she had invented the story of sexual abuse. The judge acknowledged that TB's psychiatric records were confidential but said that her rights to confidentiality were outweighed by the defendant's right to a fair trial. TB was not initially represented in court but was later called to attend. Without time to arrange legal representation, TB reluctantly consented to disclosure of her records, which showed that she had a history of self-harm and suicide attempts. TB later applied for judicial review of her case on the grounds that her right to privacy under Article 8 of the European Convention on Human Rights had been infringed because she had not been represented, and had not been able to make representations opposing the disclosure of her records. The High Court agreed with her that the existing rules, which did not oblige the court to give her notice of the summons against the NHS trust, were inconsistent with Article 8. It said that in future no such application should proceed unless the patient had been told and given adequate opportunity to make representations.[81]

In Scotland, practice is slightly different. Factual statements are taken from witnesses in advance of the trial in a system called precognition.[82] This means there may be limited disclosure of information, to both the prosecution and defence, before the court proceedings without express consent from the patient. Facts about the nature of a person's injuries can be disclosed, including the likely cause of the injury, the patient's mental state, or pre-existing conditions or health, as documented by the examining doctor.

Disclosure to solicitors

Health records required for legal proceedings are usually obtained via the Data Protection Act. In practice, most solicitors acting on a patient's behalf automatically provide a copy of that person's signed consent when requesting confidential information. If they do not, health professionals should ensure that they request and receive evidence of the patient's written consent to disclosure before proceeding. In cases of doubt or ambiguity, the solicitors should confirm that the patient understands the nature and extent of the information to be disclosed.

If solicitors acting for someone else seek information about a patient, they must first obtain the patient's consent to the disclosure. They can apply for a court order to obtain the information if the patient refuses. Standard consent forms for the disclosure of records have been drawn up jointly by the BMA and the Law Society.[83] These are applicable for cases in England, Wales and Scotland.

Disclosures in the public interest

Some disclosures of otherwise confidential information are justifiable in the public interest, without patient consent. Indeed, extreme cases arise in which health professionals are likely to be heavily criticised if they fail to act in the face of a known threat to a vulnerable person. Evidence of child abuse or neglect falls into this category (see Chapter 5). In most cases, the aim of disclosure in the public interest is to prevent or reduce a potential serious harm to someone, other than the patient (the argument being that people are entitled to harm themselves if they wish but not others). Decisions about such disclosures are made on a case-by-case basis, after weighing up all relevant factors and balancing the benefits and harms. Health professionals need to think carefully about why patient consent is not obtainable, or desirable, and whether they can justify disclosure without it, if called upon to do so by their regulatory body.

Case example – disclosure to the police

A common enquiry to the BMA is the situation in which the police, investigating a crime, approach a primary care practice. If the crime occurred in or near the practice premises, they often want a list of staff and patients who were in the building at the time and so could be a potential witness, or involved in some way. The fact that a patient attended the surgery is, itself, confidential and should not be disclosed unless the disclosure can be clearly justified. Cases need to be considered on an individual basis. As a general rule, if the crime is a relatively minor one, of theft or vandalism on a small scale, for example, disclosure is unlikely to be justifiable, but if the crime was a serious assault on someone or involved the use of knives or firearms, disclosure may well be appropriate. The other obvious option is for the practice itself to contact patients who attended on the day in question and ask if they are willing for their names to be disclosed.

A disclosure decision is relatively straightforward if speaking out would prevent or diminish a serious and imminent threat to public health or to national security, save someone's life or prevent suffering, but such cases are relatively rare. In most cases, the arguments on either side are more nuanced. General BMA advice is that threats of serious harm to people should be given more weight than crimes such as theft or risks to property, but this is not a hard and fast rule. Serious fraud or major damage to property can obviously also have a very harmful effect on people or NHS resources. Close scrutiny of the facts is needed to assess whether there is a genuine necessity for disclosure, and a balance must be drawn between the patient's right to confidentiality and the public interest. This was indicated in the *Egdell* case.

Disclosure in the public interest: *Egdell*

A man known as W had killed five people and injured two others. He was diagnosed with paranoid schizophrenia and was found guilty of manslaughter on the grounds of diminished responsibility. W was then detained indefinitely in a secure hospital. Over a decade later, plans began to be made to eventually return him to the community if he no longer represented a danger to others. The first step was the recommendation by the responsible medical officer that W be transferred to a regional secure unit. This move was vetoed by the Secretary of State, so W applied to a mental health review tribunal. To back up his application for a transfer, W commissioned a medical report from a consultant psychiatrist, Dr Egdell. In his assessment, however, the psychiatrist concluded that W was still dangerous, with a continuing interest in bomb-making. W tried to stop Dr Egdell from releasing this damning report to the medical officer at the secure hospital and made clear that he withdrew his consent to anyone seeing it.

Dr Egdell felt unable to accept W's decision, strongly believing that the report needed to be seen by the doctors treating this patient. He gave the report to the medical officer and it was later sent to the Secretary of State and the Department of Health. W initiated a legal challenge, claiming that the report about him should not have been disclosed to anyone. The Court of Appeal rejected his argument, concluding that it was necessary to balance the public interest in maintaining confidentiality against the public interest in protecting others from possible violence. Dr Egdell's action was judged appropriate in the public interest and in accordance with the advice of the GMC.[84]

Advice about the justification for disclosures in the public interest can be obtained from professional bodies, such as the BMA, indemnifying or regulatory bodies, such as the GMC, or from Caldicott Guardians. The NHS code of practice on confidentiality also confirms that disclosure can occur, without consent, if the public interest outweighs the duty of confidentiality.[85] As well as murder, manslaughter and rape, among the examples it gives are treason, kidnapping, child abuse, serious harm to state security or to public order, and crimes involving substantial financial loss. It identifies child abuse or neglect, assault, traffic accidents and the danger of infectious disease as presenting the common dilemmas for health staff. In contrast, it says that theft, fraud or damage to property, where loss or damage is less substantial, do not generally warrant a breach of confidence, although prescription fraud involving controlled drugs can be linked to serious harm for people.[86] Department of Health guidance,[87] with useful case examples, is also available to help NHS staff decide when to breach confidentiality in the public interest.

Ultimately, the health professional making a disclosure needs to be confident that the harms and benefits have been properly weighed up. Here a Caldicott Guardian or senior colleague can be helpful. Among the harms is the loss of trust on the part of the patient whose confidentiality is breached, unless that person can be persuaded to make the disclosure voluntarily. Hesitant patients can be encouraged to take responsibility for disclosure themselves, while knowing that the health professional will step in, if they do not. Where possible, encouragement to agree to disclosure should be the first option and can be successful in the sort of cases where patients represent an unwilling danger to themselves and others. A typical example includes drivers whose age or medical condition makes them a serious hazard on the road. Sometimes, patients with diabetes, epilepsy, defective eyesight or serious cardiac conditions who have been advised to stop driving continue to do so until made aware that their doctor can notify the DVLA, if they do not do so themselves.

> ### Case example – contacting the DVLA
>
> In one case raised with the BMA, a patient had been advised both by his GP and the local hospital to stop driving. Neither had actually seen his driving skills, which he insisted were fine, but his eyesight was clearly becoming more impaired. He was asked to talk to the DVLA and possibly be assessed by a medical officer there as to whether or not he could continue. The patient said this was unnecessary and kept on driving. The GP asked what he could do about it, as the patient's family was worried that he would injure himself or someone else. The BMA adviser relayed the GMC's advice that in situations where doctors cannot persuade patients to stop driving, they should contact the DVLA or the Driver and Vehicle Agency (DVA) immediately and disclose relevant information to the medical adviser.[88]

In some cases, persuasion is impractical. In the *Egdell* case for example, it seems unlikely that W would have voluntarily disclosed his bomb-making ambitions to the authorities or to the medical officer working for his release. His case shows that a breach of confidentiality is generally considered justifiable in cases where a serious threat exists and disclosure is likely to prevent it occurring.

Case example – patient with a serious communicable disease

When D was diagnosed with HIV, he was advised to inform his sexual partners and take safe sex precautions in future. It became obvious to D's GP that this advice had not been followed when P, the woman with whom D had recently begun living, told the doctor that they were trying for a baby together. The GP called D into the surgery and reminded him that, not only was he putting his partner and potential future child at risk but also that reckless transmission of HIV can amount to a criminal offence.[89]

The doctor explained that his regulatory body, the GMC, had published advice permitting him to breach confidentiality to a patient's partner if the patient had a sexually transmitted serious communicable disease and could not be persuaded to warn people with whom he had sex.[90] D was extremely upset. He said that he had attempted to broach the issue with P but failed miserably and was terrified of losing her. The GP asked if D would agree to him talking to P or to the practice counsellor raising the matter. D asked for time to think about it and promised that he would make some excuse to P to avoid unprotected sex in the meantime. Knowing that the GP would tell her if he continued to put off the discussion, D did explain the situation to P and the couple stayed together.

The confidentiality owed to deceased patients

Dead people's information is not covered by data protection legislation, but the legal and moral duty of confidentiality owed to patients does not end with their death. The policy of the BMA, GMC[91] and Department of Health[92] remains that the ethical obligation of confidentiality extends beyond a patient's death, but it is not inflexible. It needs to be balanced with other considerations, such as the interests of justice and the needs of the bereaved.

Factors to consider before disclosure

When considering requests for information from the records of a deceased patient, the GMC[91] advises doctors to take into account whether disclosure would distress or benefit the living and whether the information is already public knowledge. Attention also has to be given to the purpose of the disclosure. In some cases, it might throw light on an important genetic condition in the family and so disclosure is likely to be justified. Or the request for information may be for social reasons, such as when people want to research their family history and know more about deceased relatives whom they never met, which is unlikely to provide sufficient justification for disclosure. Any information which identifies or gives details about someone else (other than a health professional) should generally not be disclosed. In each case, the merits (or otherwise) of the disclosure need to be considered.

Information from the records of deceased patients may also be useful for research or disease surveillance. Wherever feasible, it should be used in an anonymised form and the usual safeguards applied, as previously discussed.

The needs of the bereaved

It is common for relatives to approach a deceased patient's doctor, asking for some information about their loved one's last illness. They do not have a legal right to information from the health record (other than via the Access to Health Records Act, if they have a claim arising out of the death – see Chapter 7), but doctors have always had discretion to disclose such information, when justified and for appropriate purposes.

A balance has to be kept between the ongoing duty of confidentiality and the likelihood of some disclosure putting the family's mind at rest. Relatives may feel guilty that they were not involved enough in the patient's last illness or they may want someone to blame if they think the patient was misdiagnosed or treated negligently. A blank refusal to disclose can exacerbate suspicion and result in unnecessary litigation. In some cases, it may be clear that the deceased would have wanted family members to have information. If, on the other hand, the deceased person had specified that some facts must remain private, they cannot be released to the family unless there is a legal obligation to disclose them. Few people ever do it, but in their lifetime, patients should ideally think about the possibility of relatives wanting to look at their records after death and decide whether there are specific issues they would never want known.

The interests of justice

The interests of justice were particularly highlighted by the case of GP Harold Shipman, who was found guilty in 2000 of having murdered 15 patients, although the total number of his victims was thought to be in the region of 215. Shipman had been killing patients since the 1970s, but among the factors that allowed him to do this undetected for so long were the death certification system at the time, the lack of information exchange between professionals but also the fact that relatives were unable to look at patients' records. Many were suspicious about why an apparently healthy person had gone downhill so fast under Dr Shipman's care, but they were unable to investigate the reasons. They could not even find out simple facts such as whether the patient had visited any doctor or complained of any symptom prior to death. After Shipman's trial, it was proposed that relatives should have routine access to more information about deceased patients' health management, including how often they had visited the doctor and more details about the cause of death.[93] The aim was to provide more monitoring, via the family, of mismanagement or deliberate harm.

Since Shipman, the death certification process has been reformed and a large variety of measures have been developed to identify negligence, mismanagement and near misses in health care.[94] Greater emphasis has also been placed on doctors and other health professionals talking openly to patients or their relatives about mistakes that have occurred (this is covered in Chapter 2). Identifying such events is also the aim of investigations by coroners' courts and procurators fiscal.

Investigations by a coroner or procurator fiscal

A coroner or procurator fiscal may need information in connection with an inquest or fatal accident enquiry and such requests should be complied with. There are also a limited number of additional circumstances in which the GMC advises disclosure, including for National Confidential Inquiries.[95]

Access to records in relation to claims

Unless while alive, the deceased specifically asked for some information to be kept confidential, a 'personal representative and any person who may have a claim arising out of a patient's death' has a right of access to information directly relevant to the claim.[96] Disclosure is allowed unless it would cause serious harm to someone or if it would reveal information about someone who is not a health professional. This provision is frequently used to disclose information to insurance companies in relation to a claim for life assurance.

Freedom of Information Act 2000

People may attempt to use the Freedom of Information Act to find out medical information about deceased people. In 2007, the Information Tribunal in England and Wales upheld the earlier decision of the Information Commissioner, who thought the medical records of the dead would be exempt. The IC said that most information in medical records, including those of the deceased, is likely to be confidential and exempt from disclosure under Section 41 of the Freedom of Information Act.

Freedom of information requests: *Bluck*

Mrs Bluck sought the disclosure of the medical records of her adult daughter, who had died in hospital. The hospital had admitted some liability and reached a settlement with her next of kin (her husband and children), who opposed the disclosure of the medical records. Mrs Bluck sought further information on the circumstances of her daughter's death. The Information Tribunal upheld a decision of the Information Commissioner that confidentiality in medical records should continue after the death of the patient, in part to safeguard the doctor–patient relationship and that, in this case, the records should not be released.[97]

Following the decision in this case, the Information Commissioner issued guidance to help public bodies assess requests for information about deceased individuals under the Freedom of Information Act and confirmed the exemption under Section 41.[98] The Freedom of Information (Scotland) Act 2002 contains an exemption to the disclosure of deceased patients' records.[99]

A last word on confidentiality

There seems never to be a good time to summarise where we are with legislation on patient confidentiality and information governance, since they often are in flux. This was also the situation at the time of writing, when the NHS was awaiting a new Caldicott review of information governance. The search for an appropriate balance between patient confidentiality and the effective use of health information for delivering health improvement continues. Involving patients more, and letting them know how their data can improve services and benefit other patients, is something all doctors can and should do as part of this pursuit.

References

1 General Medical Council (2009) *Confidentiality*, GMC, London, para 9.
2 Department of Health (2012) *Information: a Report from the NHS Future Forum*, DH, London.
3 Department of Health (2012) *Information: a Report from the NHS Future Forum*, DH, London, p.22.
4 General Medical Council (2006) *Good Medical Practice*, GMC, London, para 37.
5 *R v Department of Health (Respondent), ex parte Source Informatics Ltd (Appellant) and (1) Association Of The British Pharmaceutical Industry (2) General Medical Council (3) Medical*

Research Council (4) National Pharmaceutical Association Ltd (Interveners) [2000] 1 All ER 786.

6   Department of Health (2003) *Confidentiality: NHS Code of Practice*, DH, London, p.5.

7   General Medical Council Fitness to Practise Panel Hearing, 29–30 November and 13–14 December 2008 and 18 January 2009.

8   Information Commissioner (2011) *Health services must get it right on data security, says ICO*. News release, 1 July. Available at: http://www.ico.gov.uk/news (accessed 17 May 2012).

9   National Information Governance Board (2009) *NHS Care Record Guarantee*, NIGB, London.

10   These include: Department of Health (2010) *The Caldicott Guardian Manual*, DH, London; Department of Health (2003) *Confidentiality: NHS Code of Practice*, DH, London; Scottish Executive Health Department (2003) *NHS Code of Practice on Protecting Patient Confidentiality*, SEHD, Edinburgh; Department of Health, Social Services and Public Safety (2012) *Code of Practice on Protecting the Confidentiality of Service User Information*, DHSSPS, Belfast.

11   See *Ashworth Security Hospital v MGN* [2002] UKHL 29.

12   See the BMA's website for the most recent updates: bma.org.uk/ethics (accessed 26 September 2012).

13   Information Commissioner (2010) *Information Commissioner's Guidance about the Issue of Monetary Penalties Prepared and Issued under Section 55C(1) of the Data Protection Act 1998*, ICO, Wilmslow.

14   Data Protection Act 1998, Sch 1, Part 1.

15   Department of Health (2012) *The Power of Information: Putting Us All in Control of the Health and Care Information We Need*, DH, London, paras 5.24–25.

16   At the time of writing, this code of practice was being drafted.

17   In England and Wales, this is covered under the Public Health (Control of Disease) Act 1984 (as amended) and the Public Health (Infectious Diseases) Regulations 1988. In Scotland, similar provisions are contained in the Public Health etc. (Scotland) Act 2008 and in Northern Ireland in the Public Health Act (Northern Ireland) 1967 (as amended).

18   The Health Protection (Notification) Regulations 2010, SI 2010/659, Regulations 2(b) and (c); Health Protection (Notification) (Wales) Regulations 2010, SI 2010/1546, Regulations 2(b) and (c).

19   In England and Wales, doctors completing the notification form must provide a patient reference number, date of birth and postcode wherever possible as laid down in: Department of Health (2009) *Guidance Note for Completing the Abortion Notification form HSA4*, DH, London. In Scotland, doctors must give the name, address, postcode and date of birth as well as a patient reference number under: Abortion (Scotland) Regulations 1991, SI 1991/460, s 41.

20   The Reporting of Injuries, Diseases, and Dangerous Occurrences (Amendment) Regulations 1989, SI 1989/1457.

21   Care Quality Commission (2010) *Essential Standards of Quality and Safety. The Care Quality Registration Regulations*, CQC, London.

22   Gender Recognition Act 2004, s 22.

23   General Medical Council (2009) *Confidentiality: Disclosing Information about Serious Communicable Diseases*, GMC, London, pp.20–21.

24   The list of disclosures which are permitted under the 1990 Act can be found in: Human Fertilisation and Embryology Authority (2009) *Code of Practice*, 8th edn, HFEA, London, box 30A.

25   *Campbell v MGN* [2004] UKHL 22.

26   See: http://www.nigb.nhs.uk (accessed 28 September 2012).

27   National Information Governance Board (2011) *Identifying and Contacting Patients for Medical Research*, NIGB, London.

28   Further information on the Privacy Advisory Committee is available on the NHS National Services Scotland website: http://www.nhsnss.org (accessed 6 June 2012).

29   General Medical Council (2009) *Confidentiality*, GMC, London, para 25.

30   Information Commissioner (2011) *Receptionist Unlawfully Accessed Sister-in-Law's Medical Details*. News release, December 16. Available at: http://www.ico.gov.uk/news (accessed 15 May 2012).

31   Anon. (1997) GP struck off after golf club gossip. *Pulse* (Mar 8), p.12.

32   Department of Health (2009) *NHS 2010–2015: from Good to Great. Preventative, People-Centred, Productive*, DH, London, paras 2.77, 2.85 and 3.5. This stresses the importance of liaison between the NHS and adult social care services.

33   British Medical Association (2001) *Consent, Rights and Choices in Health Care for Children and Young People*, BMA, London, para 7.3.

34   General Medical Council (2007) *0–18 Years: Guidance for All Doctors*, GMC, London, para 53.

35   General Medical Council (2009) *Confidentiality*, GMC, London, paras 25–32.

36   NHS Connecting for Health. *Health and Social Care Integration programme*. Available at: http://www.connectingforhealth.nhs.uk (accessed 6 June 2012).

37   General Medical Council (2009) *Confidentiality*, GMC, London, para 12.

38   Further advice, including a chapter on the practical aspects of the assessment of capacity, is given in: British Medical Association, The Law Society (2010) *Assessment of Mental Capacity: Guidance for Doctors and Lawyers*, 3rd edn, The Law Society, London.

39   General Medical Council (2009) *Confidentiality*, GMC, London, para 33.

40   Information Commissioner (2002) *Use and Disclosure of Health Data. Guidance on the Application of the Data Protection Act 1998*, ICO, Wilmslow, p.8.

41   Department of Health (2003) *Confidentiality: NHS Code of Practice*, DH, London, p.21.

42   British Medical Association (2011) *Requests for Disclosure of Data for Secondary Purposes*, BMA, London.

43   General Medical Council (2009) *Confidentiality*, GMC, London, para 30.

44   General Medical Council (2009) *Confidentiality*, GMC, London, para 32.

45   General Medical Council (2009) *Confidentiality: Supplementary Guidance. Disclosing Information for Financial and Administrative Purposes*, GMC, London.

46   General Medical Council (2009) *Confidentiality: Supplementary Guidance. Disclosing Information for Financial and Administrative Purposes*, GMC, London, para 4.

47   Department of Health (2005) *Confidentiality and Disclosure of Information: General Medical Services (GMS), Personal Medical Services (PMS) and Alternative Provider Medical Services (APMS) Directions 2005*, DH, London; Department of Health (2005) *Confidentiality and Disclosure of Information: General Medical Services (GMS), Personal Medical Services (PMS) and Alternative Provider Medical Services (APMS) Code of Practice*, DH, London; Scottish Executive Health Department (2005) *Confidentiality and Disclosure of Information: General Medical Services (GMS), Section 17c Agreements, and Health Board Primary Medical Services (HBPMS) Directions 2005*, SEHD, Edinburgh; Scottish Executive Health Department (2005) *Confidentiality and Disclosure of Information: General Medical Services (GMS), Section 17c Agreements, and Health Board Primary Medical Services (HBPMS) Directions 2005 Code of Practice*, SEHD, Edinburgh; Welsh Assembly Government (2005) *Confidentiality and Disclosure of Information: General Medical Services and Alternative Provider Medical Services Directions 2006*, WAG, Cardiff; Welsh Assembly Government (2005) *Confidentiality and Disclosure of Information: General Medical Services and Alternative Provider Medical Services Directions 2006 Code of Practice*, WAG, Cardiff; Department of Health, Social Services and Public Safety (2006) *Confidentiality and Disclosure of Information: General Medical Services and Alternative Provider Medical Services Directions (Northern Ireland) 2006*, DHSSPS, Belfast; Department of Health, Social Services and Public Safety (2006) *Confidentiality and Disclosure of Information: General Medical Services (GMS) and Alternative Provider Medical Services (APMS) Code of Practice*, DHSSPS, Belfast.

48   Department of Health (2005) *Confidentiality and Disclosure of Information: General Medical Services (GMS), Personal Medical Services (PMS) and Alternative Provider Medical Services (APMS) Code of Practice*, DH, London, paras 30–32; Scottish Executive Health Department (2005) *Confidentiality and Disclosure of Information: General Medical Services (GMS), Section 17c Agreements, and Health Board Primary Medical Services (HBPMS) Code of Practice*, SEHD, Edinburgh, paras 29–31; Welsh Assembly Government (2005) *Confidentiality and Disclosure of Information: General Medical Services and Alternative Provider Medical Services Code of Practice*, WAG, Cardiff, paras 29–31; Department of Health, Social Services and Public Safety (2006) *Confidentiality and Disclosure of Information: General Medical Services (GMS) and Alternative Provider Medical Services (APMS) Code of Practice*, DHSSPS, Belfast, paras 30–32.

49   The NIGB has produced guidance to support both new and existing organisations during the period of transition. National Information Governance Board (2011) *Information Governance for Transition*, NIGB, London.

50   General Medical Council (2009) *Confidentiality: Supplementary Guidance. Disclosing Information for Education and Training Purposes*, GMC, London, para 3.

51   General Medical Council (2009) *Confidentiality: Supplementary Guidance. Disclosing Information for Education and Training Purposes*, GMC, London, para 17.

52   General Medical Council (2009) *Confidentiality: Supplementary Guidance. Disclosing Information for Education and Training Purposes*, GMC, London, para 13.

53   Department of Health (2010) *The NHS Constitution for England*, DH, London, p.3.

54 Department of Health (2010) *The NHS Constitution for England*, DH, London, p.7.

55 Medical Research Council (2006) *The Use of Personal Health Information in Medical Research: General Public Consultation Final Report*, MRC, London, p.55. This survey found that 79% of respondents felt that they had the right to be consulted about any use of identifiable personal data for research purposes, even if it made the research impractical; Department of Health (2008) *Summary of Responses to the Consultation on the Additional Uses of Patient Data*, DH, London, p.6. Fifty-three per cent of respondents from the general public thought that identifiable data should never be used for research purposes without consent.

56 General Medical Council (2009) *Confidentiality*, GMC, London, para 42.

57 General Medical Council (2009) *Confidentiality*, GMC, London, para 44.

58 General Medical Council (2009) *Confidentiality*, GMC, London, para 34.

59 British Medical Association, Association of British Insurers (2010) *Medical Information and Insurance*, BMA, London.

60 This is also confirmed by: Department of Health (2012) *Standard General Medical Services – Model Contract and Variation Document*, DH, London, clause 450.

61 General Medical Council (2009) *Confidentiality: Supplementary Guidance. Responding to Criticism in the Press*, GMC, London, para 3.

62 *Ashworth Security Hospital v MGN* [2002] UKHL 29.

63 Department of Health (1998) *NHS Complaints Procedures: Confidentiality, HSC 1998/059*, DH, London; Department of Health (2009) *Listening, Responding, Improving: a Guide to Better Customer Care. Advice sheet 2: Joint Working on Complaints*, DH, London; Scottish Executive Health Department (2005) *NHS Complaints Procedure Guidance – Including Statutory Directions*, SEHD, Edinburgh. Northern Ireland has not published guidance on the confidentiality aspects of complaints procedures.

64 The Data Protection Act (Processing of Sensitive Data) (Elected Representatives) Order 2002, SI 2002/2905.

65 Department of Health (2003) *Confidentiality: NHS Code of Practice*, DH, London, p.43.

66 Information Commissioner (2006) *Data Protection Technical Guidance Note. Disclosures to Members of Parliament Carrying Out Constituency Casework*, ICO, Wilmslow.

67 NHS Act 2006, Part 10, s 195–210; NHS Wales (Wales) Act 2006, s 143–158. Both the Department of Health (England) and the Welsh Assembly Government have published codes of practice for the use of these powers.

68 Health and Social Care Act 2008, s 62–64.

69 A number of the regulatory bodies who have statutory powers to require disclosure of information are listed in: General Medical Council (2009) *Confidentiality*, GMC, London, pp.33–34.

70 General Medical Council (2009) *Confidentiality*, GMC, London, para 19.

71 General Medical Council (2009) *Confidentiality*, GMC, London, paras 18 and 20.

72 General Medical Council (2009) *Confidentiality*, GMC, London, para 54.

73 Section 29 of the Data Protection Act 1998 refers to disclosures in relation in crime.

74 Crime and Disorder Act 1998, s 115.

75 Children Act 1989, s 47.

76 General Medical Council (2009) *Confidentiality: Supplementary Guidance. Reporting Gunshot and Knife Wounds*, GMC, London, paras 5–9.

77 General Medical Council (2009) *Confidentiality: Supplementary Guidance. Reporting Gunshot and Knife Wounds*, GMC, London, paras 12–15.

78 Co-ordinated Action against Domestic Abuse (2009) *CAADA – DASH MARAC Risk Identification Checklist*, CAADA, Bristol.

79 General Medical Council (2009) *Confidentiality*, GMC, London, para 51.

80 General Medical Council (2009) *Confidentiality*, GMC, London, para 63.

81 *R (on the Application of TB) v The Combined Court at Stafford* [2006] EWHC 1645 (Admin).

82 General Medical Council (2009) *Confidentiality*, GMC, London, para 23.

83 British Medical Association, The Law Society (2003) *Consent form (Releasing Health Records under the Data Protection Act 1998) – for England and Wales*, BMA, London; British Medical Association, The Law Society of Scotland, Scottish Executive Health Department (2004) *Consent Form for Access to Patients' Records by Solicitors (Releasing Health Records under the Data Protection Act 1998)*, BMA, London.

84 *W v Egdell and Ors* [1990] 1 All ER 835.

85 Department of Health (2003) *Confidentiality: NHS Code of Practice*, DH, London, p.34.

86 Department of Health (2003) *Confidentiality: NHS Code of Practice*, DH, London.

87 Department of Health (2010) *Confidentiality: NHS Code of Practice – Supplementary Guidance: Public Interest Disclosures*, DH, London.

88 General Medical Council (2009) *Confidentiality: Reporting Concerns about Patients to the DVLA or DVA*, GMC, London.

89 This was confirmed by the English and Scottish courts in the early part of the twenty-first century and as laid down in: National Aids Trust (2006) *NAT Policy Update: Criminal Prosecution of HIV Transmission*, NAT, London.

90 General Medical Council (2009) *Confidentiality: Supplementary Guidance. Disclosing Information about Serious Communicable Diseases*, GMC, London, para 10.

91 General Medical Council (2009) *Confidentiality*, GMC, London, para 70.

92 Department of Health (2003) *Confidentiality: NHS Code of Practice*, DH, London, p.13.

93 The Shipman Inquiry (2002) *Developing a New System for Death Certification*, The Shipman Inquiry Report, p.15.

94 This is covered in detail in: British Medical Association (2012) *Medical Ethics Today. The BMA's Handbook of Ethics and Law*, 3rd edn, Wiley-Blackwell, Chichester, chapter 21.

95 General Medical Council (2009) *Confidentiality*, GMC, London, para 71.

96 Access to Health Records Act 1990, s 3(1)(f); Access to Health Records (Northern Ireland) Order 1993, s 5(e).

97 *Bluck v The Information Commissioner and Epsom and St Helier University NHS Trust* [2007] EA/2006/0090; See also: *Nicholas Lewis (Claimant) v Secretary of State for Health (Defendant) and Michael Redfern QC (Interested Party)* [2008] EWHC 2196 (QB).

98 Information Commissioner (2008) *Freedom of Information Act. Practical Guidance: Information about the Deceased*, ICO, Wilmslow.

99 Freedom of Information (Scotland) Act 2002, s 38.

7: Management of health records

10 things you need to know about . . . management of health records

- The primary purpose of health records is to support direct care to the patient.
- Good quality records are factual, accurate, contemporaneous and legible.
- The same principles apply to all identifiable patient information, whether it is stored electronically, visually or on paper.
- All records must be stored and handled securely.
- Sharing the content of records with patients can help to strengthen the doctor–patient relationship and improve accuracy.
- The use of data for secondary purposes including public health, audit, teaching, NHS administration and health research is vital to the functioning of the health service.
- Where possible, records should be anonymised for secondary purposes.
- Images made for clinical care are part of patients' medical records and are subject to the same standards of confidentiality as other identifiable information.
- Individuals have a statutory right of access to their own medical records.
- NHS records should be kept for the minimum recommended retention times and thereafter disposed of securely.

Setting the scene

The majority of queries in relation to record keeping are to do with confidentiality and disclosure. The fundamental principles relating to these are covered in the previous chapter and are only briefly mentioned here. Other common uncertainties relate to what should or should not be written down, the amending of past errors and who can have access to medical records.

Common enquires about keeping medical records
- If I made a mistaken diagnosis, can I correct the record now?
- My patient and I disagree about some sensitive details in his record. He wants them deleted as out of date, but they were probably relevant for some past treatment decisions. Who is right?

(Continued)

Everyday Medical Ethics and Law, First Edition. Ann Sommerville.
© 2013 BMA Medical Ethics Department. Published 2013 by John Wiley & Sons, Ltd.

- Can I put in the record that this patient is churlish and threatening, when it is true?
- Are parents allowed to look at a teenager's record or can she stop them?
- Some of my patients are going abroad for treatment and want me to email extracts of the records to a clinic in another country. Who is liable if the information falls into the wrong hands?
- Should unsubstantiated allegations of violence be included in a patient's record?

Defining medical records

Medical records exist in various formats, including manual paper files, electronic records, X-rays, photographs, and visual and sound recordings of patients. They provide an account of patients' contact with the healthcare system. Whatever their format, if they contain identifiable information all records are confidential and subject to the same ethical principles. The Data Protection Act also applies to all identifiable material relating to living people. Such material has to be securely stored and, when appropriate, effectively destroyed. The confidentiality owed to identifiable data, and the situations when disclosure is appropriate, are discussed in Chapter 6. Key points emphasised there are that the main purpose of keeping records is to look after patients properly; their information is useful for other secondary purposes but should be anonymised, wherever feasible. If records cannot be anonymised for secondary uses, patient consent is required, unless there is a legal obligation to disclose them, or the public interest justifies it.

Manual and electronic patient records

These are the most common ways of storing patient information. Manual records are conveniently portable but not tamper-proof, nor is it necessarily obvious if information has been removed from them or changed. Electronic record systems allow health professionals to communicate quickly and find information easily, but the main advantage is the audit trail, indicating when data have been accessed and by whom. For patients wanting to restrict access to some details, most electronic systems allow data to be stored in a flagged but hidden area in the patient electronic record. Although there are still a number of practical issues that need to be resolved, the aim is to make primary care records available online for all patients by 2015. This should improve the quality of data as errors are picked up by patients, who are also expected to feel a greater sense of ownership of what is recorded. Online patient portals are being developed in England,[1] Wales[2] and Scotland.[3] Functionality varies but can include the ability for patients to view elements of their health records online, book appointments, order repeat prescriptions and input information such as blood pressure readings. Guidance is available for health professionals on patients accessing their own electronic health records in primary and secondary care.[4] The BMA has also published detailed guidance on electronic records in primary care, together with the Department of Health and the Royal College of General Practitioners.[5]

Images

Photographs are sometimes taken to record a patient's condition and monitor the stages of a disease or treatment. Like written material, the main purpose of images is to facilitate care, although the value of images in teaching, or to illustrate medical articles and textbooks, has long been recognised. Technologies such as picture messaging facilitate making, copying and transmitting images of patients, which can aid diagnosis and permit fast consultation with specialists. In order to consent to images being made, patients need to know the purpose, who will see them and how the material will be stored or erased. People with parental responsibility can authorise images made of children, and competent young people can consent, or refuse, for themselves. (Parental responsibility is explained in Chapter 5.) Some images do not need separate consent once the patient (or parent) has authorised the initial investigation or treatment. These include X-rays, images of internal organs or of pathology slides, laparoscopic and endoscopic images, ultrasound images and recordings of organ functions.[6] When used for clinical purposes, images form part of the patient's medical record and are subject to the same standards of confidentiality as other identifiable data.

Visual and sound recordings

Besides static images, other visual or sound recordings are sometimes made of patients. Although some are made as part of diagnosis or treatment (in which case they belong in the patient's record), many are intended for secondary uses such as teaching, assessment of health professionals or research. Before a recording of them is made, patients need to know its purpose and consent to it. (CCTV recordings of public areas are obviously different.[7]) Patients, including competent minors, should be assured that they can stop the recording, if they feel uncomfortable or unable to discuss things frankly during it. When a recording is finished, patients should be able to see, or listen to, it if they wish and, if necessary, to withdraw consent for its future use. It is good practice to reaffirm consent for all continued use of identifiable recordings. Patients sometimes ask if they can tape-record a consultation to help them remember what they have been told (see Chapter 2). This can be very useful for them, but they also need to understand that any recording can change the nature of the discussion.

Patients who lack capacity (including children)

If patients lack mental capacity, consent generally needs to be sought from someone lawfully authorised to give it before identifiable images or recordings are made for assessment or treatment purposes. People with parental responsibility can consent for children and young people who lack competence, but recording should stop if the patient objects to it by any means or shows distress.[8] Documenting suspected cases of child abuse sometimes involves photographic records of children's bodies. Although parental consent should normally be sought, it may not be if the recording is done under a court order and alerting the parent could put the child at risk. Particular care must be taken with such sensitive material. It must be stored safely and disclosed only for the purposes intended.

If nobody is authorised to consent for an incapacitated adult, consideration has to be given as to whether it is in the patient's best interests. (Best interest decisions are discussed in Chapter 4.) When intended to aid patients' own care, recording is likely to be in their interests (unless they show clear signs of objecting to it), but if the recording is for teaching or research, any benefit for the individual patient is less obvious. Some research on incapacitated adults involves filming how they cope in routine situations, for example, so that improvements can be made to their environment. Recording often does not benefit the individual filmed but may help others in the same situation. (Research involving incapacitated adults is discussed in Chapter 4.)

Recording telephone calls

The monitoring and surveillance of telephone calls is regulated by the Telecommunications Act 1984, which imposes a duty on anyone responsible for the call system to ensure that reasonable efforts are made to inform callers that they may be recorded. If calls to a GP practice or out-of-hours service are recorded for medico-legal purposes, callers need to know that, or the recording may be unlawful.

Making a health record

Patients' records usually include a description of their symptoms, notes made during consultations, opinions from health professionals who examine them, test results, diagnoses, recommended treatment and details of prescriptions and referrals. In addition, there may be correspondence between health professionals, X-rays, videotapes, audiotapes, photographs, tissue samples taken for diagnosis and copies of reports for third parties, such as insurance companies.

What to include in the record

Records should report investigations carried out, relevant clinical findings, decisions made and a note of drugs prescribed or other treatment provided, as well as any other actions taken and their outcomes. All notes need to be clear, accurate and legible, not least because patients have a right to read them. They should be made contemporaneously, or as soon as possible after a consultation.[9] Reasonable speculation can be included, if it has a bearing on the care recommended. Treatment is often initially based on an interim diagnosis that later investigations confirm or disprove. Health records need to show a continuous record of the action taken and its outcome. The reasons for a specific treatment decision need to remain on the record, even if later investigations show it was not the best way forward. The reasons for proposing it, given the available information at the time, can be important later.

Standardising hospital records

Standards have been published for the structure and content of medical records and communications when patients are admitted to hospital.[10] These involve 12 generic record-keeping standards, some of which (such as date and time) are automatically recorded in electronic records. The standards specify that a unique patient identifier (NHS number in England and Wales, Community Health Index in Scotland, Health and Care number in Northern Ireland) must be used on every page. Any decisions about cardiopulmonary resuscitation should be clearly recorded. Standardised headings have been drawn up for hospital admissions, hand-over and discharge communications. The content of all hospital patient records, electronic and paper, should be structured using these headings.[11] Standardised records are important not only for patient care but also for efficient NHS financial management which relies on the accurate reporting of clinical activity data, as this information directly links to the payments trusts receive for work they carry out.[12]

Recording discussion with patients and noting their wishes

A vital part of health care is the conversations between patients and health professionals. These allow patients to describe their symptoms, worries and their reasons for seeking treatment. Health professionals respond by outlining the options for care and explaining the risks and benefits of each, including the possibility of doing nothing. A summary of these discussions needs to be noted in the record so that, if necessary to check later, it is obvious why a particular course of action was taken. Recommendations for treatment should be noted, including evidence of the patient's agreement or refusal. Some patients do not want some sensitive information disclosed to anyone else and this should be noted in the record. In Chapter 6 we discuss situations where patients refuse to have information shared with other people, including other health professionals involved in their care. They need to be aware of the implications for future treatment options if they take this view and the record should indicate what they were told about that. If they have made a formal advance decision to refuse treatment, that needs to be made clear, as do any requests or specific wishes they have regarding their care, if they later become incapacitated (see Chapter 3).

Aggressive or threatening behaviour

Patients can react in an unexpectedly hostile way for various reasons, including illness or the effects of their medication. Whether or not it is worth noting an isolated incident is a matter of judgement. When patients are repeatedly aggressive or bullying to staff, this can be noted in their record. They should be made aware that such behaviour is unacceptable, and any repetition will be documented. (Management of violent patients is discussed in Chapter 2.)

What to exclude from the record

Information in patient records should be as factual as possible. Views or speculation about patients' lifestyle should not be included, unless they have some bearing on a diagnosis. Relevant information from a third party, such as a relative, can be included (but that information cannot be released to the patient if it would identify the informant, without the informant's agreement). Some of the things that relatives say about patients are unsubstantiated. Such unproven information should generally be excluded, unless there are strong reasons for noting it.

Case example – whether unsubstantiated allegations should be recorded

Difficult situations are raised with the BMA regarding serious but unproven allegations of a patient's violence or abuse, when it is unclear whether these should be recorded in the notes. Caution is needed over how allegations are noted, not least because patients have a right to look at their records and are likely to complain if there is anything untrue or potentially libellous in them. On the other hand, patterns of domestic violence and potential risks to children may only become apparent if past incidents were noted. Occasionally, unfounded allegations of violence or neglect are made when relationships break down. Ultimately it is a matter of judgment, in the individual circumstances of the case, whether an allegation should be noted. It may also be unclear *whose* record should carry the information/allegation.

In the case of adults, a verbatim note of what an informant said is likely to be appropriate, as a reported comment, on that person's own record, rather than that of the alleged (but unproven) perpetrator. If a woman says, for example, that her bruises were caused by her partner beating her, it would be appropriate to record that in *her* record as her reported speech, while also trying to persuade her to take action about it. But it may not be appropriate for this to be noted in his record, unless there is other substantive evidence that he is a danger to others or has a mental condition that needs to be treated. If there are children who may be at risk, the information should be recorded in both the child's notes and those of the alleged perpetrator. Further advice should be sought in such cases. (Reporting child abuse and neglect is covered in Chapter 5.) When patients access their own records, information that would identify another person, such as a spouse who made allegations, cannot be disclosed unless that person agrees.

Records made and shared by several professionals

Electronic record systems allow the possibility of a shared record (the 'shared detailed care record'), to which several professionals contribute their expertise for the care of a patient. Such records can be accessed by various health professionals in primary, community and secondary care, as the patient's information can be made available across organisational boundaries. In order to comply with the Data Protection Act requirement for fair processing, patients need to be aware of the sharing arrangement. They also have a right to ask for some information not to be shared. Detailed guidance is available which provides a framework within which shared electronic patient records should operate.[13] It includes some fundamental principles, such as the obligation to explain to patients who will have access to their record and to respect their wishes if they object to particular data being shared (except where disclosure is a legal requirement or justified in the public interest). The guidance also emphasises the need to have clear rules about who has responsibility for content, and for acting on the information contained in the record both within, and between, organisations.[14] Each organisation should be responsible for its own organisational shared record and there should be a guardian (or team) in each organisation with clinical and information governance responsibilities. Various UK programmes exist to deliver forms of shared electronic records for patients.[15]

National summary records

While shared detailed care records make a patient's information available to health professionals, within a local area, summary care records (SCRs) provide core health information which can be accessed anywhere in the country.[16] A summary of key data, gleaned from patients' GP records, can be accessed, where necessary, by doctors working in out-of-hours or other unscheduled care settings. Patients need sufficient information to make an informed decision about whether they want an SCR.

Changing medical records or adding to them

Disputes about accuracy

Health records need to be as accurate as possible, but sometimes mistakes occur in them or health professionals and patients simply disagree about the accuracy of an entry. The Data Protection Act gives patients a right to have inaccurate records amended. If it is clear that the details are wrong, a correction should be added (while allowing the original information to remain in an audit trail) but, if any decisions were based on the erroneous information, that too needs to be noted rather than removing all trace of the error. If no agreement can be reached about whether or not the information in the record is wrong, a note of the continuing disagreement should be made in the record.[17] If the issue concerns past treatment and the truth cannot be verified one way or the other, a summary of the patient's views should be appended so that future care providers are aware that some information may not be reliable. Advice is available for patients in such circumstances[18] and, ultimately, they can complain to the Information Commissioner's Office, if the disagreement is not resolved.

Patient requests to omit or remove some information

Sometimes there is no dispute about the truth of the details which patients ask to have omitted or removed from the record. Clinical information cannot be taken out, if relevant to the patient's past or future care. It needs to be explained to patients that records cannot be left incomplete and past treatment decisions may look arbitrary if the justifying reason for them is removed. Patients can, however, forbid the sharing of that information with other people, including other health professionals providing care (this is discussed in Chapter 6). Non-clinical information can be removed if it should never have been recorded in the first place. Often, this is an irrelevant personal remark made by an earlier contributor to the notes, or concerns social information about the patient's lifestyle or relationships which have no relevance to the individual's care. If it is not clinically relevant and both the health professional and the patient agree, it can be removed.

Some very sensitive social information may be relevant to the provision of a person's care and should be entered in read code where appropriate. The fact that a patient is on the sex offenders' register, for example, should be recorded in this way. It needs to be removed if the person is no longer on the register.

Altering or tampering

Sometimes, it becomes obvious that earlier diagnoses and recommendations were wrong and this must be reflected clearly in the notes so that future care providers do not misinterpret that person's medical history. There can be a temptation to use hindsight and alter the record to fit the current evidence. Clinically relevant information should never be changed without an explanation being added.[19] Medical defence bodies warn that doctors can face a criminal charge of attempting to pervert the course of justice, as a result of amending notes in a way which is intended to mislead.[20] Any note must clearly show the date on which it is made. Implying that the entry was made at an earlier time can lead to serious questions even if there is an innocent explanation.

Case example – tampering with records

In 2010 the GMC found a GP guilty of acting dishonestly in amending the medical records of six patients. The GP also admitted altering the medical records of 32 patients. The doctor was suspended for 12 months.[21]

Adding information later to the record

After a contemporaneous clinical note has been made, it sometimes becomes clear that more information should have been included at that point, but rather than change what is there, a fresh entry should be made and dated accordingly.

It is inadvisable to alter existing clinical data as this will be picked up through the audit trail and can look like improper tampering. Adding more information in a separate entry is preferable.

Adding or removing information when the record is shared

An audit trail always identifies where changes have been made in electronic records. Information can physically be deleted or added, but the audit trail remains, in case of any later investigation. For multi-contributory records, with different healthcare professionals adding data to the same record, it is likely that there are data controllers in common for the information held. Each organisation needs to ensure that all data protection requirements are met, which means they need to have an agreement about how their joint responsibilities will be satisfied. There are also some complexities concerning shared records and the removal of information where data are drawn from one record to construct another. The SCR, for example, is compiled from data extracted from GP practice records. The Information Commissioner has agreed that an SCR could be completely deleted at the patient's request, without keeping an audit trail of its contents, unless it has been used during the course of treatment.[22] The same information will still exist in the other electronic record systems, from which the SCR data were originally extracted. It cannot be deleted from them.

Transsexual patients

Doctors sometimes ask about how to manage the records of transsexual patients. Such patients' notes should reflect their current name and title. Once a gender recognition certificate has been obtained, new NHS numbers are available for them. Doctors sometimes ask when a patient's gender can be changed on their medical record. The BMA's understanding is that gender should not be changed until the patient has obtained a gender recognition certificate. In Scotland and Northern Ireland, NHS numbers are not changed until the patient has undergone surgery. Like any other medically relevant information, notes about gender reassignment surgery should be kept and it is inappropriate to remove all reference to a person's pre-surgery gender.

Adopted patients

The fact that a patient is adopted and not genetically related to parents and siblings is often not medically relevant. Many people who are not adopted are also not genetically related to the person they assume is their father. As the composition of 'average' families changes, with step-siblings and step-parents increasingly the norm, adoption is more openly discussed than it was in the past. Adoptive parents are always strongly encouraged to be open with children but, if adoption is mentioned in a child's notes, care needs to be taken before the notes are accessed, to verify whether the child already knows about it and does not discover it inadvertently, by asking to see the record.[23] Guidance recommends that new health records, with new NHS numbers, should be created for adopted children, unless they already know about their adoption.[24]

Tagging records

Paper records were traditionally tagged (often by coloured stickers) to draw attention to information, considered particularly important. Anyone seeing the file, and aware of the tagging system, knew immediately some facts about that patient. It might be that the person was diabetic, allergic to certain medication, or on an at-risk register. Clearly, such systems potentially compromise confidentiality and tagging records in this way is only considered acceptable when there is no effective alternative. Electronic systems have various ways of recording and displaying important coded or free-text clinical information. If important information needs to be displayed on the front page of a patient's electronic record (or tagged for paper records), patients should know about this and consent to it.

Primary and secondary uses of records

Primary uses of records

The primary function of all patient records is to support the provision of care. Information in a patient's record is often also used to provide reports that patients want for social purposes, such as employment, insurance or an application for state benefits (see Chapter 6). Patients have a statutory right to see their records, with some limited exceptions (see section on access by patients).

Secondary uses of records

In Chapter 6, we described how the patient information contained in records can have important secondary functions for the health service, in research, teaching, audit, NHS planning and administration. Wherever possible, manual or electronic records, images or recordings of patients should be effectively anonymised before being put to a secondary use. Where that is not possible, in the absence of a specific legal provision requiring identifiable data to be collected or disclosed, express consent from patients (or parents on behalf of children who lack competence) should be obtained.

Some images or recordings are specifically made for secondary uses, such as teaching, rather than for patients' care. Express patient consent is needed for this and ideally, it should be written consent.[25] Patients should be told the purpose of the recording, how it will be used, how long it will be kept and how it will be stored. They need to know that they can change their mind about being recorded and, if they do, this will not affect the quality of care they receive or their relationship with those providing care.[26] Video recordings are often used in teaching, but it can be very challenging to exercise adequate control over the material and protect it from being copied illegally. Unless the recordings have been anonymised, by obscuring or pixelating the images, consent is needed and patients ought to be able to withdraw their consent for them to be used and have the recordings destroyed. In all cases where anonymisation is carried out, it must be effective.[27] Simply blanking out part of the image or putting a bar across the eyes is likely to be insufficient. Apparently insignificant details may still identify the person.[28] Once effectively anonymised, images can be used in research, teaching or other healthcare purposes, without consent. When practicable, patients should know that they may be used in anonymised form for secondary purposes.[29]

Secondary uses of children's records

People with parental responsibility can consent to secondary uses on behalf of minors who lack competence. They can also give permission for a visual or audio recording to be used, but young people must be able to withdraw consent to its use when they have sufficient maturity to make a decision, unless the information has been effectively anonymised.

Using material in publications or other media

No identifying material may be published in textbooks or journals, or used for teaching without express patient consent, which should usually be in writing. Effectively anonymised material does not need consent, but it is difficult to completely de-identify cases given as examples or illustrative material. Express patient consent is also required to make an image or recording intended for use in public media. An identifiable recording previously made as part of patient care cannot be used for a different purpose without patient consent. Even if anonymised, it is good practice to seek consent before making a recording public in any medium.[30] Once material is in the public domain, it is virtually impossible to withdraw it from circulation. If a video recording is made for a broadcast with their consent, patients need to understand that it is very difficult to retract their permission later. If they want to restrict the use of the material, they need to get agreement in advance from the programme maker. Specific legal requirements apply to the making of recordings of adults who lack capacity, or disclosing such recordings, and legal advice should be sought.

Case example – publication of an identifiable case

In a case raised with the BMA, a middle-aged woman with an unusual gynae-cological condition had agreed to an experimental treatment for it by a specialist. The treatment was successful and the gynaecologist decided to write up the case for publication in a specialist journal. He did not seek the patient's consent but took care to exclude her name. As he thought it extremely unlikely that she would ever get to know of the article and wanted to liven it up a bit, he included details of her social background and job as a childminder on a council estate, as well as information about her childbearing history. A journalist looking for stories came across the article in a library and wrote a piece for a local free paper about the council tenant who had helped medical science through an experimental procedure. He had no trouble in tracking her down from the background details in the journal, knowing that she was a registered childminder in a relatively limited geographical area. The patient found that she had become the subject of local gossip and complained.

Giving access to patient records and reports

Health professionals are usually very willing to discuss patients' records with them informally, without requiring that the formal access procedures are carried out. Some patients prefer to read their records themselves. They are entitled to see, and have copies of, their health records, by submitting a subject access request under the Data Protection Act. Developments in electronic systems also allow some patients to have online access. Information has to be withheld if it identifies a third party (who is not a health professional) or when disclosure may cause serious harm to the patient or another person.

Ownership of records

NHS records

In law, the concept of ownership of NHS records is very underdeveloped. For most purposes, who owns them is less relevant than who has control of records and the information in them. Issues of control relate back to whether patient consent is required before data can be used, whether health professionals have discretion about that (such as when disclosure is justified in the public interest) or whether there is a legal duty to release information (see Chapter 6).

Private records

Private practitioners (or sometimes their employers) own the records they make. They have to make and keep them in accordance with the Data Protection Act, which requires that all data processing conforms with certain principles (see Chapter 6). When private practitioners retire, they usually pass their patients and the records to their successor. If there is no successor, records should be stored securely for the recommended retention period or, with the patient's consent, passed to another practitioner. Under the Data Protection Act, patients should be informed of changes in arrangements for their records.

Case example – disposing of private records

A common query to the BMA concerns the handling of records belonging to private doctors who have died or have become mentally incapacitated at the end of life. Ideally, practitioners should have left instructions but, in many cases, they have not and their relatives are left to grapple with the problem. Records could be transferred to another doctor for safekeeping. Alternatively they could be given back to the patients but, depending on the type of care provided, the records may need to be checked to ensure that third parties (apart from health professionals) are not named in them and nor is there any information that could be harmful to the patient. Ideally a registered health professional should sort through them to check these things and establish if they can be destroyed or transferred. Heirs and relatives need to ensure that the records are kept securely for the minimum retention times, but they are not allowed to look at them. Patients have rights to see their own records but may sue if someone else accesses them inappropriately.

Access by patients

Patients have a statutory right of access to information about themselves, under the Data Protection Act. This covers all health records, including reports written to satisfy the requirements of mental health legislation and medical reports written by independent doctors who have no other professional relationship with the patient. The BMA and the Department of Health publish guidance on access to health record requests.[31] Patients, including competent minors, can apply for access or authorise someone else to do so on their behalf.

They are entitled to copies of their notes if they want them, and these should be accompanied by an explanation of any difficult or arcane terms. This is a requirement of the Data Protection Act. Fees can be charged for access. These vary according to whether the records are held manually, or on computer, and whether copies are requested.[32] The Data Protection Act says that copies need not necessarily be supplied, if disproportionate effort would be needed but does not define those terms. Some patients have extremely thick files, involving many specialised terms and requiring considerable scrutiny to see whether third parties are mentioned, or potentially harmful information included. Such things are likely to be a consideration in assessing the effort involved.

Case example – third-party information in medical records

Among the common enquiries to the BMA about patient access is the question whether a GP has to go through the entire patient file before giving access to check if there is any direct or indirect comment that would identify a third party. The answer is yes. Information relating to that person either has to be removed from the copy given to the patient or consent has to be sought from the third party. Guidance about this has been issued by the Information Commissioner.[33]

Information which should not be disclosed

The Data Protection Act exempts certain categories of data from its subject access provisions. Information should not be disclosed if

- it is likely to cause serious harm to the patient or another person
- it relates to a third party (other than a health professional) who has not given consent
- it is requested by a third party but the patient had asked for information to be kept confidential
- the records are subject to legal professional privilege or, in Scotland, to confidentiality as between client and professional legal adviser (this may arise in the case of an independent medical report written for the purpose of litigation)
- it is restricted by a court order
- it relates to the keeping or using of gametes or embryos or pertains to an individual being born as a result of assisted reproduction[34] or
- in the case of children's records, disclosure is prohibited by law, for example, adoption and parental order records and records of the special educational needs of children in England, Wales, Scotland and Northern Ireland.[34]

Circumstances in which information may be withheld on the grounds of serious harm are extremely rare. It is not enough to hold it back because patients would find it upsetting. (See the section on truth-telling and good communication in Chapter 2.) When there is genuine uncertainty as to whether disclosure would cause serious harm, advice should be sought from an experienced colleague, a Caldicott Guardian or defence body. Withholding access because disclosure would be embarrassing, or may give rise to legal claims, is unacceptable.

Access by solicitors

The BMA is frequently contacted by doctors, particularly GPs, who have received requests for access to records from solicitors acting on behalf of a patient involved in a legal case. Common enquiries include cases where solicitors request the whole of the medical record and the GP is worried that the patient is not aware of the extent of the disclosure authorised. In some cases there is sensitive information the GP is concerned about releasing. In such cases it is always a good idea to check with the patient that he or she is aware that all of the information held will be disclosed. If consent is subsequently withdrawn, the solicitor should be informed of this. The BMA has worked with the Law Society[35] and the Law Society of Scotland[36] to improve communication in this area by producing a model consent form for disclosure which clearly explains that the full medical record is required.

Some GPs also ask whether original records can be sent or if the solicitor can be asked to send a member of staff to photocopy the record at the GP practice. It is not advisable to send original notes as the doctor remains responsible for their safe keeping and the BMA advises that this should only be done where copies would be illegible (and a copy of the most recent notes should be kept in case medical care is needed). GPs can invite solicitors to send someone to photocopy the records, but if the solicitor asks for copies to be made the GP is obliged to provide them. Doctors cannot refuse to comply with legitimate requests made under the terms of the legislation. The standard exemptions apply and any information that should not be disclosed (such as third-party information) must be excluded before the records are shared.

Access by people other than the subject

Patients can authorise someone else, such as a relative, to access their record on their behalf. As long as consent has been provided, these should be handled in the same way as individuals seeking access to their own records. Sometimes, however, an application for access is made without the knowledge or consent of a patient who has mental capacity. Among the examples reported to the BMA are instances when an employer wants to check up if an employee genuinely has repeated bouts of illness or a local authority wants to see if fraudulent benefit claims are being made. Patient consent would be needed before other people could have access to information in the file of an adult with capacity, unless there is a public interest justification (see Chapter 6).

Access to the records of children and young people

Competent minors (people under 16 in Scotland, under 18 in the rest of the UK) have a right of access to their own records.[37] People with parental responsibility (see Chapter 5) can also apply for access to a child's health records, unless a court has imposed conditions to the contrary or providing access would conflict with the interests of the child. Where the child or young person is competent to make a decision, the young person's consent is required before the parents can be given access. Contraceptive advice, examination for sexually transmitted infections, assistance in stopping smoking or drug abuse are among the issues that young people may wish to conceal from their parents. (Common examples of young women requesting contraception without parental knowledge are discussed in Chapter 5.) Competent children and young people should always be encouraged to involve their parents but cannot be forced to do so and are entitled to respect for their confidentiality. In exceptional cases, however, the confidentiality of any patient can be breached if there are sufficiently serious grounds to justify it.

Case example – separated parents applying for access to a child's record

Common enquiries to the BMA concern cases in which divorced or separated parents each want access to their child's record. Fathers who have parental responsibility (see Chapter 5) have the same rights as the mother and can have access to information with the consent of a mature minor or if it is in the best interests of a child who lacks the competence to consent. In these circumstances, both parents can apply for access separately and if one applies, there is no obligation to tell the other about the application. Often, one parent becomes anxious if the other has a new partner who may not get on with the child. The parent who does not live with the child may then ask to be alerted each time the child is brought to the surgery and the reason for the consultation. GPs are not obliged to issue regular bulletins in this way, nor is it reasonable to expect them to do so. Nevertheless, in some cases practices are willing to inform the parent of any significant health events.

Access to the records of incapacitated adults

Information can be shared with carers or other people close to incapacitated adults, when it is in those patients' best interests. (Sharing information with carers and relatives is discussed in Chapter 6.) Account has to be taken of any previous wishes of the patient, before capacity was lost. Information that patients wanted to be kept confidential should not be disclosed, unless there is a strong justification. Proxy decision makers or court-appointed deputies (see Chapter 4) can also seek access to the records, under the Data Protection Act. Disclosures to them should be restricted to information necessary for them to carry out their role.

Access to the records of deceased persons

The confidentiality owed to the deceased is discussed in Chapter 6. Personal representatives and other people with a claim arising from the death of a patient have statutory rights of access to some information under the Access to Health Records Act 1990 and the Access to Health Records (Northern Ireland) Order 1993.[31] Their rights are limited to information directly relevant to their claim. Chapter 6 also describes how most information in the medical records of deceased patients is likely to be exempt from disclosure under the Freedom of Information Act.[38] The Freedom of Information (Scotland) Act specifically exempts deceased patients' records from disclosure.[39]

Access to reports for insurance or employment

The Access to Medical Reports Act 1988 and the Access to Personal Files and Medical Reports (Northern Ireland) Order 1991 give patients rights to see reports written about them for employment or insurance purposes before they are sent. The legislation covers reports written by the applicant's GP or a specialist who has provided care. The extent to which occupational health physicians are subject to the legislation is a matter of debate, but the number and nature of consultations with employees are likely to be relevant. The Faculty of Occupational Medicine advises that it is for occupational physicians to determine whether their activities amount to the provision of care, as defined by the legislation.[40] Reports written by an independent medical examiner are not covered, but patients are entitled to access these reports under data protection legislation. The General Medical Council (GMC) also advises that all doctors should offer to show patients reports written about them.

The administrative requirements of the legislation fall mainly upon the organisation requesting the report (the applicant). Applicants must inform patients of their rights in writing. They must be informed when a report is sought and know that they can see it either before it is sent to the company or during the following 6 months. They have rights to instruct the doctor not to send the report or to request the amendment of inaccuracies in it. Patients also need to know that they can withhold permission altogether for the company to have a medical report, although this is likely to result in the patient not getting the job or the insurance. Patients have 21 days in which to see the report, starting from the date that they notify the doctor they want to see it, and the doctor should not send the report off during this period. If patients fail to contact the doctor within those 21 days, the completed report can be sent to the applicant. If the patient sees the report and withdraws consent for it to be sent, it must not be dispatched and the doctor should inform the applicant.

Patients are entitled to have any factual inaccuracies in the report corrected. Doctors may not agree that there is an error, in which case they have to append a note to the report about the disputed information. Patients often request that something be left out from reports, but if it is a relevant piece of information, it must either stay in or the patient can withdraw permission for the report to be sent off. Alternatively the report can be sent, but the doctor must indicate that certain relevant information has been withheld at the request of the patient.[41]

Security of data

The obligation to protect identifiable data

Maintaining patient confidentiality is a legal and moral obligation as well as being a condition of employment within the NHS. It is also a standard part of independent sector contracts. All staff and volunteers working with patients need to be aware of their responsibility to safeguard patient data and should sign a confidentiality contract agreement. Mistakes happen as human error cannot be eliminated, but they can be minimised if staff give more consideration to the routine ways they use and manage records.

Case example – misplaced records

In February 2011, Ipswich Hospital NHS Trust lost 29 patient records, after a staff member took them home to update a training log. Personal details of patients' surgery were among the lost data. The information was later recovered and the trust subsequently made data protection training mandatory for all relevant staff.[42]

All reasonable precautions must be taken to ensure that patient records or laptops holding data are kept secure, both within and outside health premises. When health professionals work at home on portable equipment, data should be encrypted. In 2010, the Information Commissioner said that the NHS was one of the worst offenders for its rates of data loss. He criticised the fact that far too much personal data were downloaded from secure servers onto unencrypted laptops, USB sticks and other portable media[43] and highlighted various cases where unencrypted USB sticks with sensitive information about patients were lost.[44] Things had not improved greatly by 2011 when more memory sticks with unencrypted data were mislaid and he said that the NHS needed 'a culture change so that staff give more consideration to how they store and disclose data'.[45]

Doctors have particular obligations for the safe storage of health information and may be held liable not only for their own breaches of confidentiality but also for those of their staff or team. They can face criminal charges if they fail to ensure the security of health information. Their obligations include both ensuring that identifiable data are protected against improper disclosure and that staff are also trained to do this.[46]

Records management policies

Health organisations handle large quantities of sensitive patient data on a daily basis. They should have robust security, information governance and records management policies in place or risk being fined by the Information Commissioner, who adjudicates serious data breaches under the Data Protection Act (see Chapter 6). Policies need to be familiar to staff and updated at regular intervals. Considerable detailed guidance is available both for hospital trusts and primary care practices[47] and includes an online *Information Governance Toolkit* in England.[48] The toolkit helps organisations assess whether data are protected from unauthorised access, loss, damage and destruction. NHS organisations in England must complete the toolkit assessment, which measures their progress against a series of standards. Other organisations, including the BMA, have collaborated in producing best practice guidelines for protecting electronic patient information.[49] Technical guidance is also available for the secure management of electronic and paper-based records.[50] Protection is needed against external hackers and inappropriate access by staff. Even simple security measures can be effective, such as regularly changing computer passwords and always clearing the screen of a previous patient's information before seeing another.

Case example – unauthorised access by staff

Among queries to the BMA are cases in which GP reception staff inappropriately access the records of friends or relatives. In one instance, it seemed that a receptionist had probably applied for the job partly with the aim of trying to change something in her son's record which she thought would prejudice his chances of future employment, if known. She had not realised that the audit trail would give her away. Strict rules against unauthorised access should be part of staff contracts, backed up by security measures to prevent any browsing of records by unauthorised staff.

Transmission of information

By fax

Although it seems self-evident, fax numbers should be checked carefully. In Chapter 6, we gave an example of the use of a wrong number being reported to the Information Commissioner, when details of patients' operations were sent to the wrong place. Checks should also be made to ensure the receiving machine is in a secure area.

NHSmail

NHSmail is an email service provided by the NHS for staff in England and Scotland. Each email is automatically encrypted during transmission. It is the only NHS email system accredited for the secure transfer of clinical data which can be emailed to colleagues who have NHSmail accounts. The service uses technology to monitor for any potential security breaches. The BMA and Connecting for Health have produced guidance on NHSmail.[51]

Transfer of information within the NHS

If records are stored remotely on a centralised server, health professionals must ensure that the remote facility has proper protection, including secure server connections and encryption technology. According to the Information Commissioner, each GP practice is not expected to develop its own IT system, but those who develop IT systems for use by GPs should build in the capability of concealing patients' identities from people who do not need to know them. He said that action could be taken against a GP (or any other data controller) who does not make use of the features available on a system for maximising patients' privacy.[52]

When transmitting patient details electronically, by fax, email, memory sticks or other portable devices, health professionals must ensure that identifiable information does not fall into the wrong hands. They must follow procedures designed to protect patients' privacy when using computer systems.[53] Whenever possible, clinical details should be separated from demographic data so that if information goes astray, it is not linked to an individual.[54] Some routine security measures are obvious, such as using an identifying number rather than the patient's name and postcode. All data transmitted in electronic format across the NHS must be encrypted.[55] Commissioning bodies, trusts and health boards should have policies in place to ensure the recommended encryption standards. Guidance is available in England, Wales and Scotland on the use of encryption to protect the transfer of sensitive data[56] and on the recommended encryption standards when it is necessary to transfer data across removable media.[57]

Transfer of GP records

When patients move between GPs, their records are transferred via the commissioning body or primary care organisation. Many transfers of electronic records between GP practices in England are completed using the 'GP2GP' system, which enables an almost instantaneous transfer of an electronic health record. If patients leave a computerised practice for a paper-based one, hard copies of their records should be sent to the commissioning body or primary care organisation, for onward transmission. The transfer of electronic patient records is discussed in detail in joint guidance from the Department of Health, the BMA and the Royal College of General Practitioners.[5]

Sending information abroad

As patients seek some private treatment overseas to cut the cost or be seen quicker, it can be necessary to send relevant extracts from their records to clinics abroad. Also some patients, such as those with kidney failure, may need to make arrangements to have dialysis while on holiday outside the UK. Information needs to be sent securely. In 2010, concern was expressed in the media that the NHS was sending millions of confidential medical notes to India for transcribing.[58] The Data Protection Act is clear that personal data must not be transferred outside the European Economic Area without adequate protection, equivalent to those provided by the Act. Data controllers must ensure that information exchanges are compliant with the Act and protection is in place.

Retention and destruction of records

Accessing records after the duty of care has ended

The main purpose of keeping health records is to provide care. For this, they have a limited shelf life but, if authorised, can still serve other useful purposes, in research, teaching and audit. As discussed above, patient consent is usually required for secondary uses unless the information has been anonymised. Some NHS professionals like to go back to patient records, long after the point at which their responsibility for the patient has ended, or to hang on to them when the records should have been either transferred to the patient's new clinician or gone back to the NHS, if the patient has died.

> ### Case example – accessing records after the duty of care has ended
>
> Among the queries to the BMA, a recurring one concerns doctors who access or keep NHS records for patients they no longer look after. Sometimes the doctor was responsible for an earlier episode of care and is anxious to check up later whether his hunch about the best treatment option turned out to be correct in the long run. In other cases, the doctor plans to write his or her memoirs when he or she retires and wants to include some memorable cases, or records are kept longer than they should be, on the off-chance that an interesting research project could be done on them one day. The GMC makes clear that only health professionals who are providing care should access patient records.[59]

Recommended retention times

There comes a time when consideration is given to whether old paper records should be destroyed. Across the UK, codes of practice give detailed guidance about the recommended retention times of paper records, to help the NHS meet its legal obligations.[60] They advise that electronic records must not be destroyed for the foreseeable future. Private practitioners are advised to follow the same rules, unless transferring patients' records to a new doctor. Although the guidance refers to *minimum* periods for which records must be retained, there may be times when they should be kept longer but it is also important to remember that the Data Protection Act (principle five) prohibits the retention of personal data for longer than necessary. Although the definition of 'necessary' varies, if records are kept longer than the periods recommended, it should be for a reason. If it is known, for example, that records are likely to be needed in litigation, they need to be kept. Private practitioners are unlikely to be criticised if they retain records for the minimum period recommended by the NHS. A basic summary of the main points follows in Table 7.1, Table 7.2 and Table 7.3.[61]

Table 7.1 Recommended minimum lengths of retention of GP records (England, Wales and Northern Ireland)

Type	Retention period
GP records	10 years after death or after the patient has permanently left the country unless the patient remains in the European Union. In the case of a child, if the illness or death could have potential relevance to adult conditions or have genetic implications for the family of the deceased, the advice of clinicians should be sought as to whether to retain the records for a longer period. Electronic patient records (EPRs) must not be destroyed, or deleted, for the foreseeable future.
Maternity records	25 years after the birth of the last child.
Records relating to persons receiving treatment for a mental disorder within the meaning of mental health legislation	20 years after the date of the last contact or 10 years after the patient's death, if sooner.
Records relating to those serving in HM Armed Forces	Not to be destroyed.
Records relating to those serving a prison sentence	Not to be destroyed.

Table 7.2 Recommended minimum lengths of retention of hospital records (England, Wales and Northern Ireland)

Type	Retention period
Maternity records (including all obstetric and midwifery records, including those of episodes of maternity care that end in stillbirth or where the child later dies)	25 years after the birth of the last child.
Children and young people (all types of records relating to children and young people)	Until the patient's 25th birthday or 26th if the young person was 17 at the conclusion of treatment, or 8 years after death.
Mentally disordered persons (within the meaning of any Mental Health Act)	20 years after the date of the last contact between the patient/client/service user and any health/care professional employed by the mental health provider, or 8 years after the death of the patient/client/service user if sooner.
All other hospital records (other than non-specified secondary care records)	8 years after the conclusion of treatment or death.

Table 7.3 Summary of minimum retention periods for personal health records (Scotland)

Type	Retention period
Adult	6 years after last entry or 3 years after the patient's death.
Records relating to children and young people (16 years on admission)	Until the patient's 25th birthday or 26th if an entry was made when the young person was 17; or 3 years after death of the patient if sooner.
Mentally disordered person (within the meaning of any Mental Health Act)	20 years after the date of the last contact between the patient/client/service user and any health/care professional employed by the mental health provider, or 3 years after the death of the patient/client/service user if sooner and the patient died while in the care of the organisation.
Maternity records	25 years after the birth of the last child.
GP records	For the patient's lifetime and 3 years after the patient's death.
	Electronic patient records (GP only) must not be destroyed, or deleted, for the foreseeable future.

Disposal of manual records

Records must be destroyed effectively and without compromising confidentiality, such as by incineration, pulping or shredding.

Storing and disposing of recordings

Recordings made as part of the patient's care are part of the medical record and must be treated in the same way as other medical records. For recordings made for secondary purposes, the GMC advises that doctors must be satisfied 'that there is agreement about the ownership, copyright, and intellectual property rights of the recording'.[62] Further advice can be sought from a Caldicott Guardian. Recordings should also be destroyed effectively.

A last word about records management

As the use of electronic records increases, it becomes easier for patients to access their own health records directly. Such direct access is intended to give them more sense of ownership of their data as well as improve accuracy. There are already some signs that patients find direct access reassuring and feel better informed about their care.[63] Experts point out, however, that 'switching on patient access alone is not enough, and potentially detrimental if appropriate support structures are not in place for patients so that they understand and know how to use the information. The planned roll-out of patient access to electronic records by the Government must acknowledge this and ensure that a support structure is in place, including a proper consent process'.[64] With the potential for patients to access their records online or via mobile devices, the health service has to adapt to new ways of working, without disadvantaging patients who are unable to use computers or other new technology and risk being left behind.

There is also increased focus on improving the quality of health records, including using insights from patients. More attention is urged for patient-generated comments via all forms of social media.[65] Improving record quality not only makes care safer for patients but also makes health data more reliable for secondary purposes that benefit everyone.

References

1   Information on how to register is available at: http://www.healthspace.nhs.uk (accessed 6 June 2012).

2   Information on 'My Health Online' is available at: http://www.wales.nhs.uk (accessed 16 August 2012).

3   Further information is available at: http://www.scotland.gov.uk (accessed 16 August 2012).

4   Royal College of General Practitioners (2010) *Enabling Patients to Access Electronic Health Records: Guidance for Health Professionals*, RCGP, London.

5   Department of Health, British Medical Association, Royal College of General Practitioners (2011) *The Good Practice Guidelines for GP Electronic Patient Records (v. 4)*, DH, London.

6   General Medical Council (2011) *Making and Using Visual and Audio Recordings of Patients*, GMC, London, para 10.

7   Information Commissioner's Office (2008) *CCTV Code of Practice*, ICO, Wilmslow.

8   General Medical Council (2011) *Making and Using Visual and Audio Recordings of Patients*, GMC, London, para 34.

9   General Medical Council (2006) *Good Medical Practice*, GMC, London, paras 3 (f) and (g).

10 Department of Health (2008) *A Clinician's Guide to Record Standards – Part 2: Standards for the Structure and Content of Medical Records and Communications When Patients Are Admitted to Hospital*, DH, London.

11 Example templates can be downloaded and used to create paper proformas that can be customised for use by individual hospitals and trusts.

12 Audit Commission, Royal College of Physicians (2009) *Improving Clinical Records and Clinical Coding Together*, Audit Commission, London.

13 Royal College of General Practitioners, Connecting for Health (2009) *Informing Shared Clinical Care: Final Report of the Shared Record Professional Guidance Project*, RCGP, London.

14 British Medical Association (2010) *Acting upon Test Results in an Electronic World*, BMA, London.

15 Detailed information can be found in: British Medical Association (2012) *Medical Ethics Today. The BMA's Handbook of Ethics and Law*, 3rd edn, Wiley-Blackwell, Chichester, pp. 240–241.

16 Information about national summary records can be found in: British Medical Association (2012) *Medical Ethics Today, The BMA's Handbook of Ethics and Law*, 3rd edn, Wiley-Blackwell, Chichester, pp. 241–242.

17 National Information Governance Board for Health and Social Care (2010) *Requesting Amendments to Health and Social Care Records*, NIGB, London, p.11; Department of Health (2010) *Guidance for Access to Health Records Requests*, DH, London, p.13.

18 National Information Governance Board for Health and Social Care (2010) *Requesting Amendments to Health and Social Care Records*, NIGB, London, p.12; Department of Health (2010) *Guidance for Access to Health Records Requests*, DH, London, p.13.

19 National Information Governance Board for Health and Social Care (2010) *Requesting Amendments to Health and Social Care Records*, NIGB, London, p.8.

20 Medical and Dental Defence Union of Scotland (2009) *Risk Alert: Altering Medical Notes* (4 June), MDDUS, Glasgow.

21 General Medical Council Fitness to Practise Panel Hearing, 22 March–5 May 2010.

22 Bowcott O. (2010) NHS patients given right to delete electronic record. *The Guardian* (May 26). Available at: http://www.guardian.co.uk (accessed 6 June 2012).

23 Adoption records are exempt from subject access requests under the Data Protection Act 1998.

24 Connecting for Health. *Adoptions*. http://www.connectingforhealth.nhs.uk (accessed 6 June 2012).

25 General Medical Council (2011) *Making and Using Visual and Audio Recordings of Patients*, GMC, London, para 24.

26 General Medical Council (2011) *Making and Using Visual and Audio Recordings of Patients*, GMC, London, para 25.

27 Further advice on anonymising information is available from the Information Commissioner's Office: Information Commissioner's Office (2007) *Data Protection Technical Guidance – Determining What Is Personal Data*, ICO, Wilmslow, section C.

28 General Medical Council (2011) *Making and Using Visual and Audio Recordings of Patients*, GMC, London, para 17.

29 General Medical Council (2011) *Making and Using Visual and Audio Recordings of Patients*, GMC, London, paras 11, 12 and 17.

30   General Medical Council (2011) *Making and Using Visual and Audio Recordings of Patients*, GMC, London, para 39.

31   British Medical Association (2008) *Access to Health Records: Guidance for Health Professionals in the United Kingdom*, BMA, London; Department of Health (2010) *Guidance for Access to Health Records Requests*, DH, London.

32   British Medical Association (2008) *Access to Health Records: Guidance for Health Professionals in the United Kingdom*, BMA, London.

33   Information Commissioner's Office (2006) *Data Protection Technical Guidance Note: Dealing with Subject Access Requests Involving Other People's Information*, ICO, Wilmslow.

34   Data Protection (Miscellaneous Subject Access Exemptions) Order 2000. SI 2000/419.

35   British Medical Association, The Law Society (2003) *Consent Form (Releasing Health Records under the Data Protection Act 1998) – for England and Wales*, BMA, London.

36   British Medical Association, The Law Society of Scotland, Scottish Executive Health Department (2004) *Consent Form for Access to Patients' Records by Solicitors (Releasing Health Records under the Data Protection Act 1998)*, BMA, London.

37   General Medical Council (2007) *0–18 Years: Guidance for Doctors*, GMC, London, paras 53–55.

38   *Bluck v The Information Commissioner and Epsom and St Helier University NHS Trust* [2007] EA/2006/0090.

39   Freedom of Information (Scotland) Act 2002, s 38.

40   Faculty of Occupational Medicine (2006) *Guidance on Ethics for Occupational Physicians*, FOM, London, para 3.41.

41   British Medical Association (2009) *Access to Medical Reports*, BMA, London.

42   Information Commissioner (2011) *Health services must get it right on data security, says ICO*. News release, 1 July. Available at: http://www.ico.gov.uk/news (accessed 15 May 2012).

43   Anon. (2010) 'Unacceptable' level of data loss. *BBC News Online* (Nov 11). Available at: http://www.bbc.co.uk/news (accessed 6 June 2012).

44   Information Commissioner (2009) *NHS staff to improve data handling after details of cancer patients go missing*. Press release, October 27; Anon. (2010) Health records found in Asda car park. *BBC News Online* (May 5). Available at: http://www.bbc.co.uk/news (accessed 6 June 2012).

45   Information Commissioner (2011) *Health services must get it right on data security, says ICO*. News release, 1 July. Available at: http://www.ico.gov.uk/news (accessed 17 May 2012).

46   General Medical Council (2009) *Confidentiality*, GMC, London, paras 12 and 15.

47   For example: Department of Health (2006) *Records Management: NHS Code of Practice*, DH, London. This sets out the standards to be included in an organisation's records management policy. The Department of Health, with the BMA and Royal College of General Practitioners, also publishes guidance on managing electronic records, information governance issues and security for GP practices. See: Department of Health, British Medical Association, Royal College of General Practition-

ers (2011) *The Good Practice Guidelines for GP Electronic Patient Records (v.4)*, DH, London.

48 Department of Health (2012) *Information Governance Toolkit*. Available at: http:// www.igt.connectingforhealth.nhs.uk (accessed 6 June 2012).

49 NHS Connecting for Health, British Medical Association (2008) *Joint Guidance on Protecting Electronic Patient Information*, BMA, London.

50 Department of Health (2007) *Information Security Management: NHS Code of Practice*, DH, London.

51 British Medical Association, Connecting for Health. *NHSmail Guidance*. Available at: http://www.connectingforhealth.nhs.uk (accessed 28 September 2012).

52 Information Commissioner's Office (2002) *Use and Disclosure of Health Data: Guidance on the Application of the Data Protection Act 1998*, ICO, Wilmslow, p.5.

53 General Medical Council (2009) *Confidentiality*, GMC, London, para 14.

54 General Medical Council (2009) *Confidentiality*, GMC, London, para 15.

55 British Medical Association (2002) *Consulting in the Modern World*, BMA, London, p.6; NHS Connecting for Health (2009) *Guidelines on Use of Encryption to Protect Identifiable and Sensitive Information*, DH, London.

56 NHS Connecting for Health (2009) *Guidelines on Use of Encryption to Protect Identifiable and Sensitive Information*, DH, London; NHS Wales, *National Encryption Framework*. Available at: http://www.wales.nhs.uk (accessed 28 September 2012); NHS Scotland, *Encryption Policy*. Available at: http://www.srr.scot.nhs.uk (accessed 24 January 2013); NHS Scotland (2008) *eHealth Mobile Data Protection Standard*, NHS Scotland, Edinburgh.

57 Department of Health (2012) *Information Governance Toolkit*, DH, London. Available at: http://www.igt.connectingforhealth.nhs.uk (accessed 6 June 2012).

58 Ungoed-Thomas J. (2010) NHS sends confidential patient records to India. *The Times* (April 4). Available at: http://www.timesonline.co.uk (accessed 6 June 2012).

59 General Medical Council (2009) *Confidentiality*, GMC, London.

60 Department of Health (2006) *Records Management: NHS Code of Practice*, DH, London; Scottish Government (2008) *Records Management: NHS Code of Practice (Scotland) Version 1.0*, Scottish Government, Edinburgh; National Assembly for Wales (2000) *Welsh Health Circular 71: for the Record*, National Assembly for Wales, Cardiff; Department of Health, Social Services and Public Safety (2005) *Good Management, Good Records*, DHSSPS, Belfast; Department of Health, Social Services and Public Safety (2000) *Preservation, Retention and Destruction of GP Medical Records Circular HSS (PCC) 2000/1*, DHSSPS, Belfast. At the time of writing, the DHSSPS was consulting on the *Good Management, Good Records* publication. The updated version will cover GP medical records as well as hospital records and will replace *Preservation, Retention and Destruction of GP Medical Records Circular.*

61 The tables quote the advice given in: Department of Health (2006) *Records Management: NHS Code of Practice*, DH, London. Similar advice is provided in the schedules relevant to each of the devolved nations.

62 General Medical Council (2011) *Making and Using Visual and Audio Recordings of Patients*, GMC, London, para 57.

63 Fisher B, Bhavnani V. (2006) How patients use access to their full health records: a qualitative study of patients in general practice. *J R Soc Med* 102(12), 539–544.

64 Department of Health (2012) *Information: a Report from the NHS Future Forum*, DH, London, p.15.

65 Department of Health (2012) *Information: a Report from the NHS Future Forum*, DH, London, p.16.

8: Prescribing and administering medication

10 things you need to know about . . . prescribing and administering medication

- The health professional who writes the prescription has clinical and legal responsibility for it.
- NHS prescribers are expected to use the most clinically and cost-effective treatment.
- NHS patients cannot insist on having specific medication.
- NHS patients have the right to medication and treatments which have been recommended by official bodies for use in the NHS if their doctor believes them to be clinically appropriate.
- When patients opt to top up their care with private treatment, they are still entitled to NHS services they would otherwise be given, on the same basis of clinical need as other patients.
- Good communication is essential when prescribing is shared between practitioners.
- Patients should be encouraged to be open with prescribers about the medications they take.
- It is unwise for prescribers to form close business connections with companies that produce, market or promote pharmaceutical products.
- Doctors must not ask for or accept any inducement, gift or hospitality which may affect or be seen to affect their judgement.
- Covert medication of patients with capacity is illegal and unethical.

Setting the scene

Prescribed medicine is the most common form of NHS intervention. With changes in the health service and the way in which health care is delivered, many of the traditional dilemmas, such as conflicts of interest, resource allocation, shared prescribing and relations with pharmaceutical companies, have taken on increased importance and greater prominence. Patients are increasingly well informed and, once they have done some internet research, often expect to have the medication of their choice within the NHS. At the same time, NHS prescribing – like other treatment decisions – has to take account of financial constraints. Tensions can arise in relationships with patients if apparently unnecessary lifestyle drugs are requested by them. The principle that

Everyday Medical Ethics and Law, First Edition. Ann Sommerville.
© 2013 BMA Medical Ethics Department. Published 2013 by John Wiley & Sons, Ltd.

prescribing should address an identified clinical need can be conflated with a more consumerist focus on what healthy patients would like in order to improve their quality of life. This raises fundamental questions about the core purpose of medicine. All of these issues we touch on in this chapter.

Common enquiries about prescribing and administering medication

- My patient thinks he is cured of his psychotic episodes and refuses the medication that keeps him stable. Can we put it secretly in his food before a crisis occurs?
- Some patients prefer their existing pain-relief pills but generic ones are cheaper for the NHS. Can I still switch the prescription, if they object strongly?
- Is it ethically acceptable to prescribe placebos?
- Is it OK to issue a prescription by email, without seeing the patient if I have treated him in the past and am generally familiar with his problems?
- Do I have to comply with the standard prescribing protocols issued to doctors in the private slimming clinic where I work? What if they seem inappropriate for some patients?
- Can I prescribe medication to treat myself or a member of my family?
- Can I accept hospitality and expenses for attending a meeting or conference sponsored by a pharmaceutical company?

Talking to patients and obtaining consent

Patients need to consent to anything done to them. In Chapter 3 we discuss the criteria that must be met in order for their consent or refusal to be valid The main requirements are that they have the necessary capacity to make the decision, have enough relevant information to make an informed choice and are not pressured to act against their will or judgement. The same considerations apply when their consent is sought for medication to be prescribed for them and when, if they agree, it is administered.

Giving information about a prescription

The professional who writes a prescription has responsibility for informing patients (or, in cases of shared care, ensuring the patient is informed) about the medicine and how to use it. Patients should be told about the product's benefits and risks, side effects, complications and, if relevant, the likelihood that it may not completely solve their problem. Pharmacists also have a responsibility to ensure patients know how to use their medication. Written patient information leaflets provide additional details, but patients often fail to read them and they are no substitute for discussion. Part of the aim of the conversation is to support patients' informed choices. Giving people choices means that some decide not to start the medication recommended, or else soon give it up. Talking to them about the reasons for taking it and involving them in the decision do not necessarily improve adherence to the recommended regime, but it can encourage them to understand better the expected benefits.

The General Medical Council (GMC) says that doctors should try to reach an agreement with patients about the medication they recommend and the management of the patient's condition.

GMC guidance on discussing prescriptions

Doctors should, where appropriate,

- establish patients' priorities, preferences and concerns and encourage them to ask questions about the proposed treatment
- discuss other treatment options with patients
- ensure that they have appropriate information, in a way they understand, about
  - any common adverse side effects
  - potentially serious side effects
  - what to do in the event of a side effect
  - interactions with other medicines
  - the dosage and administration of the medicine
- ensure that patients understand how to take the medicine as prescribed and can take it that way.[1]

Concordance/medicines adherence

Many patients do not take their medicine in the way they should, or fail to complete the full course. Some never start taking it at all, even when the consequences can be life-threatening.[2] Estimates vary but it is thought that between a third and a half of medication for long-term conditions is not taken as recommended.[3] This can obviously result in serious health problems for patients and a significant waste of NHS resources. The reasons why patients fail to take their medicines as directed can be said to fall into two groups, intentional and unintentional non-adherence.[3] Unintentional failure to stick to the regime often involves practical difficulties, such as patients' confusion over how or when to take the medicine, or their experience of unpleasant side effects. Significant intentional factors can include the value patients place on the appropriateness of taking medication and their own perceptions of the threat they face from their illness. Patients with mental capacity clearly have rights to decline medication, as long as they know the implications for themselves, even if their condition will predictably deteriorate. Where a patient decides not to take a medicine, it is important for doctors to make a note of the discussion in the medical notes and review the patient's decision on a regular basis as motivations for non-adherence can change over time.

'Concordance' describes a process of discussion and negotiation between prescriber and patient. It aims to involve patients in prescribing decisions so that their beliefs and wishes are taken into account, as well as clinical factors. It is based on a concept of partnership which highlights patients' responsibilities to maintain their own health without burdening the NHS unnecessarily, as well as their rights to choice. Detailed clinical guidelines are available on best practice in talking to patients about prescribed medicines and supporting their adherence to the medical regime prescribed.[4] Resources and learning materials are also available about how to involve patients in prescribing decisions.[5]

Taking account of patients' values and religion

Taking account of patients' beliefs and wishes regarding prescriptions can promote better medicines adherence. Vegetarians may object to taking medicines containing animal products, if there are other options. Some religious faiths also forbid the use of animal derivatives or alcohol, used in the manufacture of some medication, but religious leaders may permit their use when there is no alternative.[6] All patients must be seen as individuals, without assumptions being made about their beliefs. Patients should be encouraged to be proactive in making doctors aware of any objections they would have to taking specific medication based on their religious faith or beliefs. Doctors cannot be expected to know the constituents of all medicines they may prescribe, but where the doctor knows that the product contains ingredients to which the patient has expressed an objection, this should be discussed with the patient. In some circumstances, it may be possible for the doctor to check the ingredients of a particular medication before prescribing where this can be achieved easily and quickly. Pharmacists may also have a role in responding to specific enquiries from patients. Patients can also check the patient information leaflet for a particular product. Guidance is available about the use of drugs of porcine origin,[7] to which Muslim and Jewish patients may object.

Prescribing placebos

Ethical guidance emphasises the importance of involving patients in decisions and being frank with them, so placebos do not seem to fit well into modern medicine. They are pills or procedures, without any active pharmacological or physiological properties, or at least none specific to the condition for which they are prescribed. They usually rely on patients being unaware of that fact. For some patients, the placebo effect does work and pills with no analgesic properties, for example, can give them pain relief. Some people argue that medicine should make greater use of the placebo effect but, from an ethical perspective, the deception of patients is problematic. Deliberately deceiving them, even in their interests, not only offends the concept of respect for patient autonomy but risks damaging the doctor–patient relationship. Although studies show widespread use in some countries,[8] the BMA is opposed to the use of placebos for patients with mental capacity and a Parliamentary Committee has called for the Government to draw up clear policies on their use in the NHS,[9] but this has not yet happened.

Pressure from patients

NHS patients have the right to medication and treatments which have been recommended for use in the NHS by the National Institute for Health and Clinical Excellence (NICE) and equivalent bodies in the devolved nations, if their doctor believes them to be clinically appropriate. Beyond this, as discussed in Chapter 2, patients cannot insist that their doctor prescribes particular medication or treatments. Prescriptions should be clinically appropriate and, wherever possible, evidence based. When patients' requests are inappropriate for some reason, it is important for doctors to explain the reasons for refusing them. This can be a difficult conversation but is preferable to simply reinforcing patient's expectations, by giving in to them inappropriately.

Case example – patients insisting on having antibiotics

Among the common prescribing problems doctors face are situations in which patients visit GPs, with the expectation that they will receive a prescription, often antibiotics, irrespective of their illness. They feel short-changed if told that a prescription would not help. Although public education campaigns have raised awareness of common misconceptions about antibiotics, doctors frequently report strong pressure from patients to prescribe them for self-limiting illnesses. Some doctors may opt for writing a prescription rather than having a confrontation about it, but this contributes to the growing problem of antibiotic resistance. It also reinforces patients' expectation of getting antibiotics the next time. Patient demand and the placebo effect have been suggested as justifications for prescribing products known to be pharmacologically ineffective for the condition diagnosed. While acknowledging the pressure patients can bring to bear, the BMA emphasises that this is not good practice. The GMC also stresses that doctors should only prescribe medication to meet identified needs of patients, never for patients' own convenience or simply because patients demand them.[10]

Sometimes, patients demand a particular medicine or treatment because it has featured in high-profile reports in the media. NHS prescribers are expected to use the most clinically and cost-effective treatment available. Even if patients demand it, prescribing a more expensive branded version of the medication can only be justified if it is clinically appropriate. Patient preference and adherence to the medical regime are factors to take into account, if they contribute to a better result but they may still not warrant the cost increase for the NHS. When patients are treated privately, they can choose a more expensive option, provided the prescriber agrees to accept clinical responsibility for it.

Case example – media reports generating demand

A common example of the way demand for specific medicines often results from high-profile media reports is the way in which the decisions of NICE are reported. Media coverage can imply a sense of patient entitlement to newly approved products. Headlines stating that a particular medication has been authorised by NICE have sometimes resulted in the public assuming that all patients have an immediate and automatic right to that particular product within the NHS. In reality, much of NICE's guidance recommends that a particular treatment be available for certain categories of patient and commissioning bodies may be disinclined to fund it for other groups.

Patients' requests for complementary and alternative medicines (CAMs)

Some patients request complementary therapies such as homeopathy, herbal medicine and acupuncture either in addition to, or instead of, conventional medicine. Many self-refer for private treatment or ask their GP for a referral to a CAM practitioner. Some GPs are trained to offer these services themselves or employ therapists to provide them. If registered doctors prescribe or administer complementary or alternative medicines, they are accountable to the GMC, as for any other prescribing or treatment decision.

The NHS funds some complementary and alternative therapies, but this is controversial. Much debate has focused on homeopathy and whether there is enough evidence of efficacy to justify using public resources to fund it. Supporters of homeopathy, including doctors who offer it, argue that some patients benefit from it and allowing access to homeopathy is in line with maximising patient choice in the NHS. Critics claim that the lack of scientific evidence for its efficacy means that scarce NHS resources should not be spent on homeopathy. In 2010, the House of Commons Science and Technology Committee investigated the evidence base and discussed whether homeopathy should be NHS-funded. It concluded that the theoretical basis for it was weak and scientifically implausible, and that the evidence from systematic reviews and meta-analyses showed that homeopathic products perform no better than placebos.[9] The Committee argued that NHS funding of homeopathy was equivalent to endorsing it, so that patients might assume that it is an evidence-based treatment. It recommended that NHS funding for homeopathy be withdrawn. The Government responded saying that treatment decisions, including those about complementary therapies, should be made by clinicians, not by the Department of Health.[11] In 2010, the BMA's policy-making body, the annual representatives meeting, voted to oppose the provision of homeopathy on the NHS.

Sometimes, it is doctors rather than patients who suggest the use of complementary or alternative medicines. Medical recommendations should always be evidence based and when discussing alternative or complementary therapies with patients, doctors must be objective. Patients should be informed where such practices have been objectively assessed and approved (such as NICE's recommendation for the use of acupuncture in the treatment of non-specific lower back pain[12]). Doctors should not allow their personal beliefs to influence the treatment they offer or to pressure patients to accept their view.

Case example – failure to tell patients about lack of evidence

A GP was found guilty of serious professional misconduct for failing to obtain the informed consent of patients before prescribing homeopathic or natural remedies for them. None of the patients had requested homeopathic treatment. The doctor failed to explain the rationale for using dowsing in selecting a remedy and was found to have pressured a child's parent to consult a geopathic stress therapist. She did not tell the parent that this therapist was not medically qualified and implied that geopathic stress gridlines near the family house could cause cot death. The GP was suspended from the medical register for 3 months. The GMC's Professional Conduct Committee strongly recommended that she used the time to consider the effect on her patients of her use of alternative medicine and ensure that, in future, her personal beliefs did not prejudice her patients' care.[13]

Requests for repeat prescriptions

Repeat prescribing accounts for the majority of prescriptions written by GPs. It makes life easier for patients and doctors by reducing consultations. When they become accustomed to the ease of phoning or emailing for a repeat prescription, patients can be reluctant to turn up for regular clinical assessments when they need them. Doctors must resist pressure to prescribe larger doses of medication than are clinically appropriate or for repeat prescriptions without appropriate clinical review. Detailed guidance on repeat prescribing is available.[14]

Dilemmas also arise from patients trying to insist on the continuation of a prescription that can no longer be justified. They may have faith in a product prescribed for them in the past and be reluctant to admit that it is no longer helping. Often, they think that they cannot manage without it. Dealing with the situation requires patience and tact. The doctor may know that the medicine is no longer appropriate because either it is unable to achieve the objective of stabilising or improving the patient's condition or it may be creating dependency. Patients' views need to be heard and doctors need time to explain why the product is no longer good for the patient. If appropriate, alternative options should be discussed.

Doctors should also ensure that their repeat prescribing systems are updated to prevent unnecessary repeat prescriptions being generated.

Case example – demand for inappropriate repeat prescriptions

Common examples of patient demand for inappropriate repeat prescriptions include requests for hypnotics and anxiolytics, which may have been prescribed to enable the patient to deal with an emotionally painful situation. Patients often underestimate or disregard the possibility of creating a physical or psychological dependence, particularly when they are feeling in control of their medication. Non-pharmaceutical alternatives, possibly including counselling, may need to be discussed with patients, with the aim of reaching an agreement about how they can achieve their goals by other means.

Among the most difficult cases are situations where patients have a life-threatening condition and the medication that alleviated their symptoms or achieved a remission of the disease in the past is no longer effective. When told that fact, patients can feel abandoned or that the health service is giving up hope, even if high-quality palliative alternatives are offered. When patients are approaching the end of their life, it may be tempting to concede to their wishes, even when these involve continuing an ineffective medication, and such cases require very careful handling. It is important to involve patients as much as possible in any decision to change a prescribing pattern upon which they may have come to rely emotionally, as well as clinically.

The BMA and the GMC have published detailed advice on withholding or withdrawing treatment at the end of life, as well as on other aspects of terminal care.[15]

Case example – request for past prescribing to continue

Mr and Mrs H were a childless couple in their early 60s when Mrs H was diagnosed with breast cancer. After a double mastectomy, part of her

(Continued)

ongoing treatment was a regular prescription for tamoxifen. Her overall treatment was successful in extending her life beyond initial expectations. A decade later, Mrs H had outlived her husband and siblings and was still taking tamoxifen. It was evident, however, that due to a combination of other problems, her health was irrevocably deteriorating. Her specialist talked to her about the importance of making a new care plan, with a different medication. Mrs H was extremely upset to know that the tamoxifen would no longer be prescribed. She had great faith in the medication and, although it had been only one facet of treatment, she attributed her 10-year survival to it alone. Having experienced several major bereavements, the proposed change in regime seemed to her another loss of something she relied on. She argued strongly for tamoxifen to be continued. Much effort was put into explaining to Mrs H that a change of medication was important to keep her functioning and comfortable for as long as possible. Reluctantly at first, she gradually became involved in drawing up a personalised palliative care plan which she eventually recognised was a more effective way of managing her symptoms.

'Lifestyle drugs'

Medication is prescribed when clinicians consider it necessary for the patient, but views of what is necessary differ greatly. Concepts of *need* have become increasingly interchangeable with *wants* or *desires*, and patient demand for so called 'lifestyle drugs', which seek to improve quality of life rather than alleviate or cure symptoms of disease, has grown significantly in recent years. Improving the quality of life is a legitimate aim of the health service but where boundaries should be drawn remains a matter of debate. Among the medications commonly requested are hair loss treatments, which illustrate how perceptions of clinical need have altered over time. Some clinicians question the use of therapeutic products for patients' social convenience. For example, an analysis of the prescribing of norethisterone in one area over a 3-year period showed significant peaks during the holiday seasons, which researchers concluded was likely to have been caused by patients delaying menstruation during their holidays. The authors of the study questioned whether norethisterone was being used as a lifestyle drug, and if so, was that appropriate within the NHS.[16] Responses to the study argued, among other things, that 'health is not merely the absence of disease, but a positive concept of wellbeing'.[17] In most cases, it is for prescribers to decide what is appropriate in individual cases, apart from those medicines which are prohibited or restricted within the NHS.[18] Part of this assessment should include considering whether the benefits the patients will, or believe they will, derive outweigh any risks associated with the medication.

Case example – drugs to improve exam performance

An increasing trend has been identified for students and other people under pressure to perform well intellectually to buy prescription-only medication from illegal online pharmacies.[19] They seek the performance-enhancing effect some products can have on healthy people. Examples include the off-label use of modafinil (Provigil) and methylphenidate (Ritalin) to improve cognition. The medication alters the chemical balance of neurotransmitters in the brain and is used therapeutically to treat narcolepsy and attention deficit hyperactivity disorder (ADHD) but have also been shown to improve concentration and alertness for people with otherwise normal cognitive functioning. Such 'smart drugs' are popular as study aids and reports suggest that demand is growing quickly in this demographic, although there are also concerns that some students may feel coerced into taking them to remain competitive.

Although much of the debate has focused on using smart drugs to improve academic performance, the issues raised could have much wider ethical and practical implications for society. On the one hand, for example, it has been argued that cognitive enhancement could potentially help tackle the inequalities that exist within society, counteracting the disadvantages many face in learning and development as a result of environmental and economic factors beyond their control. Widespread use of psycho-pharmaceuticals could, however, also negatively impact on the psychological and physical health of society and reinforce a culture of competitiveness and individualism.

There are also safety concerns associated with people buying medication over the internet from unknown sources and without appropriate medical advice. The medication obtained may be counterfeit or of substandard quality and the long-term effects on the brain of sustained use of smart drugs are also unknown.

Choosing the right product for the patient

Responsibility for prescribing

Prescribers have clinical and legal responsibility for their decisions and must be prepared to justify them, if called upon to do so. They should only prescribe products when they believe them to be clinically appropriate for the patient. The GMC publishes general guidance on prescribing.[20] Doctors should only prescribe medication or treatment when they have 'adequate knowledge of the patient's health, and are satisfied that the medication or treatment serve the patient's needs'.[21]

Clinical freedom

Deciding what to prescribe is a matter of clinical judgement, based on training, experience and published guidance. Decisions are made on the basis of appropriateness, effectiveness, safety, economy and the patient's individual circumstances. The range of medication available is constantly changing, so it is important that all prescribers have access to up-to-date guidance.[22] In some circumstances doctors can prescribe unlicensed medicines and medicines outside the terms of their licence (off-label). This is discussed later. In theory, doctors can prescribe any appropriate and approved medicine but, in practice, resource constraints can limit their clinical autonomy in the NHS.

Prescribing errors

The complexity of modern pharmacology is among the contributory factors for prescribing errors. In 2009, a study into the prevalence of medication errors in hospitals found that such errors were the result of a range of interconnected factors.[23] These included the complexity of the system in which the errors were made, problems related to the working environment, and with the interaction and communication within the medical team. The study also found that medication errors occurred across all clinical grades, including consultants. A 2012 study of prescribing errors in general practice found the following:

- prescribing errors in general practice are common, although severe errors are unusual
- prescribing or monitoring errors were detected for one in eight patients, involving around one in 20 of all prescription items
- prescribing or monitoring errors were not associated with the grade of GP or whether prescriptions were issued as acute or repeat items
- a wide range of underlying causes of error were identified relating to the prescriber, patient, the team, the working environment, the task, the computer system and the primary/secondary care interface.[24]

Although the primary responsibility for ensuring prescriptions are correct lies with the prescriber, other health professionals and pharmacists also play a vital role in checking prescriptions and picking up errors. In order to minimise the risk of errors, it is important that prescribers are receptive to such interventions and that healthcare organisations develop a culture within which such questioning is encouraged. Electronic prescribing systems, used mostly in primary care, can also help reduce errors at all stages of the prescribing process, by giving doctors access to clinical decision support systems to help identify potential adverse drug interactions or patient allergies.

Case example – failure to prescribe correctly

A doctor was found guilty by the GMC of serious professional misconduct for a series of failings in relation to his prescribing of phentermine, the licence for which had already been withdrawn when he prescribed it for three women attending his private slimming clinic. The prescriptions were judged by the GMC to be inappropriate, unjustified, not in the patients' interests and contrary to accepted medical practice. The doctor had failed to warn the patients of the risks of taking the medication nor had he told them that it was unlicensed. He had not carried out an adequate physical examination of the patients nor talked to them about the nature of obesity and its dangers. The patients were not asked about their GPs nor advised to keep them informed. The doctor did not discuss follow-up review with the patients nor make any arrangement to see them again, and he did not record the dosage of phentermine prescribed. His registration was restricted to practice within the NHS, and not in a single-handed general practice either as a principal or a locum, for a period of 3 years.[25]

Pressure from employers

Doctors can sometimes come under pressure to adopt a standard pattern of prescribing, rather than consider the case of each patient individually. As they are personally responsible for their prescribing decisions, doctors need to exercise independent clinical judgement, regardless of the organisation's policies. They should not agree to employment contracts that imply their freedom to prescribe is restricted by the employer's instructions, when these run contrary to patients' interests. The fact that an employer issues such instructions and tells doctors to implement prescribing policies does not mitigate their duty to assess each case individually and to advise patients accordingly.

Case example – pressure from employers

Among the common queries raised with the BMA are situations where doctors are employed on a sessional basis in health facilities, such as private slimming clinics. The clinic management sometimes has standard policies about the medication that it instructs doctors to supply to the patients they see. In some cases, this has appeared to be regardless of the weight loss the patient needed to achieve. Indeed, in some cases, patients who presented for treatment were not significantly overweight. In its advice, the BMA emphasised that such pressure to follow standard, predefined prescribing policies must be resisted and reminded doctors that they were entirely responsible for the prescribing decisions they made. If a patient suffered harm as a result of the product prescribed or the dosage used, the prescriber would be legally liable and would have to justify the decision.

Complying with official guidance

Since the late 1990s new treatments, and some established ones, as well as devices and drugs, have been subject to formal assessment for clinical efficacy and cost-effectiveness. Different national bodies are responsible for this role in England and Wales, Scotland, and Northern Ireland.

NICE (England and Wales)

NICE aims to provide authoritative and reliable guidance on current best practice for the health service, patients and the public. Its formal remit extends only to England and Wales, but its guidelines are influential throughout the UK. NICE is responsible for collecting and evaluating all relevant evidence and considering its implications for clinical practice, with reference to both clinical effectiveness and cost-effectiveness. Its appraisals focus primarily on pharmaceutical products but also include medical devices, diagnostic techniques, health promotion and surgical procedures. Guidance results from the appraisal, which indicates whether, and, if so, in what circumstances, it would be appropriate to use the technology in the NHS. There are two types of technology appraisal. Single technology appraisals evaluate an individual medicine for a particular condition, whereas in a multiple technology appraisal, NICE compares several different types of treatment resulting in more detailed guidance. NICE produces clinical guidelines which are not binding on health professionals but give recommendations on the management of particular diseases and clinical conditions, based on the best available evidence. Among the topics covered by its guidance are cancer services, diagnostic technologies, interventional procedures, medical technologies and public health issues.

Where NICE guidance applies in the UK[26]

England
- Clinical guidelines
- Single and multiple technology appraisals
- Interventional procedures
- Public health guidance
- Medical technologies guidance

Wales
- Clinical guidelines
- Single and multiple technology appraisals
- Interventional procedures
- Public health guidance has no formal status but is regarded as a useful source of reviewed evidence

Northern Ireland
- Clinical guidelines (subject to general review)
- Single and multiple technology appraisals (subject to local review)
- Interventional procedures
- Public health guidance (subject to local review)

Scotland
- Multiple technology appraisals (with advice on implementation from Healthcare Improvement Scotland)
- Interventional procedures
- Public health guidance (subject to local review)

NICE evaluates the cost-effectiveness of new treatments, bearing in mind the significant pressures on NHS resources. If it has approved the use of a drug, in a technology appraisal, commissioning bodies are required to provide funding for it in the NHS, within 3 months. Recommendations not to fund, or to restrict access to medicines, have been subject to intense scrutiny in the media. NICE has often faced intense public criticism and pressure from pharmaceutical companies and patient support groups. In 2010, significant changes were proposed to the role of NICE[27] and, from April 2013, it will be re-established as the 'National Institute for Health and Care Excellence (NICE)' and, for England, its remit will be extended to include children's and adults' social care.

Comparable arrangements for technology evaluation in Scotland

Healthcare Improvement Scotland (HIS) provides advice to Scottish health boards about new and existing technologies. Its guidance may be based on NICE recommendations or on separate health technology assessments. HIS also supports the Scottish Medicines Consortium (SMC), which advises NHS boards about the efficacy of all newly licensed medicines, all new major formulations of existing medicines and any major new indications of established medicines. HIS evaluates the multiple technology appraisals published by NICE for their applicability in Scotland. Where it validates a positive NICE multiple technology appraisal, NHS boards in Scotland are required to make these medicines available. Single evaluations of newly licensed drugs are performed by the SMC. Health boards in Scotland are expected to ensure that the drugs or treatments recommended by the SMC are made available to meet clinical need, but doing so is not mandatory. Doctors in Scotland also have guidance from the Scottish Intercollegiate Guidelines Network (SIGN), which comes under the remit of HIS. SIGN aims to improve the quality of care for patients in Scotland, by reducing variations in practice and outcomes, through the development of national clinical guidelines on good practice.

Arrangements for technology appraisals in Wales

NICE appraisals apply in Wales, but the All Wales Medicines Strategy Group (AWMSG) also plays a role in the approval of high-cost cardiac and cancer medicines. This guidance may be issued either before NICE has published advice or in the absence of NICE comments.[28] AWMSG appraisals are intended to complement those from NICE, which remain the primary source of guidance on new medicines and ultimately take precedence if the two sets of guidance differ. Local health boards and trusts are required to follow the recommendations of AWMSG within 3 months.

Arrangements for technology appraisals in Northern Ireland

In Northern Ireland, a formal link exists between the Department of Health, Social Services and Public Safety and NICE through which guidance produced by NICE is subject to either general or local review before its implementation in Northern Ireland.

Prescribing and monitoring resources

In theory, doctors can prescribe any appropriate and approved medicine but, in practice, their clinical autonomy is limited. Within the NHS, the state keeps a close eye on their prescribing habits. Huge variations exist in the volume and cost of NHS prescribing, in different geographical areas and between individual prescribers. Inevitably, resources are limited and there are various ways in which this can create ethical dilemmas for doctors.

Case example – Viagra

The case of sildenafil (Viagra) was the first time the NHS refused to fund a licensed drug with proven benefits to a large number of people. Sildenafil was licensed in September 1998 to treat patients with erectile dysfunction. A huge demand was anticipated for the product and the Government was worried about the financial implications. Estimates at the time calculated that the annual bill for Viagra would exceed £1 billion, if it were prescribed for all men who might benefit.[29] The Department of Health's Standing Medical Advisory Committee told doctors not to prescribe it until definitive guidance was available.

After months of debate, guidance was issued, rationing access to sildenafil on the basis of the aetiology of the condition, rather than according to clinical need or via the waiting list system. In the NHS, sildenafil and other treatments for erectile dysfunction were restricted to patients who were already receiving treatment for impotence at the time the licence was issued or suffered from one of a range of specific conditions, such as diabetes, multiple sclerosis and prostate cancer. Patients were also eligible for the medication if they were receiving treatment for renal failure or had undergone surgery, such as prostatectomy, radical pelvic surgery or a kidney transplant.[30] It was agreed that treatment would be available to other men, in exceptional cases of severe distress. The BMA opposed this rationing on the basis of the cause of the underlying condition rather than according to clinical need, which, it argued, made an 'inequitable distinction between acceptable and unacceptable forms of impotence'.[31]

'Topping up' NHS treatment

In Chapter 2 we discuss how NHS patients need to be aware of treatments that could benefit them which are only available in the private sector and how they can choose to transfer between the NHS and private treatment. Patients in England and Scotland can also supplement or top up care they receive in the NHS with treatment or medication in the private sector. They can pay for medication to supplement their care, when those medicines have been rejected for use in the NHS on grounds of clinical or cost-effectiveness. Guidance is available on the circumstances in which it is acceptable to combine NHS and private healthcare services.[32] The Scottish[33] arrangements and those for the rest of the UK[34] are based on some fundamental principles. All possibilities of NHS funding for a particular medicine should have been considered and exhausted. NHS resources should not be used to subsidise private treatment, so the patient must bear the full cost of that and a clear distinction must be kept between the NHS and private care provided. Patients who combine NHS and private care are entitled to NHS services on the same basis of clinical need as any other patient. Health professionals should inform patients about the possibility of topping up their care, when it may be appropriate.

Patients who want to supplement their NHS care with medication unavailable on the NHS often ask their GPs to prescribe them privately. This can result in GPs being asked to prescribe and supervise products with which they are not familiar. Doctors should not prescribe medicines unfamiliar to them and about which they lack expertise, unless they have reliable advice and support from a colleague which gives them sufficient confidence to proceed and take responsibility for the prescription. Examples are discussed later of situations where prescribing is shared between doctors, such as between a GP and consultant. In such cases it should always be clear who retains overall clinical responsibility for prescribing.

Generic prescribing

The vast majority of prescriptions are for generic medicines.[35] Doctors are encouraged to prescribe generic alternatives wherever possible because they are considerably cheaper than branded drugs. NHS managers and doctors sometimes reduce costs by switching patients from branded drugs to generic substitutes with the same active ingredient. GPs can also be pressured, or offered incentives, to do this. With some drugs, such as statins, the savings are significant. Ethical problems arise, however, when all of a GP's patients are automatically switched from a specific branded drug to a generic. Although, where possible, less-expensive products are to be preferred, the process by which patients are transferred should be carefully considered. It can, for example, take some time to stabilise patients on particular drugs, and there is at least anecdotal evidence that generic substitutes can act in subtly different ways because of variations in bioavailability which may have an impact on patient tolerance of the active ingredient. Where dosages or packaging differ, or the drugs seem very unlike those with which they have become familiar, some patients may struggle with the new regime, which raises the possibility of negative outcomes.

Drug switching

Drug switching is where a drug is switched for a therapeutic substitute which has a different active ingredient but a similar therapeutic purpose. Clearly, therapeutic substitutes may have different biological pathways and different side effects and these aspects need to be carefully discussed with patients.

Any major change in medication, whether from branded to generic drugs or drug switching to a therapeutic substitute, should involve informed discussion with patients so that they are involved in the decision. Those patients likely to need more support should be identified at an early stage. Some may be unable to cope with a new regime and switching would not be in their best interests. Pressure to switch drugs for such patients should be resisted.

Off-label prescribing and unlicensed drugs

When deciding what medicine to prescribe, the primary consideration should be the individual needs of the patient. In most cases, this need is fulfilled with a licensed medicine on label, but if that is not possible, then a licensed medicine off-label can be used. Only if neither of these is available should an unlicensed medicine be considered. The licensing process tests the safety, efficacy and quality of drugs for a specific indication and ensures that they are manufactured to appropriate quality standards. Prescribing drugs that have not undergone these checks places more responsibility on the prescriber. Nevertheless, off-label prescribing is common and often unavoidable, particularly in specialities such as paediatrics. GMC guidance[36] emphasises that in prescribing an off-label drug, doctors must be satisfied it would better serve the patient's needs than an appropriately licensed alternative. Decisions to prescribe an off-label or unlicensed drug should be based on sufficient evidence or experience which demonstrates its safety and efficacy. Doctors take responsibility for the prescription and for overseeing the patient's care, including monitoring and follow-up treatment. Where prescriptions deviate from established practice, doctors should record in the patients' notes the reasons for choosing it. They 'must explain the reasons for prescribing a medicine that is unlicensed or being used outside the scope of its licence where there is little research or other evidence of current practice to support its use, or the use of the medicine is innovative'.[37] The GMC advises that where drugs are used routinely outside the scope of their licence, it may be unnecessary to draw patients' attention to the licence.[38]

Prescribing drugs off-label to save money

The question of whether doctors are permitted to prescribe off-label, or unlicensed drugs, where there is a suitable licensed alternative is currently the subject of debate. The dilemma often arises because the off-label drugs are considerably cheaper than the licensed alternative. In some cases, following a review of the evidence, NICE has recommended, in its clinical guidelines, the use of off-label drugs, in preference, or as an alternative, to a more expensive licensed product.[39] The most high-profile case of prescribing off-label to save money involves Lucentis and Avastin for the treatment of wet age-related macular degeneration (see below).

Case example – prescribing off-label on cost grounds

In 2008, NICE recommended Lucentis for the treatment of wet age-related macular degeneration. Prior to Lucentis being licensed, ophthalmologists had been using a much cheaper drug, Avastin, which was licensed but only as a cancer treatment. In 2011, a primary care trust (PCT) gave local NHS ophthalmologists the option of using the much cheaper product (Avastin) off-label, which, it calculated, would save £5 million a year. The drug company marketing Lucentis in the UK sought a judicial review of the PCT's decision, arguing that Lucentis was safer for patients.[40] While the case was ongoing, the PCT withdrew its guidance for a range of reasons including that very few ophthalmologists had taken up the option to prescribe the cheaper drug.[41]

Prior to this legal challenge the issue had been raised as part of the GMC's consultation on its new prescribing guidance. Some bodies, such as the Medicine and Healthcare products Regulatory Agency (MHRA) and the Association of the British Pharmaceutical Industry (ABPI), argued strongly against this practice on the grounds that it undermined the licensing process which is intended to ensure patient safety. When the BMA's ethics committee considered the issue, it recommended that doctors should be able to prescribe off-label in preference to an appropriately licensed alternative medication, on cost grounds, but only when authoritative clinical guidance supported that choice. At the time of writing this issue was still unresolved. Any further information that becomes available will be reported on the BMA's website.

Reporting adverse drug reactions and adverse incidents

Drugs are assessed over time by any evidence of previous patients' adverse reactions being reported. The Yellow Card Scheme helps to monitor and investigate such reports, relying on information supplied on a voluntary basis by doctors, dentists, pharmacists and coroners. Pharmaceutical companies have statutory obligations to report adverse reactions.[42] Patients can also report any suspected adverse reaction to a drug using the scheme. Health professionals and patients are particularly encouraged to report all suspected reactions to drugs that are newly licensed for use in the UK, known as 'Black Triangle' medicines, which are closely monitored for any rare or long-term adverse effects that may not be identifiable during clinical trials. Safety updates are published that give health professionals the latest drug safety information and guidance.[43] The National Reporting and Learning System (England and Wales) collects information about adverse incidents and near misses, including those involving medication.[44] NHS staff are encouraged to report all patient safety incidents irrespective of whether they result in harm.

Shared prescribing and continuity of care

Increasingly, treatment is delivered by a team of health professionals working together, but it should always be clear who is responsible for the overall management of a patient's care. That clinician needs to be able to oversee all prescriptions. This can prove difficult. As well as different prescribers recommending different medications for the episodes of care they manage, many patients use over-the-counter products and some buy medication over the internet, without keeping their doctor informed. When several health professionals are involved, effective liaison and communication are essential, but patient consent is needed. Patients should be encouraged to be open with clinicians about the medication they take and also allow information about them to be shared with others involved in their care. (Confidentiality and patient consent to information sharing, within the health team and beyond it, are discussed in Chapter 6.) If patients refuse to allow information to be shared, they need to understand the risks and the implications of that decision. It may result in some doctors deciding not to prescribe for patients, when their existing medication is not fully known.

Prescribing shared between different doctors

Prescribing shared between primary and secondary care

GPs usually take over prescribing for ongoing conditions, once patients are discharged from hospital or are being treated as outpatients. When a patient's condition is stable, consultants ask the GP to agree to a shared care arrangement, in which the GP is advised which medicine to prescribe. If an unusual product is recommended, the dosage, manner of administration and any potential adverse drug reactions must be explained by the consultant so that the GP, if agreeable, can monitor it. If the drug is unlicensed for a particular indication, the GP (as well as the patient) needs to understand why it is recommended. Doctors agreeing to prescribe products suggested by a colleague need to remember that they have full clinical responsibility for the prescription. They have to be satisfied that the drug and dosage are correct for the patient and be prepared to take responsibility for monitoring both. It must be clear which clinician has responsibility for continuing the treatment. If problems arise or there is disagreement about the medication or dose which cannot be resolved, GPs should not agree to a shared prescribing arrangement but must ensure that the patient continues to receive appropriate care. The BMA publishes guidance for GPs on shared care, which outlines other common problems and gives examples of best practice.[45] Other detailed guidance is also available on the transfer of prescribing responsibility between hospitals and GPs.[46] This can help doctors decide whether shared prescribing is appropriate. It makes clear that consultants have full responsibility for prescribing for inpatients and for treatments administered in outpatient clinics. The guidance states that at least a week's supply of medication should be given to inpatients when discharged (although in practice a longer period may be better for the patient) and outpatients need a minimum of 2 weeks' supply (unless, of course, the medication is not required for that long). The GP into whose care the patient is returning needs notification in good time of the diagnosis and medication regime and, if there is a delay, the patient should be given a longer supply of medication by the hospital. If the medication is part of a hospital-based clinical trial, responsibility for prescribing rests with the consultant and, in other cases where the medication is not normally dispensed in the community, there needs to be ongoing liaison between the hospital and community pharmacist to ensure continuity.

In Northern Ireland[47] and in some areas of the rest of the UK, a local traffic light system exists, which classifies medicines to help identify where responsibility lies for prescribing different medication. Consultants are responsible for prescribing drugs on the red list and GPs for those on the green list. Responsibility for amber list drugs may be transferred to primary care with GPs' agreement and where shared care arrangements are developed locally.

Prescribing shared between the NHS and the private sector

When patients opt for private treatment or assessment, they are still entitled to NHS services and may ask their GP to prescribe medication they need as part of private care. These requests have often caused concern for GPs, who worry that they appear unsupportive if they refuse but are reluctant to accept legal, financial and ethical responsibility for a course of medication that they have not initiated. The decision is more straightforward in cases where they do not consider the medication to be clinically necessary. In such cases, they should not agree. Similarly, for very unusual medication, GPs may not have the specialised expertise to take responsibility for the prescription and should refuse such requests, unless they are able to come to an arrangement with relevant specialists which makes them confident that they can prescribe and monitor safely.

Case example – shared care

A common query raised with the BMA concerns patients receiving private treatment but requesting that medication associated with it is supplied by the NHS. If NHS GPs consider that the medication is clinically necessary, they are required under their terms of service to prescribe it within the NHS, even if the assessment which identified the need for it took place in the private sector. In order to agree to prescribe it, GPs must be willing to accept clinical responsibility for the medication recommended by another doctor. A contractual obligation to prescribe does not arise if the medication is not clinically necessary, or if it is generally not funded by the NHS. A common example is fertility treatment, where patients seek in vitro fertilisation in the private sector and ask their GP to issue NHS prescriptions for the medication. The decision about whether to comply with such requests rests with the individual GP or, where the medication is not generally funded on the NHS, the commissioning body.

Many problems concerning shared prescribing between the private sector and the NHS can be avoided by good communication. NHS GPs should not be put in a position where patients automatically expect them to prescribe products related to private treatment. Specialists should tell patients that GPs are not obliged to prescribe the medication, or else they could sound out the GP's views first, with patient consent.

Patient group directions (PGDs)

Traditional arrangements, whereby health professionals prescribe for, and have clinical responsibility for, individual patients, are generally seen as the best way of providing people with the medicines they need. An alternative option is available for some limited situations, where it is consistent with appropriate professional relationships and accountability.[48] PGDs allow named registered health professionals to supply and administer medicines to patients, without the need for an individual prescription. They are drawn up by multidisciplinary groups and are signed by a senior doctor and a senior pharmacist. PGDs must comply with certain legal requirements. The provision of emergency hormonal contraception is an example of their use. PGDs are used in the NHS and for NHS-funded services, provided by the private, voluntary or charitable sector. Independent hospital agencies and clinics registered with the Care Quality Commission (CQC) on or before 30 September 2010, and which continue to be registered, are also permitted to use PGDs, as are prison and police health-care services and defence medical services. Doctors should not sign PGDs if they have any doubts about the safety or efficacy of the medication, or uncertainties about the ability of any named health professionals to assess patients' suitability for the treatment. The BMA has published guidance on the use of PGDs in general practice[49] and NICE's Medicine and Prescribing Centre also has guidance for health professionals and organisations that use PGDs.[50]

Prescribing shared between doctors and other health professionals

Supplementary prescribing and independent non-medical prescribers

Current prescribing arrangements often involve various members of the health team, so that patients can access medicines more conveniently and the prescribing burden on doctors is reduced. Some health professionals can be trained to operate either as independent, or supplementary, prescribers.

Supplementary prescribing is a voluntary prescribing partnership between a doctor and a supplementary prescriber to implement an agreed patient-specific clinical management plan, with the patient's agreement. Nurses, podiatrists or chiropodists, optometrists, physiotherapists, radiographers and pharmacists can train and register as supplementary prescribers. Supplementary prescribers can prescribe any licensed or unlicensed medicine listed on the plan, including controlled drugs.

Nurses, pharmacists and optometrists can also train and register as independent prescribers. Nurse and pharmacist independent prescribers are able to prescribe any medicine for medical conditions that fall within their level of competence and area of expertise. From April 2012, this included any controlled drug listed in schedules 2–5 of the Misuse of Drugs Regulations 2001, except diamorphine, cocaine and dipipanone for the treatment of addiction. Optometrist independent prescribers can prescribe any licensed medicine for ocular conditions affecting the eye and surrounding tissue but cannot prescribe any controlled drug or medicines for parenteral administration. Community practitioner nurse prescribers have more limited prescribing responsibilities. They can prescribe preparations specified in the *Nurse Prescribers' Formulary for Community Practitioners.*[51]

With any shared prescribing arrangement, collaborative working is essential to ensure patient safety. Prescribing activity should be recorded in a way that is easily accessible to all prescribing members of the team.

Prescribing shared with practitioners of complementary therapies

In any situation where treatment is provided by more than one practitioner, patients need to keep all therapists informed to minimise risks of harmful interaction between the preparations recommended. Particular concerns can arise when patients' treatment is shared between conventional health professionals and complementary practitioners, to whom patients often self-refer. Doctors often express anxiety if patients postpone or refuse orthodox treatments, while they explore other therapies, or combine complementary and orthodox medicine. Among the complementary therapies available, the evidence of efficacy varies considerably. Doctors who are registered with the GMC and who provide complementary therapies are obliged to share with a patient's GP 'the results of any investigations, the treatment provided and any other information necessary for the continuing care of the patient, unless the patient objects'.[52] Some patients are reluctant to discuss complementary therapies with their GP. Research on the attitudes of health professionals to herbal medicines showed that a significant proportion (73%) of those surveyed were worried that their patients would take herbal medicines and not inform them.[53] GPs should always encourage patients to tell them about such treatment, and if a complementary therapy appears to be harming patients, this should be sensitively explained to them.

Continuity of care

Exchange of information between doctors in referrals and discharge summaries

Prompt exchange of information about patients' medication is essential when they transfer from one clinical setting to another. Hospitals need to be aware of patients' existing medication to avoid incompatibility with new treatment and, when patients are discharged, GPs need to be informed promptly of any changes to patients' medicines. The CQC has looked at medicines' management, focusing on the information shared on admission to, and discharge from, hospital.[54] It found that good systems were in place to ensure the quality of repeat prescribing and medication reviews of high-risk patients, but raised concerns about some routines. It discovered that almost a quarter of GPs surveyed did not systematically provide information on patients' co-morbidities, allergies and drug reactions when their patients were admitted to hospital. The provision of information to hospitals in emergencies also tended to be too slow. Such problems were partly alleviated by schemes, such as 'patients' own drug' (POD) and 'green bag' arrangements, that encourage patients to bring their existing medication with them into hospital. Deficiencies were also found in the quality of information provided in discharge summaries, particularly with respect to medicines prescribed on discharge. Over 80% of GPs responding said that the details of prescribed medicine were incomplete or inaccurate in the majority of cases. The CQC recommended the use of standard referral forms to cover elective and emergency admissions and that GPs carry out a higher proportion of medication reviews with the patient present. It also advised acute trusts to remind clinicians of their responsibilities regarding the timely completion of discharge summaries.

Prescribing for people at a distance – internet, email or telephone

Email consultations and internet prescribing have grown in popularity. While these are a useful addition to the services on offer, doctors still need to ensure that patients consent, have mental capacity and receive enough information to make informed decisions. Normal standards of record keeping should be maintained (see Chapter 7) and attention must be given to confidentiality and security arrangements when communicating electronically (see Chapter 6). The BMA issues guidance for GPs on the advantages and disadvantages of various means of electronic communication.[55]

Consultations conducted remotely have limitations, not least when prescribing decisions are made for patients who are unseen and not physically examined. Repeat prescribing is relatively unproblematic and remote prescribing can also work in a limited number of other situations. The GMC suggests that such occasions are most likely to occur if doctors have sole responsibility for patients or are deputising for another doctor who does. It can also be appropriate when doctors are familiar with patients, have prior knowledge of their condition and can access their medical record. In such cases, doctors must ensure that they

- establish the patient's current medical conditions and history and concurrent or recent use of other medications including non-prescription medicines
- carry out an adequate assessment of the patient's condition

- identify the likely cause of the patient's condition
- ensure that there is sufficient justification to prescribe the medicines or treatment proposed and discuss other treatment options with the patient where appropriate
- ensure that the treatment and/or medicines are not contraindicated for the patient
- make a clear, accurate and legible record of all medicines prescribed.[56]

Particular caution is needed for remote prescribing when doctors lack prior knowledge of the patient and they need to consider very carefully whether a prescription can be issued safely. They also need to bear in mind that it may be impossible to verify who the patient is or whether the medical complaints described are genuine. Although the GMC does not rule out prescribing remotely in such cases, it specifies that doctors must provide the patient with their name and GMC number. They must also explain to patients the processes involved in remote consultation and establish a dialogue with them, using a questionnaire, to ensure that they have enough information to prescribe safely. They must make arrangements to check patients' progress, monitor the effectiveness of the treatment and/or review the diagnosis. If the patient consents, they should also inform the patient's GP.[57] If doctors cannot satisfy these requirements, the GMC advises that they should not prescribe remotely.

In July 2012 the GMC published new guidance on remote prescribing which states that '[y]ou must undertake a physical examination of patients before prescribing non-surgical cosmetic medicinal products such as Botox, Dysport or Vistabel. . . . You must not therefore prescribe these medicines by telephone, fax, video-link or online'.[58]

Case example – failings in internet prescribing

A GMC fitness to practise panel found a doctor guilty of serious professional misconduct in 2009 for prescribing medication to patients through his online company in a way that was judged 'irresponsible, not in the best interests of patients and below the standard expected of a registered medical practitioner'.[59] The doctor had prescribed the powerful analgesic dihydrocodeine for one patient remotely, without taking an adequate history. He did not ask if she had a GP, nor advise her to inform her GP of the repeat prescriptions for dihydrocodeine, which he continued to write for her for about 16 months, without examining her, monitoring her condition or contacting her GP himself. The doctor was judged to have put the patient at risk by not assessing her condition. He was unable to judge whether the information the patient gave him was true and she was later arrested for attempting to forge more prescriptions, as she was addicted to the drug.

(Continued)

The doctor was also found guilty of involvement in the inappropriate prescribing of Viagra and the weight loss pill Reductil to other patients. The same doctor had been brought before the panel 2 years' previously when he was described as having a cavalier attitude to prescribing. On that occasion, he was also found guilty of serious errors of conduct in relation to prescribing. One of the earlier cases was that of a 16-year-old psychiatric patient who had informed the doctor that he had suicidal thoughts and had previously attempted suicide. This patient was still prescribed potent medicine and later took an overdose of the beta-blocker propranolol, which the doctor had prescribed. The GMC panel found that the doctor had put his business interests ahead of patient safety and he was erased from the medical register.

Prescribing for patients abroad

Among the enquiries doctors raise with the BMA are questions about issuing private prescriptions for people living abroad (such patients are not entitled to NHS prescriptions). These may be a GP's own previous patients who have retired to another country or current patients asking for a prescription for their relatives abroad. An urgent decision is sometimes needed if the person living overseas is seriously ill and unable to obtain a prescription locally. If doctors agree to prescribe, they cannot examine the patient but have full clinical responsibility for the medication. Many refuse for this reason but some agree to help if they can. Such situations are fraught with difficulty, but if doctors wish to pursue the matter, they should try to obtain as much factual information about the patient as possible. If feasible, this should be from the patient's own doctor abroad. Such cases virtually amount to shared prescribing, with the prescriber relying heavily on the opinion of the examining doctor. For some patients, the dangers of not obtaining appropriate drugs can be greater than the risks of a prescribing error, but it is not a situation for doctors to enter into lightly. Among the hurdles to be considered is how the medication, once prescribed and privately dispensed, can be transported. Many countries restrict the medication that can be imported and any medication posted overseas is subject to customs labelling and postage regulations. Advice may need to be sought from the relevant embassy. Before prescribing for patients who are overseas, doctors should also ensure that they have adequate indemnity cover.[60]

Prescription-only medicines on the internet

Many online pharmacies have grown up to meet the public's demand for easy and convenient methods of obtaining medicines. Some offer over-the-counter and prescription-only medications direct to patients via the internet. Online providers also offer greater accessibility to pharmacy services for people who are housebound or have limited mobility, but there are also risks involved in buying pharmaceuticals online. Over two million people are estimated to purchase medication regularly via the internet.[61] As well as using legitimate online pharmacies, they may also contact websites abroad, which offer prescription-only medication direct to patients, without a prescription. Some people like the level of privacy this method of purchase provides. Popular prescription medicines bought online are lifestyle drugs, such as sildenafil, fluoxetine, methylphenidate and modafinil. Prescription-only analgesics, including controlled opioids, can also be obtained online without prescription.[62]

Risks associated with purchasing medication from unregulated suppliers include the possibility that the medication may be substandard, out of date, unlicensed or banned in the UK. Consumers may receive counterfeit drugs containing toxic substances or unknown amounts of active ingredients. Medication may also be supplied without information about dosage or potential side effects. Ultimately, patient safety in relation to prescription medication can only be assured if a medical consultation takes place. For patients who take medication without clinical advice, there are the risks of contraindications or adverse reactions that they are then reluctant to report, even when they cause significant health problems.[63] A 2009 survey of GPs found that a quarter of those who replied had treated patients for adverse reactions from medicines bought over the internet.[64] If they do not seek medical advice first, patients may be self-medicating for the wrong diagnosis and, as a main motivation for online purchasing is secrecy, they are unlikely to talk to their GP about what they buy. Doctors may prescribe other products, without knowing what the patient is already taking.

The MHRA regulates the safety, efficacy and quality of medicines in the UK, and all pharmacies in England, Scotland and Wales, including internet pharmacies, have to register with the General Pharmaceutical Council (GPhC). To help the public identify safe, legitimate online sites, the GPhC runs an internet pharmacy logo scheme which identifies pharmacies registered with the GPhC and compliant with its standards.[65] Regulation of pharmacies in Northern Ireland is the responsibility of the Pharmaceutical Society of Northern Ireland, which sets out how internet pharmacies registered in Northern Ireland must operate.[66]

Prescribing for different patient groups

Controlled drugs and prescribing for addicts

The way that controlled drugs are prescribed, dispensed and stored came under intense scrutiny when GP Harold Shipman was found guilty, in 2000, of having murdered many of his patients over a long career, during which he hoarded controlled drugs. An Inquiry, chaired by Dame Janet Smith, looked at the issues raised by the case, including how Dr Shipman acquired large quantities of diamorphine over 20 years, without being detected. The Inquiry published six reports, the fourth of which focused on drug regulation[67] and made a series of recommendations. Dame Janet's aim was to tighten up the handling of controlled drugs to prevent future misuse by health professionals, without unnecessarily hindering the supply to patients.

Her fourth report said that a key area that needed strengthening was the way that information was collected about private prescriptions for controlled drugs. Following her recommendations, a number of legislative changes and other requirements were introduced. These govern current practice and include the following:

- the use of special forms for private prescriptions of schedule 2 and 3 controlled drugs under the Misuse of Drugs Regulations 2001
- the requirement that patients (or others who collect their prescriptions for controlled drugs) must sign for them
- the validity of prescriptions for schedule 2, 3 and 4 drugs is limited to 28 days
- private prescribers of controlled drugs must be issued with a unique identifying number
- prescriptions for controlled drugs written by private prescribers in a certain area should be subject to external monitoring
- prescriptions for controlled drugs must be signed by the prescriber
- prescriptions for schedule 2, 3 and 4 drugs should be limited to a quantity necessary for up to 30 days' clinical need
- all healthcare providers who keep controlled drugs on site must comply with the terms of a standard operating procedure.

Doctors who prescribe for drug addicts must be familiar with the regulations and guidance.[68] To prescribe, administer or supply diamorphine, dipipanone or cocaine in the treatment of drug addiction, doctors must hold a general licence issued by their health department. Other practitioners must refer addicts requiring these drugs to a treatment centre. Controlled drugs commonly prescribed to addicts, such as methadone, have a high street value and may be sold on, by patients. To limit this possibility, dispensers in England, Scotland and Wales are required to check who collects a prescription for a schedule 2 controlled drug. Although it is not a legal requirement, dispensers also have the discretion to request proof of identity and can refuse to supply the drugs if they are not satisfied as to the person's identity.

Prescribing strong opioids for pain in adult palliative care

Pain is common in the late stages of various diseases, including cancer, heart failure, kidney, liver and respiratory disease, as well as some neurological conditions, but many clinicians are reluctant to use strong opioids. This can result in the systematic under-treatment of severe pain in some patients. For example, it is estimated that almost 'half of patients with advanced cancer are under-treated for their pain, largely because clinicians are reluctant to use strong opioids for effective analgesia'.[69] Some commentators have seen this wariness about opioid use as another one of the unfortunate legacies of the Shipman case, as Shipman used diamorphine to murder his victims.[70] Uncertainty about opioid use led NICE to issue guidelines on the most commonly used drugs – morphine, diamorphine, buprenophine, fentanyl and oxycodone.[71] NICE points out that misunderstandings have surrounded the use of such strong opioids for decades, and prescribing advice has sometimes been conflicting, resulting in some patients being underdosed and suffering avoidable pain, while others are overdosed and experience distressing adverse effects. The NICE guidelines cover the use of strong opioids and management of side effects associated with them. They encourage good communication with patients about issues such as the possibility of addiction, recommending frank face-to-face discussion, backed up by information leaflets.

Use of opioids and the principle of double effect

Prescribing of strong analgesia may also have been inhibited by doctors' uncertainty about the so-called principle of 'double effect'. This allows the provision of drugs which have both bad and good effects, as long as the intention is to provide an overall good effect. Sedatives and analgesics can be given with the intention of, and in proportion to, the relief of suffering, even if as a consequence the patient's life risks being shortened. Prescribing drugs which might hasten death is lawful and ethical when patients are terminally ill or dying, the drugs are in their best interests and the motive for giving them is the relief of suffering, rather than to cause the person's death. The dosage must be recognised as reasonable and proper within the profession. Severe mental distress, as well as physical symptoms, can be managed by the appropriate use of medication. The case of Annie Lindsell highlighted the legal situation even though it did not proceed through the courts.

Case example – Annie Lindsell and double effect

Annie Lindsell had motor neurone disease and sought a declaration from the court that it would not be unlawful for her GP to administer medication

(Continued)

for the relief of her mental distress when she became unable to swallow. Having seen others die of the disease, she was fearful of having to go through the final stages of choking and being unable to speak. Her GP had been warned by the Medical Protection Society that he might face a murder charge if he carried out her wishes to medicate her to relieve her distress. She asked the High Court to confirm that mental distress, as well as physical pain, could be treated with medication that could have the incidental effect of shortening her life. The GP said that he was not proposing to 'anaesthetise her to death' but he did believe 'in forthright and unhesitating relief of distress and pain, with no half measures'. Experts in palliative care told the court that the regime proposed by the GP was in accordance with best medical practice. Annie Lindsell withdrew her application after her doctor's plans for her care were supported by the medical experts; a declaration was therefore not required. This case merely restated the existing legal position on double effect.[72]

Prescribing for older people

Patients over the age of 60 receive more prescriptions than any other age group, but prescribing for them can present challenges. Physiological changes associated with ageing can have effects on both pharmacokinetics and pharmacodynamics. Changes to renal clearance, liver size and body mass can all affect how drugs are distributed, metabolised and cleared from the body. Older patients are also more sensitive to the effects of medication and more susceptible to idiosyncratic and adverse reactions. Polypharmacy is also common in older people, with patients often requiring a number of prescriptions to address co-morbidities, which can leave them at greater risk of adverse drug interactions.[73] These difficulties can contribute to the high prevalence of drug errors that occur among patients in this age group but so can other factors. A study into the use of medicines in residential and nursing homes found that over two-thirds of residents experienced medication error, which occurred in the prescribing, monitoring, administration and dispensing of medication.[74] Communication problems and systemic problems, such as a lack of integration and coordination between the different elements of care, were among the factors contributing to the errors.

Involving older people in concordance

There can sometimes be an assumption that older people have less desire for information than younger patients or that they may be overwhelmed by receiving too much. Often the contrary is the case. Older people in care homes and hospitals often complain that they are not told the reason behind their medication and had no choice or active involvement in the prescribing decision.[75] They need to be actively engaged in prescribing choices. This might include advising them that taking products such as antidepressants, if they need them, should not be seen as stigmatising. Doctors should ensure that all patients receive enough information about their medication to make a valid decision, including what it is used for and what side effects patients may experience. Where any information is provided, it should be in a form best suited to the needs of individual patients.

There is conflicting evidence as to whether older people are more or less likely to be non-compliant than other age groups.[76] A 2009 survey showed that nearly half of over-65s take more than five medicines at any one time, and a fifth of these patients do not take their medicines as prescribed.[77] As in other patient populations, some older people decide not take, or not to finish, a particular course of medication, but for others, forgetfulness, confusion or the fact that they have multiple medications may be the cause. Various strategies have been developed to help them remember what to take when. Among the obvious steps are Medicines Use Reviews to minimise polypharmacy and, where appropriate, avoiding medication that itself can cause confusion, if other alternatives are available. Dosette boxes, prepared by pharmacists, group medications in separate daily doses and simple calendars can remind older patients of the correct medication and dosage to take. Supervised medicine taking in care settings also helps.

Over-medication of older people

The over-medication of older people in institutional settings has given repeated cause for concern. In 2004, the House of Commons Health Committee published its report on the prevalence and causes of elder abuse. One of the main types of physical abuse the report focused on was the over-medication of older people in care homes. The committee heard evidence that neuroleptics or antipsychotics were often used to sedate people with dementia in care homes as a management tool to prevent residents wandering, or to deal with uncooperativeness. In its recommendations, the committee concluded that 'the incorrect prescription of medication is a serious problem within some care homes, and that medication is, in many cases, being used simply as a tool for the easier management of residents'.[78] Five years later, a study looked again at the use of antipsychotic medication for patients with dementia.[79] It highlighted that UK care systems deliver a largely antipsychotic-based response to deal with some behavioural problems, common in dementia patients, even though the drugs appear to have only a limited positive effect and can cause significant harm. Of the 180,000 dementia patients estimated in the study to be treated annually by the NHS, using antipsychotics, only up to 36,000 may derive benefit from the treatment. It recommended changes across all care settings, with the aim of reducing the rate of use of antipsychotic medication by two-thirds, especially when alternative approaches can be used.

Prescribing for children

A challenge for doctors prescribing for children is the lack of medication specifically licensed for them. Most medicines used in the UK are only licensed for adults. In paediatric care, doctors often have to prescribe unlicensed or off-label medicines. Among factors that need to be taken into account when prescribing are changes in pharmacokinetic and pharmacodynamic maturity, which mean that 'standard doses' rarely exist for minors as they do for adults.[80] In the past, the pharmaceutical industry was reluctant to develop paediatric medicines as the market for them is relatively small. Although this is changing as new paediatric products are tested and marketed, prescribing off-label is often still necessary. Since 2005, the *British National Formulary for Children (BNFC)*[81] has been available, which includes advice on prescribing outside a medicine's product licence. Consent issues for children and young people have been discussed earlier (see Chapter 5), and when specifically seeking consent to medication, the fact that a medicine is prescribed off-label or is unlicensed may need to be discussed, along with other relevant information. (The GMC advises that when the off-label use is current practice, it may not be necessary to draw attention to the licence when seeking consent; see section on off-label prescribing and unlicensed drugs). The Medicines for Children website has a series of online patient information leaflets for a range of medicines, which are specifically related to their use in children. These give information about dosage, side effects, the different formulations available and how the medicine should be taken.[82]

Prescribing for oneself, friends or family

In Chapter 2, we discuss the reasons why health professionals should not normally treat themselves, their family, friends or colleagues, for anything other than trivial conditions. The same prohibition applies to prescribing as to other forms of care, but it is particularly emphatic in the case of prescribing controlled drugs. In its prescribing guidance, the GMC says that doctors should not prescribe controlled drugs for themselves or anyone close to them, unless no other person with the legal right to prescribe is available and to delay would put the patient's life or health at risk or cause the patient unacceptable pain. If doctors prescribe controlled drugs to someone close to them, they must be able to justify their action. They must make a record of the relationship they have with the patient and the reasons why it was necessary to prescribe.[83] The GMC makes clear that 'objectivity is essential in providing good care; independent medical care should be sought whenever you or someone with whom you have a close personal relationship requires prescription medicines'.[84]

Conflicts of interest

Prescribing decisions should be made on the basis of the individual needs of the patient. Doctors must not be (or give reason to be thought to be) influenced in prescribing matters by the offer of any financial or other incentives. The offer of financial or other incentives from the manufacturers of particular drugs would clearly raise questions about the motivation of a doctor who prescribed that drug in preference to one produced by a competitor. Even if the doctor sincerely believed the former drug to be the best option for the patient, it would be difficult to prove that his or her judgement had not been affected by personal gain. All doctors need to be alert to any actual, or perceived, conflicts of interest and to take steps to manage them appropriately.

Financial interests in health-related products or services

In Chapter 2, we discussed various conflicts of interest that health professionals may have, including when they have shares in a pharmaceutical company.

> **Case example – the influence of financial investments**
>
> Prescriptions must be based on the best interests of the patient. Common enquiries to the BMA concern the propriety of prescribing medicines marketed by pharmaceutical companies in which doctors or their family have a significant financial interest. Sometimes the financial interest has been acquired *after* patients have been prescribed a long-term course of a medication that suits them and is marketed by the company in which the doctor has investments. In such cases, it is unlikely that any objection would be raised about it. Changing a patient's medication, however, from an established regime to a different product in which the doctor has a financial interest would be highly questionable. It would be unethical to do so, if the motive was financial benefit.

Health professionals should tell patients if they have a financial interest in a health facility or service, which they want to recommend to them. A declaration of a financial interest, however, does not provide sufficient safeguard in the case of prescribing since the patient is usually not in a position to exercise an informed choice about other medicines available as suitable alternatives. This is why the BMA believes it is generally unwise for doctors to form close business relationships with companies producing, marketing or promoting such products.

Ownership of pharmacies

Patients are free to choose which pharmacy they use. Doctors must not direct a patient to use a particular pharmaceutical outlet, particularly if it is one in which they have a financial interest. If doctors do own or have a financial interest in a pharmacy, they must make their patients aware of this[85] but must not direct, encourage, induce or otherwise persuade their patients to use it, nor must doctors discourage patients from using other pharmacies. The freedom of patients to choose where they have their medicines dispensed must be respected at all times.

Dispensing doctors

GPs serving patients who live in more rural areas, where there may be fewer pharmacies, can be authorised to dispense NHS prescriptions to their eligible patients. Dispensing doctors are under the same ethical obligations as all doctors to act in the best interests of patients and to use NHS resources cost-effectively. Dispensing doctors must not seek to influence or persuade their dispensing patients that they may only receive dispensing services from the practice. A dispensing doctor must not unreasonably refrain from issuing (or indeed refuse to issue) a prescription for a patient who wishes to have it dispensed elsewhere.

Gifts and hospitality from pharmaceutical companies

Doctors are not permitted to accept gifts or hospitality from pharmaceutical companies, and representatives of pharmaceutical companies are not permitted to offer them. The GMC reminds doctors that they must always act in their patients' best interests when making referrals and providing treatment. They must not ask for, or accept, any inducement, gift or hospitality which may affect or be seen to affect their judgement.[86] Doctors who have financial or commercial interests in pharmaceutical or other biomedical companies must not let these affect how they prescribe for, treat or refer patients.[87]

Regulations specifically forbid the offer or acceptance of 'any gift, pecuniary advantage or benefit in kind, unless it is inexpensive and relevant to the practice of medicine or pharmacy'.[88] Standards for the pharmaceutical industry, published by the ABPI, go even further and prohibit the provision of any promotional aids, such as pens, pads and mugs, to healthcare professionals and administrative staff. Inexpensive items that are to be passed on to patients, as part of a formal patient support programme, and which directly benefit patient care, are permitted. Medical and educational goods and services may also be provided, but not for the personal benefit of individuals and only when it is in the interests of patients or will benefit the NHS while maintaining patient care.[89]

The ABPI code of practice covers the ways in which prescription-only medicines can be made known to prescribers. It also sets out the requirements that must be met for industry sponsorship of meetings and any hospitality provided. In the past, pharmaceutical companies were allowed to arrange lavish events in exotic locations, where it may have seemed that the main purpose of the meeting was drug promotion rather than being educational. This practice generated perceived conflicts of interest for health professionals attending such events, even if they did not believe that their judgement would be influenced. Now health professionals can be offered travel costs for attendance at meetings and hospitality at events hosted or sponsored by a pharmaceutical company, provided that the meeting has a clear scientific or educational content. It must also be held at an 'appropriate' venue and the cost of the hospitality should not exceed what participants would normally pay for themselves. The hospitality should be subordinate to the purpose of the meeting and should only be provided to participants, not their spouses or other accompanying people. Meetings centred around sporting or social events are prohibited. If events organised by pharmaceutical companies take place abroad, they must meet the criteria mentioned above. Valid reasons should exist for the meeting to be held in that location so that the travel is not seen as an incentive for doctors to attend.[90] The ABPI code permits companies to use health professionals as consultants and advisors for purposes such as chairing sessions or speaking at them, but they should meet certain criteria. Doctors who act as consultants must be contractually obliged to declare the arrangement whenever they write or speak in public on any issue relating to the company.[91]

Pharmaceutical companies sometimes offer to pay for a nurse, or other member of staff, to carry out audit or to review prescribing patterns in primary or secondary care. It has been suggested that acceptance of such offers could be interpreted as a gift or benefit in kind. Concerns are also expressed about the motive for such offers, which could put indirect pressure on doctors to change their prescribing patterns. If they accept the offer, doctors must ensure that they can justify the decision and can demonstrate that their prescribing is not influenced in the company's favour. A detailed written protocol should specify the terms of the agreement. The ABPI code of practice says that therapeutic reviews, intended to ensure patients receive optimum treatment following clinical assessment, are a legitimate activity for pharmaceutical companies to support, providing they do not solely serve the interests of the company and its products.[92]

Case example – meeting with pharmaceutical company representatives

In the past, the BMA received enquiries about the rules concerning meeting with representatives from pharmaceutical companies. It is unacceptable for doctors to demand or receive payment for meeting and listening to pharmaceutical representatives. Nor are they allowed to charge a fee for the use of a room for such a meeting. It is also contrary to the ABPI's code of practice for industry representatives to offer any inducements in return for an interview.[93]

Participation in market research

Doctors are sometimes invited to participate in market research carried out by an independent organisation on behalf of a pharmaceutical company. This can include questionnaires, interviews, or focus group work to ascertain doctors' views about certain generic drugs. Usually, doctors invited to participate are unaware which company has sponsored the research. The ABPI code of practice makes it clear to pharmaceutical companies that market research should simply involve the collection and analysis of information and must be unbiased and non-promotional.[94] There is no problem with doctors participating in such research, provided that patients' confidential information is not disclosed without their consent. Doctors must also be able to demonstrate that their participation, and the payment they receive for it, does not influence their prescribing decisions, nor could be perceived as doing so. Guidance is available on appropriate levels of remuneration for participating in market research.[95]

Administering medication

Any suitably trained member of staff within health or social care can administer medicines prescribed by an authorised prescriber. Health professionals who are responsible for administering medication must ensure that they have the necessary knowledge and expertise to do so safely and effectively. Medical students must be properly supervised and trained in any procedures they are expected to undertake. Any health professional in doubt about the method of administration of a particular drug, or the correct procedures to be followed, should seek prompt advice from a senior colleague or from a pharmacist. Similarly, the advice of a pharmacist should be sought if there is uncertainty about the appropriate dosage of a drug for a particular patient. As for any other treatment, valid patient consent needs to be obtained before medication can be administered.

Following guidance and protocols

Protocols should be in place in all hospitals, setting out clearly the checking procedures that must be followed to ensure that the dose and strength of a drug are those prescribed and that the medication is administered in the correct way. It is important that adequate training, supervision and safeguards are in place to guard against potential medication errors. Doctors should not feel pressured to carry out procedures they feel are beyond their training or capability, and it is their responsibility to speak out about any concerns (see Chapter 2).

Case example – lack of protocols for administering medication

In 2001, a young man known as WJ attended Queen's Medical Centre, Nottingham, for chemotherapy, as part of his medical maintenance programme after successful treatment of leukaemia. He was due to receive cytosine by intrathecal injection and, on the following day, he was to receive vincristine intravenously. Owing to a series of errors and the lack of training and experience of the doctors concerned, the vincristine was administered on the same day and also by intrathecal injection. This error is almost always fatal and, despite emergency treatment being provided, WJ died a few weeks later. An inquiry was carried out, which concluded that his death 'was not caused by one or even several human errors but by a far more complex amalgam of human, organisational, technical and social interactions'.[96] Among the failings highlighted in the report were the lack of explicit written protocols, the lack of formal training for the doctors concerned, and the unwillingness of the senior house officer to mention his doubts about the treatment to his senior colleague.

When medication needs special safeguards

Some drugs carry significant risks, require particularly rigorous safeguards and should be administered according to standard operating procedures. Because of the potency of the drugs involved in chemotherapy, for example, a set protocol should exist for their use and the drugs should be administered only by those who have received specific training. This should include how to make up the drugs, the nature of the agents, including their danger to the administering health professional and other employees, and their administration. The individual administering the medication should also be aware of the appropriate procedures to follow in the event of spillage or a failure in clinical technique during administration, as well as procedures for the safe disposal of any unused drugs and the containers and instruments used in administration. Where necessary, supervision and advice should be available from a more senior colleague and doctors must not be afraid to seek help. Doctors have an ethical responsibility to be satisfied that they have the necessary competence and support to undertake these procedures.

Covert medication

Patients with capacity

Covert medication for a person with capacity is illegal and unethical. As it involves deliberate deception, covert medication breaches the principle of informed consent. Refusal of treatment by an adult with capacity is legally and ethically binding. The only exceptional situation (see Chapter 3) concerns patients who have mental capacity but still fulfil the legal requirements for compulsory treatment under mental health legislation and so can be detained and treated for their mental disorder despite a refusal.

Case example – covert medication of people with capacity

The question of covert medication commonly arises in the context of the residential care of older people, people with learning disabilities or patients with challenging behaviour. In some cases raised with the BMA, no formal assessment of patients' capacity has been undertaken, but it is assumed that their age, diagnosis or medical condition necessarily means that they cannot, or need not, give consent. Until there is evidence to the contrary, all adults should be assumed to have capacity and despite their impairments, many of the patients in institutions have sufficient capacity to understand the purpose of medication and so must be asked to consent to it. In some cases, drugs are administered covertly to disguise the fact that they are intended to facilitate patient management rather than being necessary in the patients' interests.[78] Health professionals must seek consent from individuals with capacity and ensure that an assessment of capacity is carried out in cases of doubt. They must not mislead patients about the purpose of their medication, nor should they fail to answer their questions, on the grounds of lack of time or difficulties in communicating.

Patients who lack mental capacity

When patients lack capacity to take decisions about their care, they should be treated with the authorisation of an appointed healthcare proxy, or in their best interests (in Scotland, under the general authority to treat or be treated in a way that benefits them). All of these issues are covered in Chapter 4. There may be exceptional cases in which incapacitated patients require medication and their interests would be best served by giving this in the least distressing manner, which could be covertly. Any such decision must be made on an individual basis. Blanket rules must not be applied to particular categories of patient. Covert administration of medication is never justified for the convenience of those providing treatment. Even if judged to be in the best interests of incapacitated patients, covert medication should not be routine. Any decision to administer it should be taken by the clinician in overall charge of the patient's care, in consultation with the care team. The reasons for a decision to give medication covertly should be recorded in the patient's care plan and regularly reviewed. In making the decision, consideration should be given to whether the patient genuinely lacks capacity to consent to or refuse treatment, why covert medication is proposed, whether it is in the patient's best interests and whether there are feasible alternatives that are more respectful of the individual. Detailed guidance is available in Scotland on the use of covert medication in relation to adults lacking capacity.[97]

A last word about prescribing and administering medicine

Prescribing medication is the most common NHS intervention but, as briefly mentioned in this chapter, it also raises difficult issues about patient choice and rationing. It plays a significant role in preventative care as well as the treatment of illness. Increasingly, it also offers healthy people opportunities to improve aspects of their cognition or general quality of life. As more people want to take up such options, traditional ideas about the core purpose of medicine are challenged. Lifestyle drugs and smart drugs may also make us rethink where boundaries should be drawn in terms of NHS funding.

A significant proportion of people never complete, and some never even start, the medication regime prescribed for them. Huge efforts are made to improve concordance and medicines adherence, but still the level of wastage in the NHS remains massive and the avoidable damage to patients' health is also difficult to comprehend. Involving patients at all stages of the prescribing decision, so that they feel ownership of it, is seen as a major part of the way forward, but that requires time, patience and persistence.

The ways in which patients obtain medication are also changing. Many drugs are purchased over the internet, where patients and prescribers never meet. Medication can be bought from websites which offer no guarantees about the quality or the authenticity of the product. Patients like the privacy and sense of control this gives, although the level of control they think they have is sometimes illusory. Only if a situation can be created where there is trust, frankness and excellent communication between prescribers and patients can the potentially harmful effects of this unrecognised polypharmacy from multiple prescribers be mitigated.

References

1 General Medical Council (2008) *Good Practice in Prescribing Medicines*, GMC, London, para 5c.
2 Carter S, Taylor D, Levenson R. (2005) *A Question of Choice – Compliance in Medicine Taking*, 3rd edn, Medicines Partnership, p.7. Available at: http://www.keele.ac.uk/pharmacy/npcplus (accessed 30 April 2012).
3 National Institute for Health and Clinical Excellence (2009) *Medicines Adherence – Involving Patients in Decisions about Prescribed Medicines and Supporting Adherence CG76*, NICE, London, p.4.
4 National Institute for Health and Clinical Excellence (2009) *Medicines Adherence – Involving Patients in Decisions about Prescribed Medicines and Supporting Adherence CG76*, NICE, London.
5 The National Prescribing Centre learning resources are available at: http://www.npci.org.uk (accessed 1 May 2012).
6 Robinson K, Hoey M. (2009) Religion and drugs. *Stud BMJ* 17, b4453.
7 Mynors G, Ghalamkari H, Beaumont S, *et al.* (2004) *Informed choice in medicine taking: drugs of porcine origin and their clinical alternatives*, Medicines Partnership, London.
8 Tilburt J, Emanuel E, Kaptchuk T, *et al.* (2008) Prescribing 'placebo treatments': results of a national survey of US internists and rheumatologists. *BMJ* 337, a1938; d'Arcy Hughes A. (2011) Half of German doctors prescribe placebos, new study shows. *The Guardian* (Mar 6). Available at: http://www.guardian.co.uk (accessed 28 September 2012).
9 House of Commons Science and Technology Committee (2010) *Evidence Check 2: Homeopathy – Fourth Report of the Session 2009–10*, The Stationery Office, London.
10 General Medical Council (2008) *Good Practice in Prescribing Medicines*, GMC, London, para 3.
11 Department of Health (2010) *Government Response to the Science and Technology Committee report 'Evidence Check 2: Homeopathy'*, The Stationery Office, London.
12 National Institute for Health and Clinical Excellence (2009) *Low Back Pain: NICE Guidance CG88*, NICE, London.

13   GMC Professional Conduct Committee hearing, 13–17 January 2003.

14   National Prescribing Centre (2004) *Saving Time Helping Patients: a Good Practice Guide to Quality Repeat Prescribing*, NPC, Liverpool.

15   British Medical Association (2007) *Withholding and Withdrawing Life-Prolonging Medical Treatment*, 3rd edn, Blackwell, Oxford; General Medical Council (2010) *Treatment and Care towards the End of Life: Good Practice in Decision-Making*, GMC, London; British Medical Association (2012) *Medical Ethics Today. The BMA's Handbook of Ethics and Law*, 3rd edn, Wiley-Blackwell, Chichester, chapter 10.

16   Shakespeare J, Neve E, Hodder K. (2000) Is norethisterone a lifestyle drug? Results of a database analysis. *BMJ* 320, 291.

17   Bryant G, Scott I, Worrall A. (2000) Is norethisterone a lifestyle drug? Health is not merely the absence of disease. *BMJ* 320, 1605.

18   Schedule 1 of the National Health Service (General Medical Services Contracts) (Prescription of Drugs etc.) Regulations 2004. SI 2004/629. This provides for a list of drugs and other substances that are not to be prescribed within the NHS, also frequently referred to as the 'blacklist'. Schedule 2 drugs are a small list within the drug tariff of drugs to be prescribed within the NHS only in certain circumstances.

19   For a detailed discussion of different forms of cognitive enhancement and the issues it raises, see: British Medical Association (2007) *Boosting Your Brainpower: Ethical Aspects of Cognitive Enhancement*, BMA, London.

20   General Medical Council (2008) *Good Practice in Prescribing Medicines*, GMC, London.

21   General Medical Council (2006) *Good Medical Practice*, GMC, London, para 3b.

22   The British National Formulary is regularly updated. Joint Formulary Committee (published biannually) *British National Formulary*. British Medical Association and Pharmaceutical Press, London. Authoritative guidance is also available from national advisory bodies (where available) and other organisations, such as the National Prescribing Centre.

23   Dornan T, Ashcroft D, Heathfield H, *et al.* (2009) *An In-depth Investigation into the Causes of Prescribing Errors by Foundation Trainees in Relation to Their Medical Education – EQUIP Study.* Available at: http://www.gmc-uk.org (accessed 23 January 2013).

24   Avery T, Barber N, Ghaleb M, *et al.* (2012) *Investigating the Prevalence and Causes of Prescribing Errors in General Practice: the PRACtICe Study. A Report for the GMC*, GMC, London.

25   GMC Professional Conduct Committee hearing, 23–25 September 2002.

26   National Institute for Health and Clinical Excellence (2010) *Nice and the NHS*, NICE, London.

27   Department of Health (2010) *Equity and Excellence: Liberating the NHS*, The Stationery Office, London.

28   All Wales Medicines Strategy Group (2010) *Appraisals*. Available at: http://www.wales.nhs.uk (accessed 18 January 2012).

29   Brooks V. (1998) Viagra is licensed in Europe but rationed in Britain. *BMJ* 217, 765.

30   NHS Executive (1999) *Treatment for Impotence HSC 1999/115*, DH, Leeds.

31   Chisholm J. (1999) Viagra: a botched test case for rationing. *BMJ* 318, 273–274.

32   Department of Health (2009) *Guidance on NHS Patients Who Wish to Pay for Additional Private Care*, DH, London; Scottish Government Health Directorates (2009) *Arrangements for NHS Patients Receiving Healthcare Services through Private Healthcare Arrangements*, SGHD, Edinburgh.

33   British Medical Association (2009) *The Interface between NHS and Private Treatment: a Practical Guide for Doctors in Scotland*, BMA, London.

34   British Medical Association (2009) *The Interface between NHS and Private Treatment: a Practical Guide for Doctors in England, Wales and Northern Ireland*, BMA, London.

35   NHS Information Centre (2010) *Prescriptions Dispensed in the Community, England – Statistics for 1999 to 2009*. Available at: http://www.ic.nhs.uk (accessed 23 January 2013), p.8; Statistics for Wales (2010) *Prescriptions by General Medical Practitioners in Wales 2009–10*. Available at: wales.gov.uk (accessed 23 January 2013), p.20; Information Services Division Scotland (2010) *Generic Prescribing*. Available at: http://www.isdscotland.org (accessed 23 January 2013).

36   General Medical Council (2008) *Good Practice in Prescribing Medicines*, GMC, London, paras 18 and 20.

37   General Medical Council (2008) *Good Practice in Prescribing Medicines*, GMC, London, para 23.

38   General Medical Council (2008) *Good Practice in Prescribing Medicines*, GMC, London, para 22.

39   See, for example: National Institute for Health and Clinical Excellence (2010) *Neuropathic Pain: the Pharmacological Management of Neuropathic Pain in Adults in Non-specialist Settings*. CG96, NICE, London.

40   Torjesen I. (2012) Novartis takes legal action over trusts' advice to use bevacizemab for wet AMD to save money. *BMJ* 344, p.1.

41   NHS Southampton, Hampshire, Isle of Wight and Portsmouth (2012) *Board decision over wet AMD Policy*. Press release, July 25. Available at: http://www.southamptonhealth.nhs.uk (accessed 29 September 2012).

42   Medicines for Human Use (Marketing Authorisations etc.) Regulations 1994, SI 1994/3144, Regulation 7.

43   For more information, see the MHRA website: http://www.mhra.gov.uk (accessed 23 January 2013).

44   For further information, see the National Reporting and Learning Service website at: http://www.nrls.npsa.nhs.uk (accessed 23 January 2013).

45   British Medical Association (2007) *Prescribing and the Primary and Secondary Care Interface*, BMA, London.

46   NHS Management Executive (1991) *Responsibilities for Prescribing between Hospitals and GPs (EL(91)127)*, Department of Health, London.

47   Department of Health, Social Services and Public Safety (2003) *The regional group on specialist drugs – implementation of red/amber lists – 1 May 2003 (HSS(MD)16/2003)*, DHSSPS, Belfast.

48   General Medical Council (2008) *Good Practice in Prescribing Medicines*, GMC, London, para 28.

49   British Medical Association (2010) *Patient Group Directions and Patient Specific Directions in General Practice*, BMA, London.

50 National Prescribing Centre (2009) *Patient Group Directions – a Practical Guide and Framework of Competencies for All Professionals Using Patient Group Directions*, NPC, Liverpool.

51 Nurse Prescribers' Formulary Subcommittee (published biannually) *Nurse Prescribers' Formulary for Community Practitioners*, British Medical Association and Royal Pharmaceutical Society of Great Britain in association with Community Practitioners' and Health Visitors' Association and the Royal College of Nursing, London.

52 General Medical Council (2006) *Good Medical Practice*, GMC, London, para 52.

53 Anon. (2010) Herbal medicines – what do clinicians know? *Drug Ther Bull* 48, 4.

54 Care Quality Commission (2009) *Managing Patients' Medicines after Discharge from Hospital*, CQC, London.

55 British Medical Association (2001) *Consulting in the Modern World – Guidance for GPs*, BMA, London.

56 General Medical Council (2008) *Good Practice in Prescribing Medicines*, GMC, London, para 40.

57 General Medical Council (2008) *Good Practice in Prescribing Medicines*, GMC, London, para 41.

58 General Medical Council (2012) *Remote Prescribing via Telephone, Fax, Video-Link or Online*, GMC, London.

59 General Medical Council, Fitness to Practise Hearing, 24 August–2 September 2009.

60 General Medical Council (2008) *Good Practice in Prescribing Medicines*, GMC, London, para 43.

61 Royal Pharmaceutical Society of Great Britain (2008) *Millions risk health buying drugs online*. Press release, January 10.

62 Raine C, Webb DJ, Maxwell SRJ. (2008) The availability of prescription-only analgesics purchased from the internet in the UK. *Br J Clin Pharmacol* 67(2), 250–254.

63 Nuffield Council on Bioethics (2010) *Medical Profiling and Online Medicine: the Ethics of 'Personalised Healthcare' in a Consumer Age*, NCB, London, p.109.

64 Moberly T. (2009) 1 in 4 GPs report online drug concerns. *GP* (Apr 17), p.4.

65 General Pharmaceutical Society (2010) *Standards for Pharmacy Owners and Superintendent Pharmacists of Retail Pharmacy Businesses*, GPhC, London.

66 Pharmaceutical Society of Northern Ireland (2009) *Professional Standards and Guidance for Internet Pharmacy Services*, PSNI, Belfast.

67 The Shipman Inquiry (2004) *The Shipman Inquiry, Fourth Report: The Regulation of Controlled Drugs in the Community*, The Stationery Office, London.

68 Department of Health (England) and the devolved administrations (2007) *Drug Misuse and Dependence: UK Guidelines on Clinical Management*, Department of Health (England), the Scottish Government, Welsh Assembly Government and Northern Ireland Executive. Available at: http://www.dh.gov.uk (accessed 30 May 2012).

69 Bennett MI, Graham J, Schmidt-Hansen M, *et al.* (2012) Prescribing strong opioids in adult palliative care: summary of NICE guidance. *BMJ* 344, 42.

70 Walsh F. (2012) NICE releases new pain relief guidelines. *BBC News* (May 23). Available at: http://www.bbc.co.uk/news (accessed 23 May 2012).

71 National Institute for Health and Clinical Excellence (2012) *Safe and Effective Prescribing of Strong Opioids for Pain in Palliative Care of Adults (Clinical Guideline 140)*, NICE, London.

72 Dyer C. (1997) Court confirms right to palliative treatment for mental distress. *BMJ* 315, 1177.

73 British Medical Association (2007) *Evidence-Based Prescribing*, BMA, London, p.10.

74 Barber ND, Alldred DP, Raynor DK, *et al.* (2009) Care homes' use of medicines study: prevalence, causes and potential harm of medication errors in care homes for older people. *Qual Saf Health Care* 18, 341–346.

75 British Medical Association (2009) *The Ethics of Caring for Older People*, Wiley-Blackwell, Chichester, p.15.

76 Carter S, Taylor D, Levenson R. (2005) *A Question of Choice – Compliance in Medicine Taking*, 3rd edn, Medicines Partnership, London, p.94.

77 Royal Pharmaceutical Society of Great Britain (2009) *Royal Pharmaceutical Society calls for older people to review their medicine with a pharmacist.* Press release, July 29.

78 House of Commons Health Committee (2004) *Elder Abuse: Second Report of Session 2003–04 Vol. 1*, The Stationery Office, London, para 65.

79 Banerjee S. (2009) *The Use of Antipsychotic Medication for People with Dementia: Time for Action*, DH, London.

80 Sammons H, Conroy S. (2008) How do we ensure safe prescribing for children? *Arch Dis Child* 93, 98–99.

81 Paediatric Formulary Committee (published annually) *BNF for Children*, BMJ Publishing Group, Pharmaceutical Press and Royal College of Paediatrics and Child Health Publications, London.

82 For more information, see: http://www.medicinesforchildren.org.uk (accessed 23 January 2013).

83 General Medical Council (2008) *Good Practice in Prescribing Medicines*, GMC, London, paras 13–15.

84 General Medical Council (2008) *Good Practice in Prescribing Medicines*, GMC, London, para 4.

85 General Medical Council (2008) *Good Practice in Prescribing Medicines*, GMC, London, para 10.

86 General Medical Council (2006) *Good Medical Practice*, GMC, London, para 74.

87 General Medical Council (2006) *Good Medical Practice*, GMC, London, paras 75–76.

88 The Medicines (Advertising) Regulations 1994, SI 1994/1932, Regulation 21(1).

89 Association of the British Pharmaceutical Industry (2011) *Code of Practice for the Pharmaceutical Industry 2011*, ABPI, London, clause 18.

90 Association of the British Pharmaceutical Industry (2011) *Code of Practice for the Pharmaceutical Industry 2011*, ABPI, London, clause 19.

91 Association of the British Pharmaceutical Industry (2011) *Code of Practice for the Pharmaceutical Industry 2011*, ABPI, London, clause 20.

92 Association of the British Pharmaceutical Industry (2011) *Code of Practice for the Pharmaceutical Industry 2011*, ABPI, London, clause 18.4.

93 Association of the British Pharmaceutical Industry (2011) *Code of Practice for the Pharmaceutical Industry 2011*, ABPI, London, clause 15.3.

94   Association of the British Pharmaceutical Industry (2011) *Code of Practice for the Pharmaceutical Industry 2011*, ABPI, London, clause 12.2.

95   British Healthcare Business Intelligence Association (2009) *The Legal & Ethical Guidelines for Healthcare Market Research*, BHBIA, St Albans.

96   Toft B. (2001) *External Inquiry into the Adverse Incident That Occurred at Queen's Medical Centre, Nottingham, 4th January 2001*, DH, London.

97   Mental Welfare Commission for Scotland (2006) *Covert Medication: Legal and Practical Guidance*, MWCS, Edinburgh.

Index